# FIRST AID AND EMERGENCY CARE WORKBOOK

**THIRD EDITION**

**Brent Q. Hafen • Keith J. Karren**

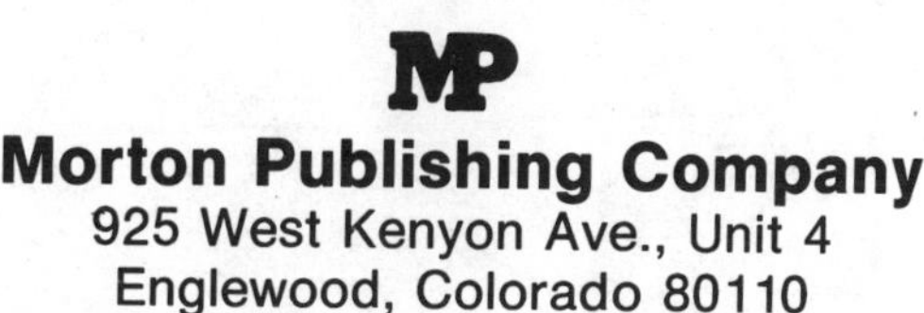
**Morton Publishing Company**
925 West Kenyon Ave., Unit 4
Englewood, Colorado 80110

**ISBN: 0-89582-114-1**

# Contents

# Preface

Sudden illnesses, injuries, and accidents often happen with little or no warning. In many cases, prompt and efficient action on the part of the first person to help the victim may mean the difference between a speedy recovery and chronic disability (or even death).

Prompt and efficient action goes far beyond calling for an ambulance or a doctor. A certain amount of time lapses before professional medical help arrives; offering prompt and effective emergency care, then, includes providing life-support measures and stabilizing the victim while waiting for help to arrive.

If effective first aid is not performed at the scene of the accident, a victim who is not breathing may die before the ambulance arrives; a bleeding victim may die from loss of blood; a heart attack victim may die from the lack of the pumping ability of his/her heart; or a closed fracture may be converted to an open fracture. In these and many other situations, the life and health of the victim depends on the training of those who render emergency first aid.

The purpose of this text/workbook is to provide instruction in emergency first aid procedures.

The authors recognize that training and practice are the keys to efficiency. We have, therefore, organized each section of the text/workbook according to the following format:

1. Content
2. Work Exercises
3. Self-test

It may be used without any supplemental materials. However, it has been designed to supplement the American Red Cross first aid books.

Each chapter of the text/workbook contains a list of corresponding chapters and page numbers from the American Red Cross first aid texts (Standard and Advanced).

Terms that appear in boldface in the text are defined in the glossary at the end of the book.

Corresponds with:
**American Red Cross**
**Standard First Aid & Personal Safety**
Chapter 1, pages 11-17
and
**Advanced First Aid & Emergency Care**
Chapter 1, pages 17-23

# 1 Introduction to First Aid and Emergency Care

## EMERGENCIES IN AMERICA

One of the most critical and visible health problems in America today is the sudden loss of life and disability from catastrophic accidents and illnesses. While facts and figures are not essential to the preparation of emergency rescuers, they do paint a picture of the great need for properly prepared First Aiders to the accident situation. Consider the following:

- Over 70 million Americans receive hospital emergency care each year.
- Over 150,000 people die each year from trauma, and 400,000 permanent injuries are caused, making trauma the fourth largest killer in the United States.
- There are 1.4 million injuries occurring on American highways, resulting in 51,900 traffic deaths and permanent disability to 150,000.
- Each year there are 2 million burn accidents, 1.5 million heart attack victims (50 percent of these dying within two hours of onset), and 5 million poisonings, 90 percent of these victims being children.

## EFFECTIVE CARE

Too often, those who arrive first at the scene of an accident, and even some ambulance personnel, are not sufficiently trained to give proper, on-the-scene emergency care or in-transit emergency assistance. Often, too much time passes after an accident before proper emergency care is given and victims who might have been saved die because of lack of necessary care.

## NEED FOR WELL-TRAINED FIRST AIDERS

Remarkably, studies suggest that 15 to 20 percent of accidental highway deaths could be avoided if prompt, effective emergency care was available at the scene. The old philosophy of "load and go" is just not acceptable. The Maryland Institute for Emergency Medical Services discusses the time immediately after an accident has occurred as the "Golden Hour," when lives that hang in the balance can be saved through the administration of proper first aid and emergency care.

The first people on the scene, the First Aiders, can properly initiate lifesaving procedures, such as:

- Airway and respiratory intervention.
- Cardiopulmonary resuscitation.
- Bleeding control.
- Special wound care (such as head, chest, and abdominal wounds).
- Stabilization of spinal injuries.
- Splinting fractures.

You will become a very important part of the emergency care team as you properly prepare

LITHO'D IN CANADA

70 MILLION — EMERGENCY CARE

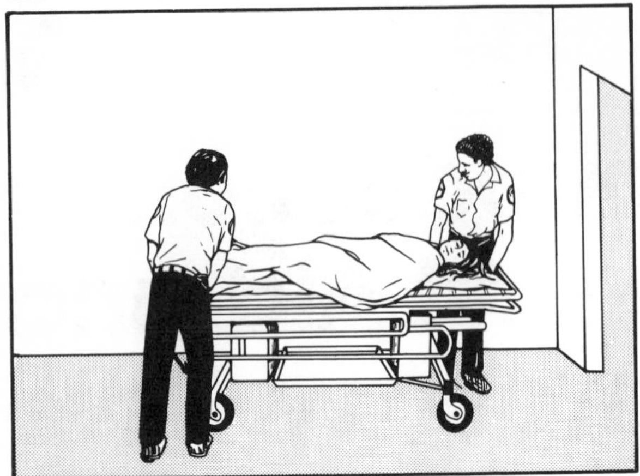

150,000 DEATHS

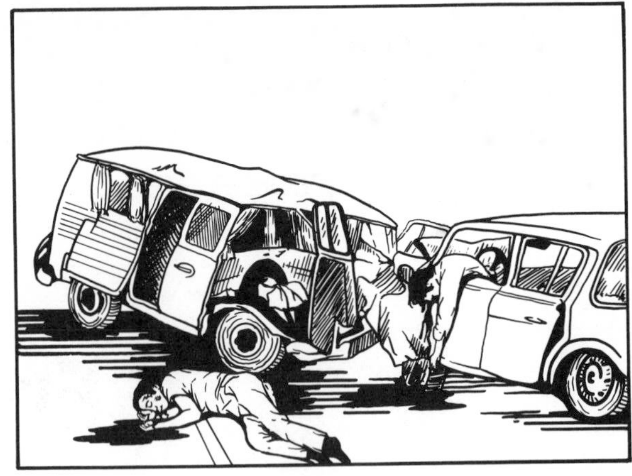

1.4 MILLION INJURIES

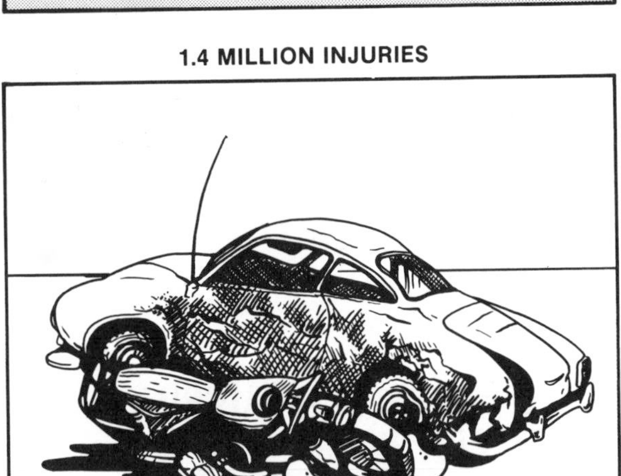

2 MILLION BURNS

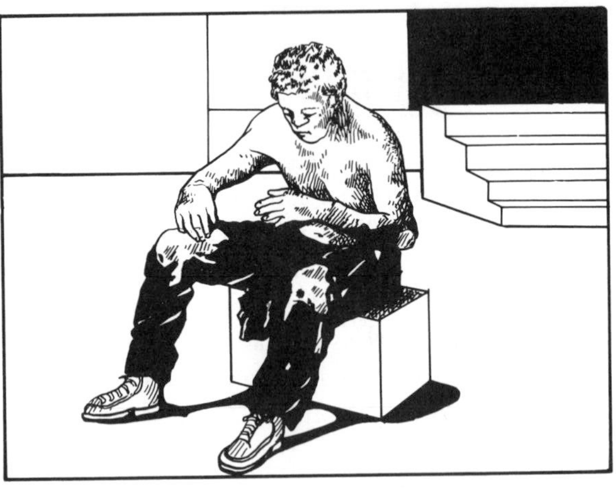

These facts and figures illustrate the need for properly prepared First Aiders at the scene of an emergency.

with the right knowledge and practical skills to render appropriate, lifesaving care.

## WHAT IS FIRST AID?

First aid is the temporary and immediate care given to a person who is injured or suddenly becomes ill. First aid also involves home care if medical assistance is delayed or not available. First aid includes recognizing life-threatening conditions and taking effective action to keep the injured or ill person alive and in the best possible condition until medical treatment can be obtained.

First aid does not replace the physician, nurse, or paramedic. One of the primary principles of first aid is to obtain medical assistance in all cases of serious injury.

The principle aims of first aid are as follows:

- To properly prepare so as to avoid errors and know what NOT to do as well as what to do.
- To care for life-threatening conditions.
- To minimize further injury and complications.
- To make the victim as comfortable as possible to conserve strength.
- To minimize infection.
- To transport the victim to a medical facility, when necessary, in such a manner as not to complicate the injury or subject the victim to unnecessary discomfort.

A part of proper preparation is to become more safety conscious. This will help to reduce the number of accidents and potential first aid situations. Three key terms in the promotion of safety awareness are **cause, effect,** and **prevention.**

The major cause of accidents is human failure. Mechanical or structural failures can also cause accidents. It is essential that every possible hazard be eliminated, controlled, or avoided.

The effects of an accident or a sudden illness may change the body's function and structure. The goal of first aid is to not allow these changes to cause death or permanent injury. The prevention of untimely accidents and illnesses directly saves suffering and loss of lives.

First aiders should know how to recognize life-threatening problems, to supply artificial ventilation and circulation, to control bleeding, to protect injuries from infection and other complications, and to arrange for medical assistance and transportation. When first aid is properly administered, the victim's chances of recovery are greatly increased.

First aiders must be able to take charge of a situation, keep calm while working under pressure, and organize others to do likewise. By demonstrating competence and using well-selected words of encouragement, first aiders should win the confidence of others nearby and do everything possible to reassure the apprehensive victim.

## GENERAL DIRECTIONS

The First Aider is generally involved in a sudden injury or illness situation that requires fast thinking and action. This necessitates a plan of action.

- Observe the accident scene as you approach it.
- If necessary, direct others to direct traffic and position safety flares, keep bystanders at a safe distance, make essential telephone calls, turn off engines that may be still running, etc.
- Provide basic life support to those whose lives are threatened, the most serious given emergency care first.

## EVALUATING THE SITUATION

When a person is injured, someone must (1) take charge, (2) administer first aid, and (3) arrange for medical assistance.

### Arranging for Medical Assistance

During the first minutes after an accident, it is essential that the Emergency Medical Services System is activated. If a victim has suffered a heart attack, the First Aider activates the EMS system as soon as he finds the victim is pulseless. In other situations where victims have a pulse and are breathing, they should be stabilized while one of the First Aiders finds a telephone to activate the EMS system.

In the majority of urban and in some rural areas in the United States, the First Aider can activate the EMS system by telephoning 911. Other areas will have a local emergency number. If the emergency number is unknown, the First Aider should dial 0 (zero or operator). After the proper connection is made, the First Aider should give to the dispatcher the following information:

- The exact location, such as the correct and complete address, the number of the floor or office in the building, or any other information which will identify the exact location of the victim.
- A correct phone number where the First Aider may be reached.
- The name of the First Aider.
- Any necessary information which will help the dispatcher send the appropriate personnel and equipment.

The First Aider should send any responsible bystander to telephone with the above information. If the First Aider is alone, he should perform the ABCs of emergency care for one minute, then quickly telephone for help. If no telephone is available, the First Aider should continue giving emergency care until a bystander is available to activate the Emergency Medical System. First aiders should take charge with full recognition of their own limitations, and, while caring for life-threatening conditions, direct others briefly and clearly as to exactly what they should do and how to secure assistance.

## FIRST AIDER SKILLS

Some of the skills that you have or will need to acquire as a First Aider have already been discussed. The following is a basic list of skills that form the core of the First Aid course. Other skills may be added to the course by your instructors. You may want to check these skills off as you master them. At the conclusion of your First Aid course, you should be able to:

- Control the accident scene so that further injury will not occur.
- Gain access to victims in the easiest and safest way possible.
- Effectively and quickly evaluate the accident scene for cause and control for safety.
- Obtain information from bystanders and the victim(s) of the accident or sudden illness.
- Perform quick, effective primary and secondary victim surveys, including taking of vital signs (breathing, pulse, skin temperature).
- Determine any diagnostic signs and relate those to possible injuries or sudden illnesses that require emergency care.
- Perform the necessary ABCBs of emergency care.

  **A** — Open airway.
  **B** — Breathing (breathlessness — provide artificial ventilation).
  **C** — Circulation (pulselessness — provide one- and two-rescuer cardiopulmonary resuscitation).
  **B** — Bleeding control (hemorrhage controlled by direct pressure and elevation, pressure points, and tourniquets).

- Detect and care for shock.
- Detect and care for soft tissue and internal injuries, including basic dressing and bandaging techniques.
- Detect and care for open and closed fractures, sprains, strains, and dislocations, including cold treatment and basic splinting techniques.
- Detect and care for poisoning, including alcohol and drug abuse.
- Detect and care for heart attack, stroke, diabetic coma, insulin shock, and epileptic or other seizures.
- Detect and care for facial and head injuries, neck and spinal injuries, and chest injuries, including fractured ribs, flail chest, and penetrating chest wounds.
- Detect and care for first-, second-, and third-degree burns and smoke inhalation.
- Detect and care for exposure to heat and cold, which includes heat cramps, heat exhaustion, heat stroke, hypothermia, and frostbite.
- Assist in childbirth and care of the newborn.
- Give psychological and proper emergency care to victims of crisis and disasters.
- Perform non-emergency and emergency moves and other proper transportation techniques.

## THE LEGAL ASPECTS OF FIRST AID

It is natural for a First Aider to wonder if he or she can safely give a victim emergency care and be free from liability or litigation. Legally, you are not forced to give emergency care, but becoming a First Aider indicates that you choose to do so.

In certain instances, a victim may feel justified in (or may simply try to justify) suing a First Aider for the way in which the victim was handled during emergency care. In order to protect health care personnel from being sued, states have inacted Good Samaritan laws. These laws indicate that the practitioner (First Aider) is not held liable for his actions as long as he does not do anything that can be defined as grossly negligent or that constitutes willful misconduct. Because of these laws, lawsuits against emergency medical personnel (such as First Aiders) have become extremely rare. Good Samaritan laws provide some guidelines for personnel rendering aid and make it difficult for one who is aided to sue.

If such a case *is* taken to court, the case is prosecuted as a tort proceeding — a civil court proceeding designed to determine whether the natural rights of an individual have been violated. A tort action is not a criminal action nor one involving a broken contract or failure to pay a debt.

In tort proceedings involving emergency medical personnel, the First Aider must be accused of negligence — carelessness, inattention, disregard, inadvertence, or oversight that was accidental but avoidable. In a tort proceeding there are three categories of negligence:

1. Nonfeasance: the First Aider failed to perform his duty.
2. Misfeasance: the First Aider failed to perform his duty properly.
3. Malfeasance: the First Aider performed his duty without consent.

In order to establish negligence, the court must decide that:

- The victim was injured.
- The First Aider actions or lack of action caused or contributed to the injury.
- The First Aider had a duty to act.
- The First Aider acted in an unusual, unreasonable, or imprudent way.

It is essential that the First Aider receive consent to care for a victim. The four types of consent are:

1. **Actual Consent.** To be effective, it must be an informed consent. Oral consent is valid. A consent form does not eliminate the need for conversation.
2. **Implied Consent.** In a true emergency in which there is a significant risk of death, disability, or deterioration of condition, the law assumes that the victim would give his consent.
3. **Minor's Consent.** The right to consent is usually given to the parent or other person so close to the minor as to be treated as a parent.
4. **Consent of the Mentally Ill.** The situation is similar to that for minors.

A competent adult has the right to refuse treatment for himself or a minor due to religious or other reasons.

Critical to the First Aider's defense is the "reasonable man" test: did the First Aider act the same way that a normal, prudent person would have acted under the same circumstances if that normal, prudent person had the First Aider's background and training? The First Aider usually has the support of expert witnesses who are called to testify about how a person with training and background would have acted under those circumstances.

The jury then decides six critical issues:

1. Did the First Aider act, or fail to act?
2. Did the victim sustain physical, psychological, or financial injury?
3. Did the action or inaction of the First Aider cause or contribute to that injury?
4. Was the victim guilty of contributing to his own injury?
5. Did the First Aider violate his duty to care for the victim?
6. If the victim proves his case, what damages should be awarded?

In any court case of this kind, the burden of proof is on the victim. The only time that the First Aider *can* be prosecuted is when he is guilty of gross negligence, recklessness, willful or wanton conduct, or intentional injury to the victim.

Basically, the First Aider's duty legally can be defined as follows:

- The First Aider should not interfere with the first aid help that is being given by others.
- The First Aider should follow the directions of a police officer and do what a reasonable First Aider would do under the circumstances.
- The First Aider should not force his help on a victim unless the situation is life-threatening (such as severe bleeding, attempted suicide, poisoning, cardiac arrest, and so on). When the victim is unconscious, consent is automatic (by law). If the victim is not in a life-threatening situation and if he resists care, the First Aider can be charged with battery (physical contact of a person's

body or clothing without consent) if care is forced on the victim without consent.

- Once a First Aider has voluntarily started care, he should not leave the scene or stop the care until a qualified and responsible person relieves him; if he does, it constitutes abandonment.
- The First Aider should follow accepted and recognized emergency care procedures taught in this and other First Aid texts.

## Work Exercises

### Safety Awareness

Safety awareness prevents accidents and, therefore, saves lives. What are the three key terms in the promotion of safety awareness?

1.

2.

3.

The following is a list of First Aid and Emergency Care skills. Read them through and indicate if you feel prepared to perform them by checking the appropriate column.*

| First Aid Skills | Yes | No |
|---|---|---|
| 1. Control the accident scene so that further injury will not occur. | | |
| 2. Gain access to victims in the easiest and safest way possible. | | |
| 3. Effectively and quickly evaluate the accident scene for cause and control for safety. | | |
| 4. Obtain information from bystanders and the victim(s) of the accident or sudden illness. | | |
| 5. Perform a quick, effective primary and secondary victim survey including vital signs (breathing, pulse, skin temperature). | | |
| 6. Determine any diagnostic signs and relate those to possible injuries or sudden illnesses that require emergency care. | | |
| 7. Perform the necessary ABCBs of emergency care. A — Open Airway. B — Breathing (Breathlessness — provide artificial ventilation). C — Circulation (Pulselessness — provide one and two rescuer cardiopulmonary resuscitation). B — Bleeding Control (Hemorrhage controlled by direct pressure and elevation, pressure points and tourniquets). | | |
| 8. Detect and care for shock. | | |
| 9. Detect and care for soft tissue and internal injuries, including basic dressing and bandaging techniques. | | |
| 10. Detect and care for open and closed fractures, sprains, and dislocations, including cold treatment and basic splinting techniques. | | |
| 11. Detect and care for poisoning; including alcohol and drug abuse. | | |

*Check this list again at the end of your course to measure improvement in your preparation.

## Legal Questions

Liability is always a concern in the medical field, and first aid and emergency care is no exception. Proper knowledge, good skills, and common sense will protect you, the first aider.

If a First Aider is sued, the case is prosecuted as a ____________________ proceeding.

Is this a criminal action? ________ Yes ________ No

There are three categories of negligence in a tort proceeding. (Please fill in the following table):

| **Category of Negligence** | **Definition** |
|---|---|
| Nonfeasance | |
| Misfeasance: | |
| Malfeasance: | |

To establish negligence by a First Aider the court must determine the presence of four conditions. Name these four conditions.

1. The victim was injured
2. 
3. 
4. 

Critical to the defense of a First Aider is the "reasonable man" test. What does this mean?

## SELF-TEST

### Part I: True and False

If you believe the statement is true, circle the T. If you believe the statement is false, circle F.

T F 1. Accidents are the leading cause of death among those aged one to thirty-eight, and twice as many women die from accidents as do men.

T F 2. As the population has increased, so have numbers of doctors, nurses, and other health care workers.

T F 3. An injured person should not be moved immediately unless a specific hazard — such as fire, spilled chemicals, or noxious fumes — is present.

T F 4. You should loosen all constricting clothing for a victim, including the necktie and belt.

T F 5. As a First Aider, you should prepare to give a diagnosis to medical personnel who arrive on the scene.

T F 6. A very important value of First Aid Training is self-help.

T F 7. A first aider should explain the victim's probable condition to concerned bystanders.

T F 8. The first thing to do for an injured person is to control bleeding.

T F 9. One of the main concerns of a first aider is to prevent added injury or death.

T F 10. It is as important to know what NOT to do as well as what to do.

T F 11. The First Aider should not worry about activating the emergency medical services system until all possible emergency care has been given.

T F 12. An important part of first aid is to control the accident scene.

T F 13. A person who receives first aid training is required by law to stop and help at an accident scene.

### Part II: Multiple Choice

For each question, circle the answer that best reflects an accurate statement.

1. Accidents are the leading cause of death for which age group:
   a. 1-38 years old
   b. 40-45 years old
   c. 46-69 years old
   d. 70-90 years old

2. First aid is the immediate action taken to
   a. care for the injured until medical help is available
   b. supplement proper medical or surgical treatment
   c. preserve vitality and resistance to disease
   d. rescue and transport the injured

3. When administering first aid, the condition that should be cared for first is:
   a. the most painful one
   b. the most life-threatening one
   c. the most obvious one
   d. bleeding

4. Avoid moving an injured victim until all injuries are identified so that:
   a. investigating authorities can know what happened when
   b. the victim will not suffer unnecessary pain
   c. the victim can be stabilized before being moved
   d. the victim will not suffer further injury
   e. it is not necessary to identify injuries before moving a victim

5. If you can't feel a victim's pulse at his wrist, the easiest alternate place to check is:
   a. the side of the neck
   b. the inside of the thigh
   c. the ankle
   d. the temples

6. In a dark-skinned victim, check for bluish signs of lack of oxygen by examining:
   a. palms of the hands
   b. skin behind the ears
   c. mucous membranes inside the mouth
   d. skin between the toes

7. By definition, first aid is:
   a. immediate care given to someone who is ill or injured
   b. care administered at home
   c. self-help
   d. all of the above

8. Which of the following is an immediate priority?
   a. determining the cause of injury
   b. controlling severe bleeding
   c. taking measures to keep the victim warm
   d. all of the above

9. Under normal circumstances, the best first contact for help in case of accident is:
   a. the hospital emergency room
   b. the fire department
   c. the police or highway patrol
   d. an ambulance service

10. If the First aider is alone, what should he do about telephoning for help?
    a. he should quickly telephone and then begin emergency care
    b. he should perform the ABCs of emergency care for one minute, then phone
    c. he should concentrate on emergency care and not take time to phone
    d. he should stabilize victim and then phone

11. The "reasonable man" test is the test that is:
    a. administered to a First Aider to test his skills in practical logic before he is allowed to begin victim care
    b. administered to a normal, prudent person to determine what personality traits a First Aider should have
    c. administered to the First Aider to ascertain if his actions during a given victim care experience were fair, reasonable, and unbiased
    d. to determine if the First Aider acted as a normal, prudent person with First Aider training would have acted

12. What can the First Aider be charged with if he administers care when the victim is not in a life-threatening situation and refuses care?
    a. negligence
    b. battery
    c. abandonment
    d. assault

13. What has first priority in emergency care?
    a. open airway
    b. control hemorrhage
    c. determine if there is a pulse
    d. stabilize any possible head, neck, or back fractures

American Red Cross
does not cover this subject.

# 2

# Victim Assessment and Vital Signs

It's after five, and the sidewalks aren't nearly as crowded as they were earlier in the day. As you round a corner near a large department store, you almost stumble over a woman who has fallen to the sidewalk. You kneel quickly beside her; you want to help, but where do you begin? How can you find out, in the few seconds you have before treatment is needed, what is wrong with this woman?

The ability to assess a victim — whether conscious or unconscious — is one of the most important and critical parts of first aid. Without the ability to assess at least roughly, you can't possibly know where to begin or what care to give the victim. Along with the ability to assess is the ability to monitor vital signs — critical in a life-threatening emergency.

## VITAL SIGNS

Two important indicators that may tell us about the seriousness of the victim's condition are signs and symptoms. A sign is something visual — such as an injury you can see; for example, a deformity caused by a fractured limb or bleeding from a wound. A symptom is a victim's complaint that you, the First Aider, cannot readily see; for example, a stomach pain or a headache.

Vital signs are visual signs that tell us the condition of the victim. They include:

1. Breathing rate, and if the victim is breathing
2. Pulse rate
3. Pupil reaction
4. Level of consciousness
5. Skin temperature
6. Skin color
7. Ability to move
8. Reaction to pain.

## PRIMARY SURVEY

Several conditions are considered life-threatening, but four in particular require immediate action:

- Respiratory arrest.
- Circulatory failure.
- Severe bleeding.
- Poisoning, which threatens life.

Respiratory arrest and/or circulatory failure can set off a chain of events that will lead to death. Severe and uncontrolled bleeding can lead to an irreversible state of shock in which death is inevitable. Poison can stimulate or depress the central nervous system dangerously, or its corrosive action can eat holes in the oral cavity, esophagus, and stomach. Death may occur in a very few minutes if an attempt is not made to help the victim in these situations. The First Aiders should perform the primary survey to determine the extent of the problem as soon as the victim is reached, and if any of the life-threatening conditions are found, begin first aid procedures without delay.

In checking for adequate breathing, an open airway must be established and maintained. If there are no signs of breathing, artificial ventilation must immediately be given.

If a victim experiences circulatory failure, a person trained in cardiopulmonary resuscitation (CPR) should check for a pulse, and, if none is detected, should start CPR at once.

A careful and thorough check must be made for any severe bleeding. Serious bleeding must be controlled by proper methods.

1

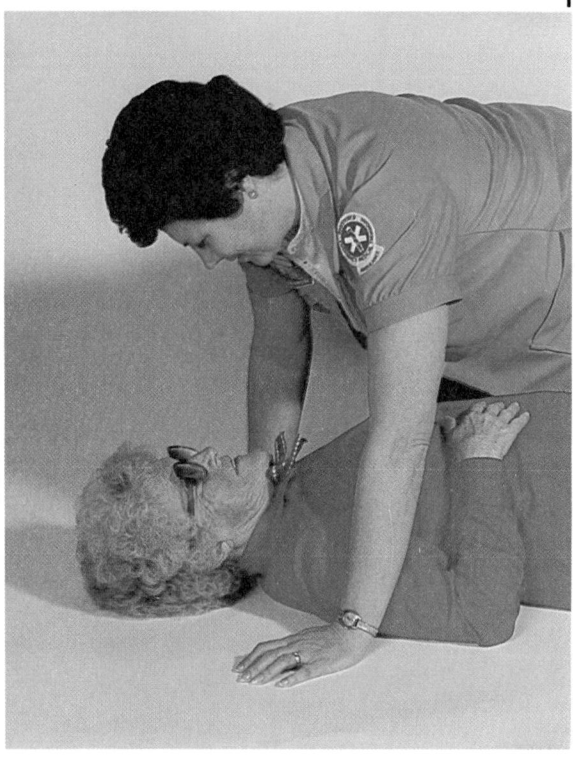

Approach the victim, determine consciousness, and if conscious, reassure.

2

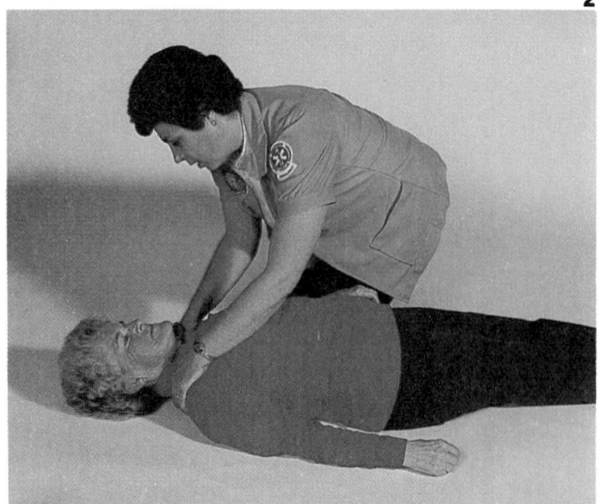

Establish unresponsiveness by the "shake and shout" method.

3

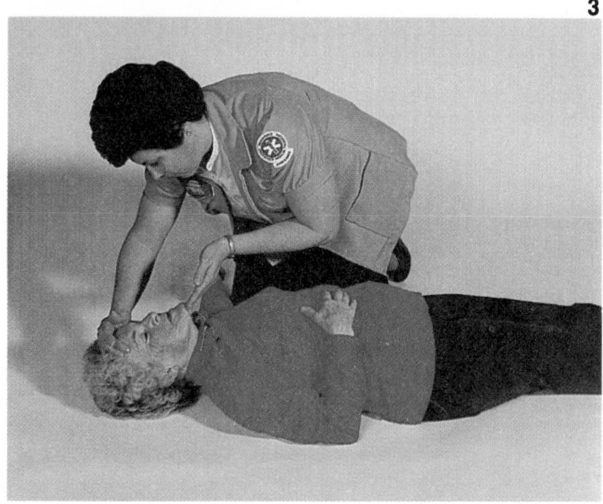

Assure an open airway with the head tilt-neck lift method (above) or the head tilt-chin lift method (below).

4

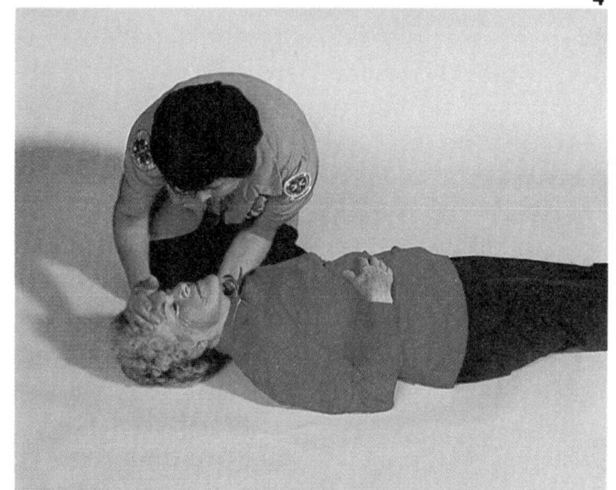

5

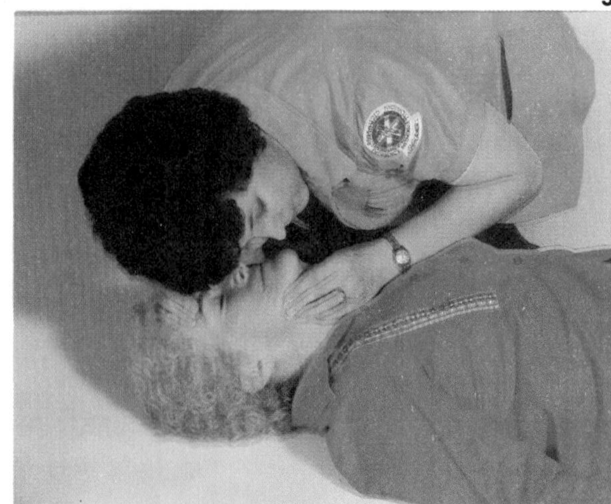

Assess for adequate breathing by: Look — for chest rising; Listen — for breathing sound; and Feel — for breath against the cheek.

6

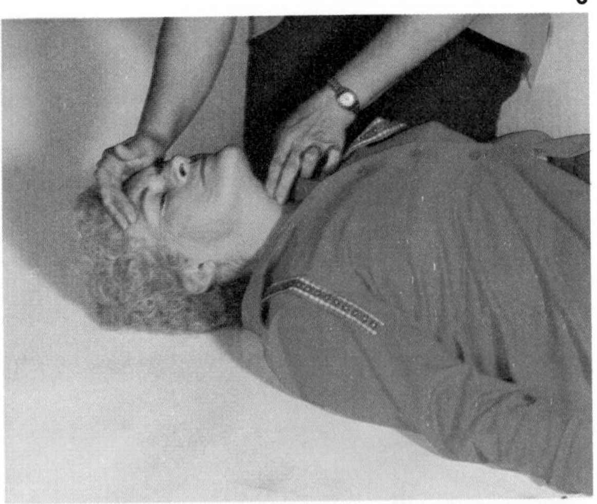

Assess for pulselessness and bleeding by taking the carotid pulse. If the victim is breathless and/or pulseless, send someone for emergency assistance.

7

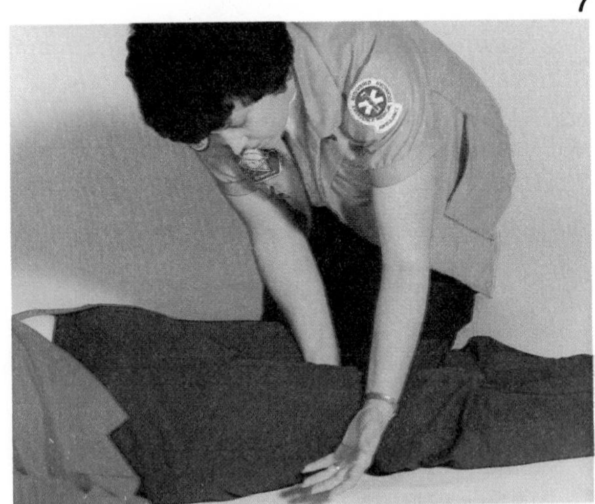

Observe and palpate for bleeding.

8

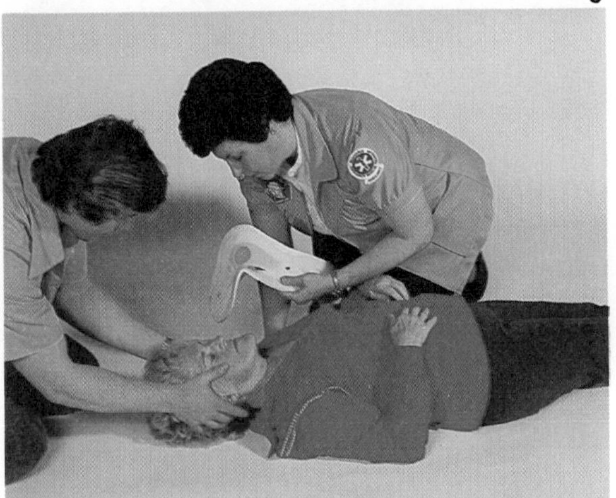

9

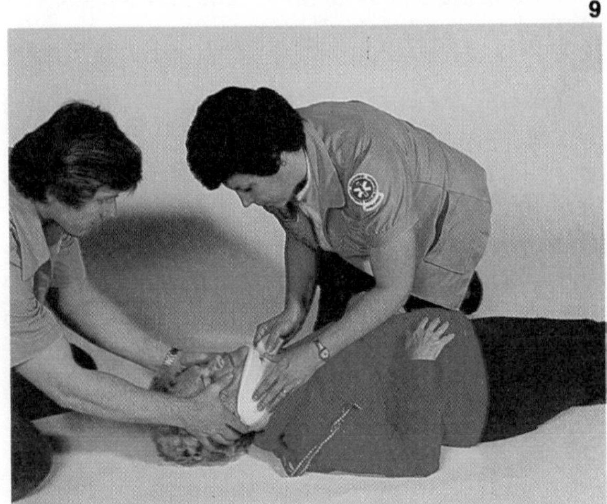

If you suspect that the victim may have a spinal fracture, stabilize the neck by applying a cervical collar or other stabilization method.

A poisoning victim needs to have the poison diluted and possibly emitted from the stomach.

In making the primary survey, the First Aider must be careful not to move the victim any more than is necessary to support life. Rough handling or any unnecessary movement might cause additional pain and aggravate serious injuries that have not yet been detected.

## SECONDARY SURVEY

When the life-threatening conditions have been controlled, the secondary survey should begin. While doing the secondary survey, be on the lookout for a *Medic Alert* tag, necklace, or bracelet. This medical identification may give important information about the victim. The secondary survey is a head-to-toe examination to check carefully for any additional unseen injuries that can cause serious complications. This body survey should be conducted quickly, not to exceed two to three minutes. It is conducted by examining for the following:

- Scalp lacerations and contusions. Without moving the head, check for blood in the hair.
- Skull depressions. Gently feel for possible bone fragments or depressions.
- Constricted, dilated, or unequal pupils may indicate possible injury or drug use.

- Loss of fluid or bleeding from the ears and nose may indicate possible skull fracture and damage to the brain.
- Broken teeth or foreign objects may obstruct the airway.
- Spine fractures, especially in the neck area. Gently feel and look for any abnormalities. If a spinal injury is suspected, stop the secondary survey until the head can be stabilized with sandbags or with rolled blankets or towels.
- Chest fractures and penetrating (sucking) wounds. Observe chest movement. When the sides are not rising together or one side is not moving at all, there may be lung and rib damage.
- Abdominal spasms and tenderness. Gently feel the abdominal area.
- Fractures in the pelvic area. Check for grating, tenderness, bony protrusions, and depressions.
- Fractures or dislocations of the extremities. Check for discoloration, swelling, tenderness, and lumps.
- Paralysis of the extremities. This condition indicates spinal cord damage. Paralysis in the arms and legs indicates a broken neck. Paralysis in the legs, but not arms, indicates a broken back. The three checks used to determine this are as follows:

  First, check the lower extremities for paralysis. If the victim is conscious, determine the following:

  1. Whether the victim can feel your touch to his/her feet.
  2. Whether the victim can wiggle his/her toes and then can raise his/her legs.
  3. Whether the victim can press against your hand with his/her feet.

  Second, check the upper extremities for paralysis. If the victim is conscious, determine the following:

  1. Whether the victim can feel your touch to his/her hands and arms.
  2. Whether the victim can wiggle his/her fingers and then raise his/her arms.
  3. Whether the victim can grasp your hand and squeeze.

If the victim is unconscious, perform the following tests for paralysis.

1. Stroke the soles of the feet or the ankles with a pointed object; if the spinal cord is undamaged, the foot will react.
2. Stroke the palm of the hand with a pointed object; if the spinal cord is undamaged, the hand will react.

10

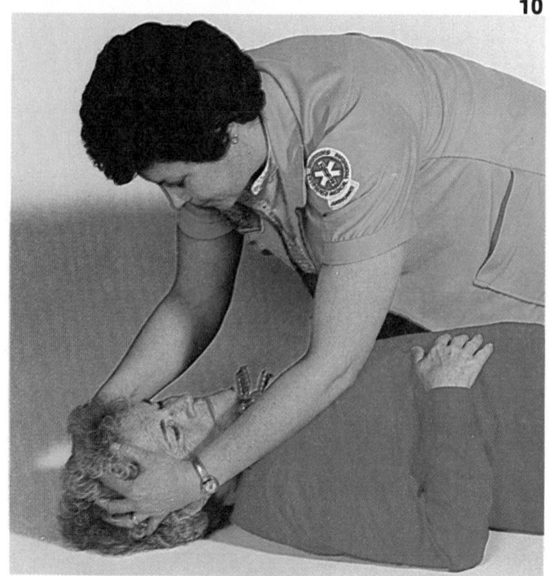

Check the head for scalp wounds and depressions.

11

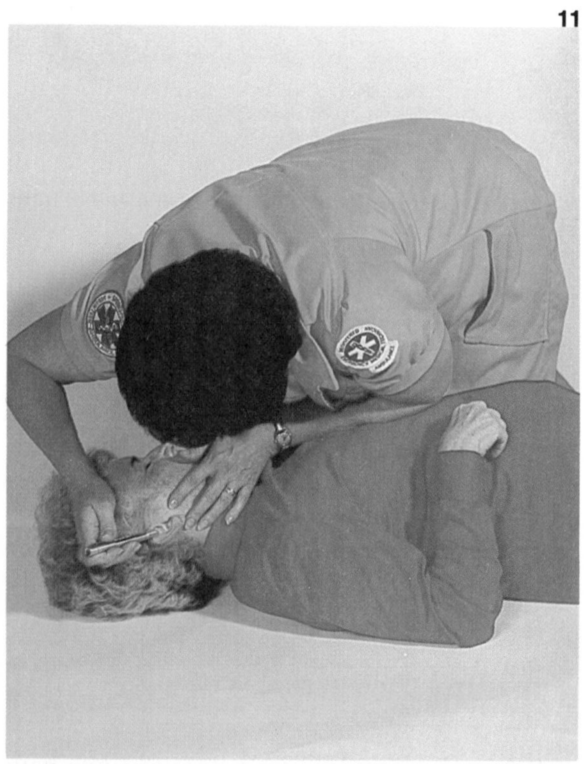

Check the ears and nose for fluid discharge, because this indicates skull fracture. If available, a penlight makes it easier.

12

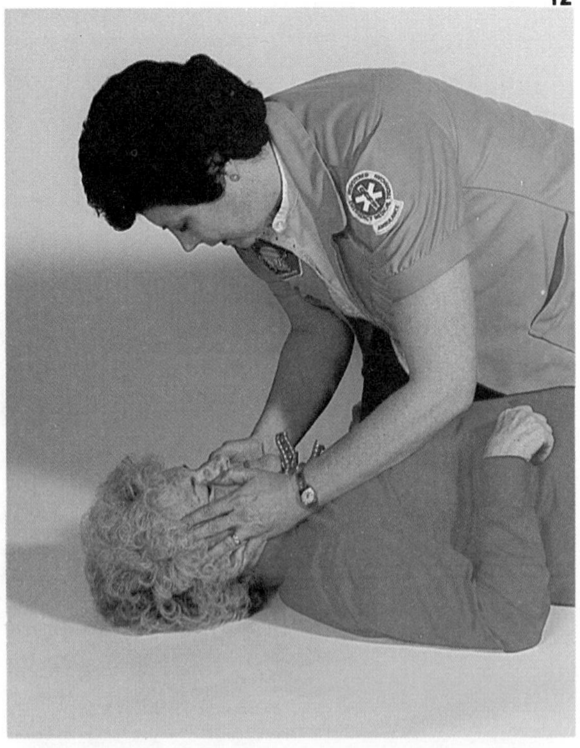

Check the facial bones for pain and possible fractures.

14

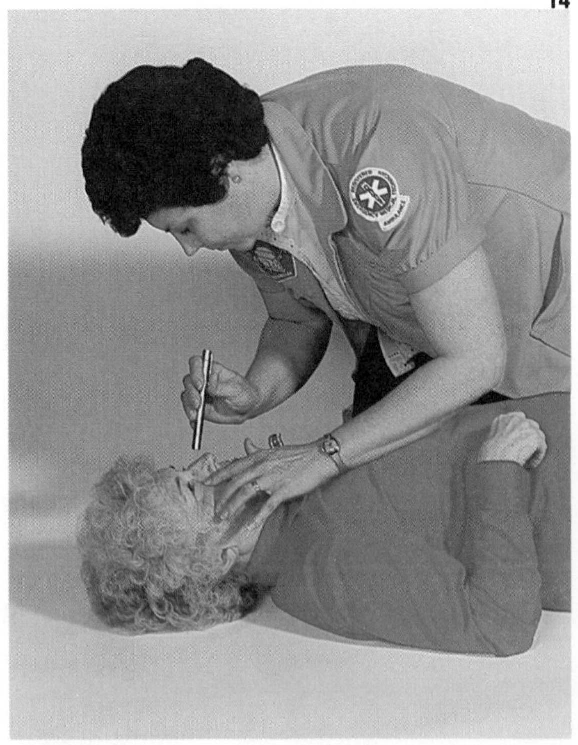

Check the eyes for reactive pupils and for possible damage.

13

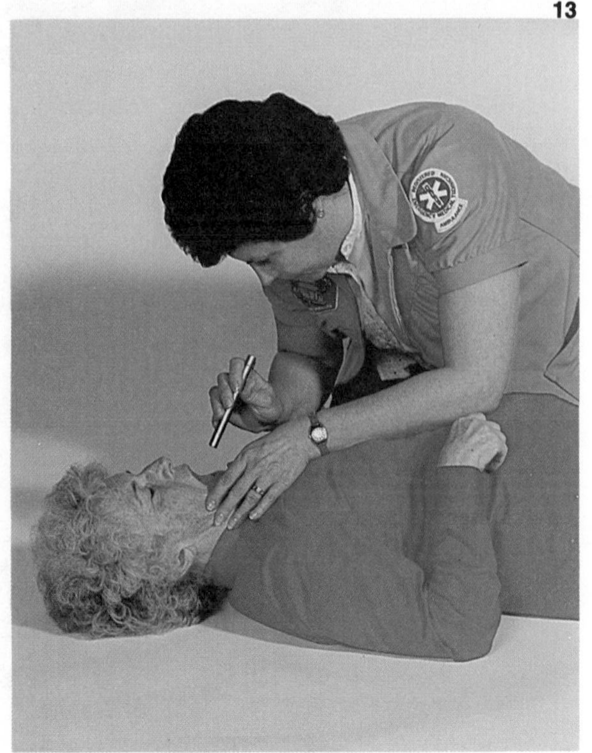

Check the mouth and jaw for possible fractures and obstructions.

15

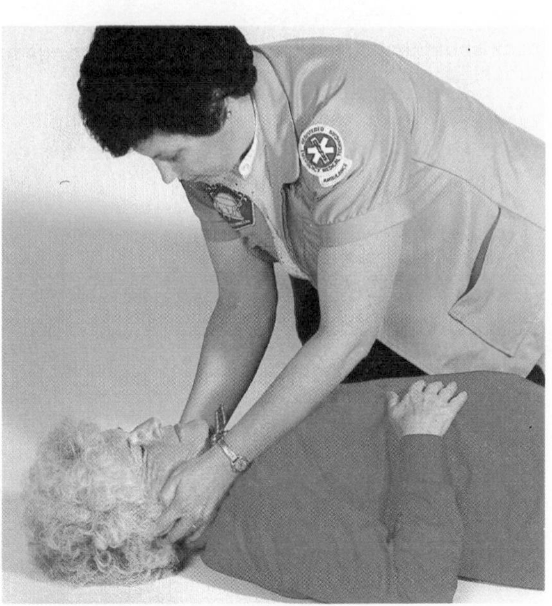

Feel the head and neck for wounds, pain, and deformities that may indicate skull or spinal injury.

16

Check the collarbone and shoulder girdle for possible injury.

17

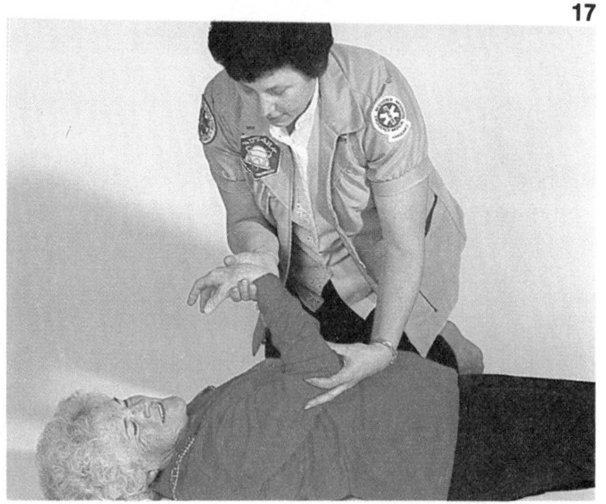

Check shoulders, arms, elbows, wrists, and hands for injuries. Establish a radial pulse for each arm.

18

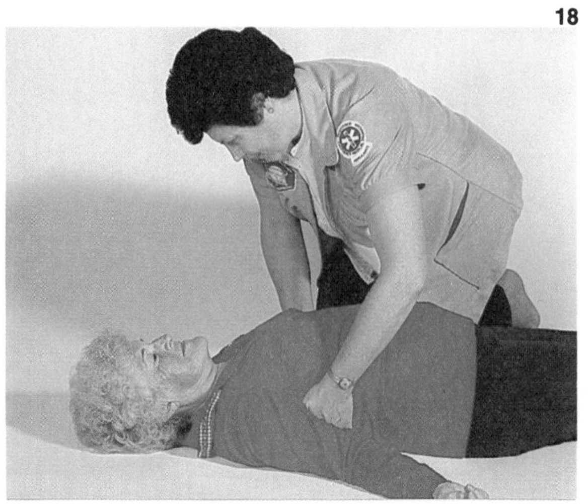

Check the rib cage for pain and deformity.

19

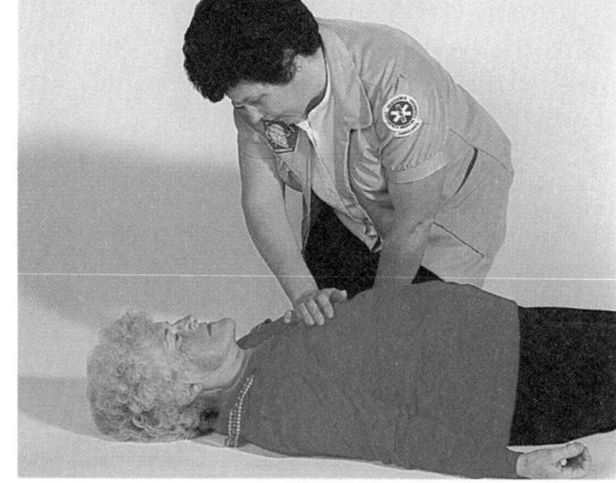

Check the sternum for pain and deformity.

20

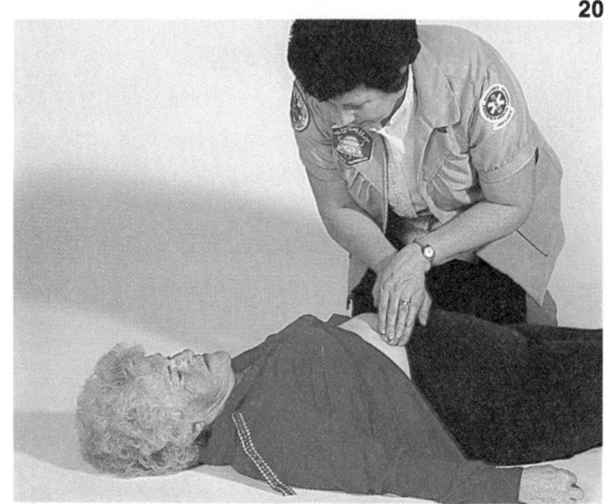

Check the abdomen for tenderness, rigidity, and deformity.

21

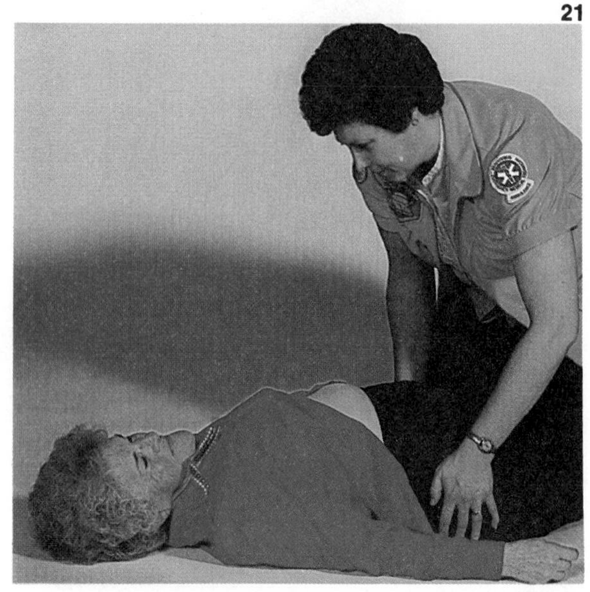

Check the pelvis for pain, injury, and deformity.

22

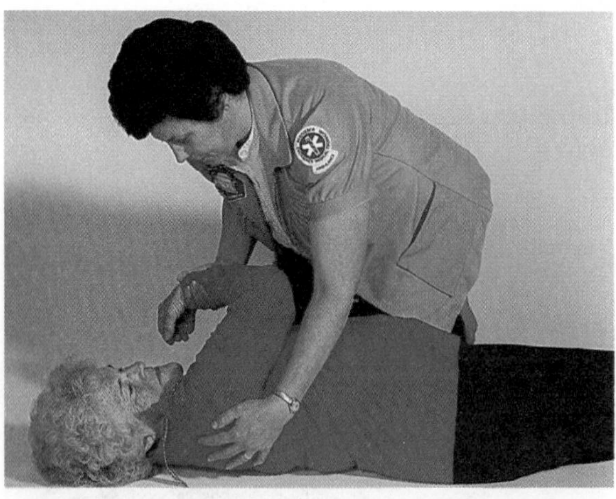

Check the upper and lower back for bleeding, deformity, and pain.

23

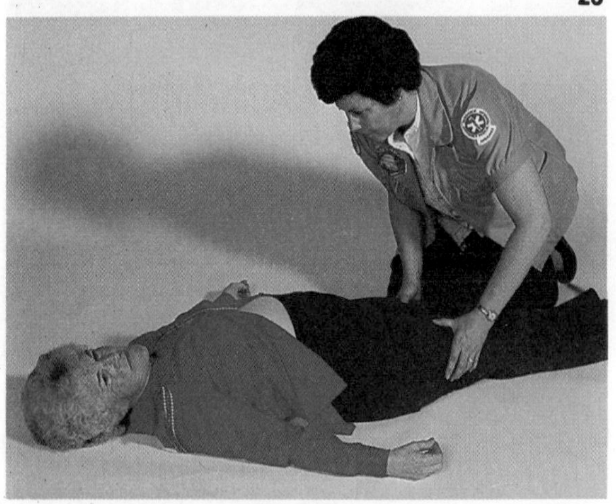

Check the legs and feet for bleeding, pain, and deformity.

24

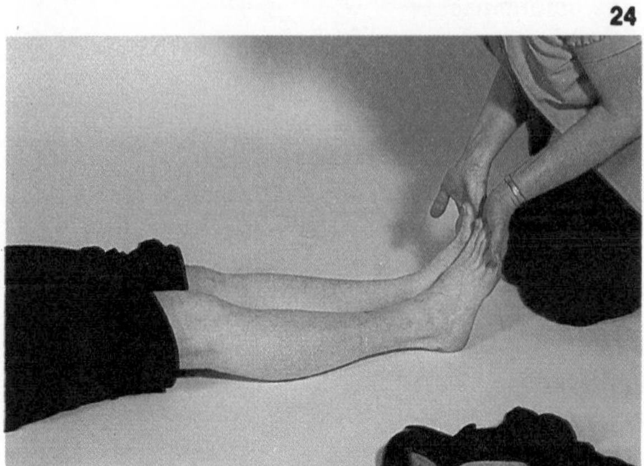

If the victim is conscious, see if he/she can feel your touch to his/her feet, then press against your hand with his/her feet. Can the victim wiggle his/her toes and raise the legs?

25

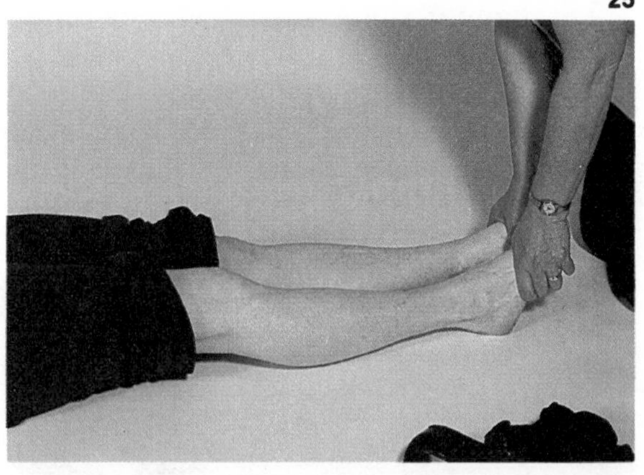

Have the victim pull his/her feet up against your hand.

26

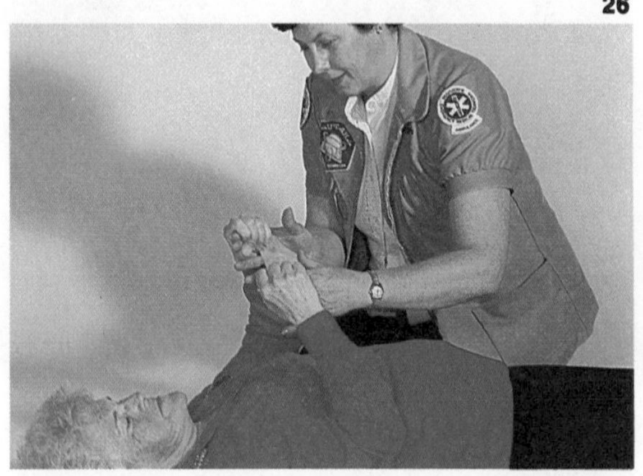

If the victim is conscious, see if he/she can grasp your hand and squeeze it.

27

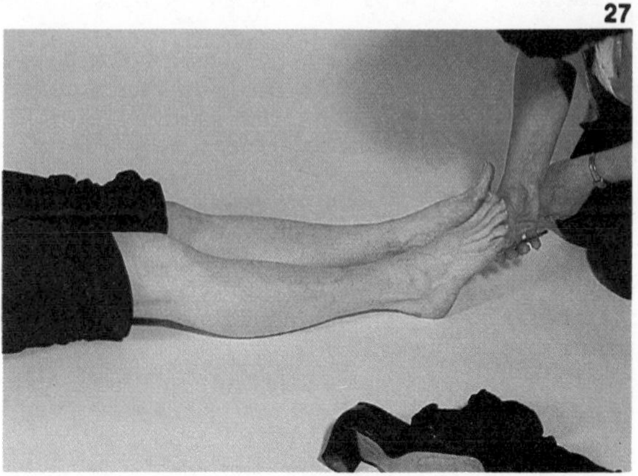

If the victim is unconscious, stroke the soles of the feet with a pointed object. If the spinal cord is **not** damaged, the foot will react.

Throughout the examination, you should briefly and in a general way explain what you are doing, why you are doing it, and what should be done about it. This will help alleviate the concern of the victim and involved bystanders. It will help you and other First Aiders know what should be done and in what order. If the victim is conscious, ask questions about what he/she feels as you proceed.

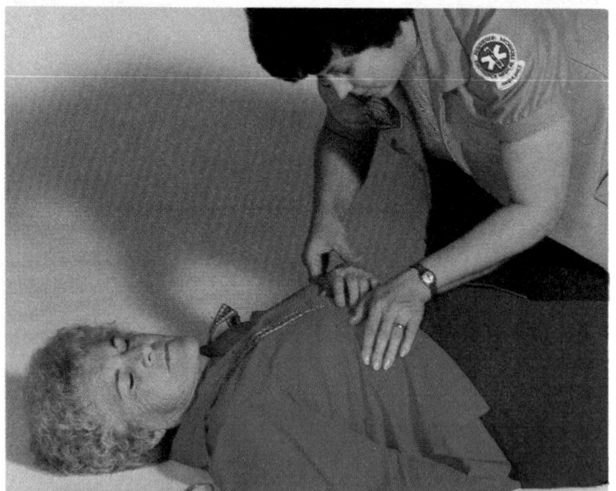

Taking respirations

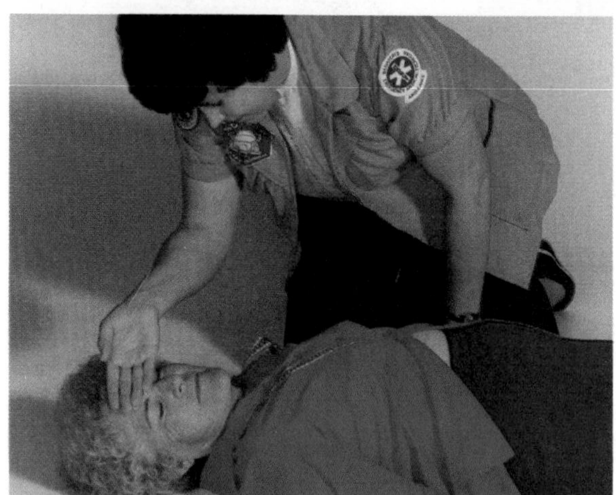

Taking a skin temperature

## Secondary Victim Assessment

It is not necessary to perform the following sequentially, but the First Aider should be consistent with a specific plan. The head-to-toe exam should take only one to two minutes unless emergent injuries are found.

### Physical Examination

**Head:** Observe skin color, lacerations, contusions, facial symmetry.
Assess level of consciousness.
Check pupils.
Palpate gently for depressions in the skull.
Check ears and nose for fluid or blood.
Check mouth for foreign objects and bleeding if necessary.

**Neck:** Observe and palpate areas of tenderness and deformities.

**Arms:** Palpate entire length for pain, wounds, deformity, and sensation.
Ask about pain, tingling, numbness, and movement.

**Chest:** Palpate clavicles and shoulders.
Observe for wounds and that both sides of the chest expand normally upon inspiration.
Perform rib spring on sternum to check for pain.
Press gently on lateral ribs, checking for integrity of ribs.

**Abdomen:** Observe for distention or wounds.
Palpate four quadrants for tenderness and rigidity (rebound tenderness technique).

**Pelvis:** Palpate iliac crest and pubis for pain.
Observe for incontinence (loss of bowel or bladder control).

**Spine:** Palpate for tenderness, wounds, and deformity from shoulders to buttocks.

**Legs:** Palpate entire length for pain, deformity, wounds, and sensation.
Ask about pain, tingling, numbness, and movement.

**Table 2-1**

| CHECK | OBSERVE | SIGNS | POSSIBLE PROBLEMS/CAUSES |
|---|---|---|---|
| **BREATHING** | Watch and feel for chest to rise and fall; listen for breathing; check skin color | No respiration; cyanotic; ashen-gray color or general death-like appearance | Respiratory arrest |
| | | Rapid, shallow breathing | Airway obstruction; heart failure; shock |
| | | Deep, gasping, labored, choking breathing | Hypertension, pain, hyperventilation |
| | | Frothy blood at nose and mouth; coughing | Lung damage; fractured ribs; foreign bodies (bullets); pulmonary edema; severe lung contusions |
| **PULSE** | Feel carotid artery | Absent | Cardiac arrest; death |
| | | Rapid, strong | Fright; heat stroke; hypertension; apprehension |
| | | Rapid, weak | Shock; heat exhaustion; bleeding (hemorrhage); diabetic coma |
| | | Slow, strong | Stroke; concussion |
| **BLEEDING** | Look for wounds<br>Check body openings<br>Feel clothing<br>Feel body | Serious | Hemorrhage; shock |
| | | Minor | Wound |
| | | Internal | Closed wound |
| **POISONING** | Look in mouth<br>Look for container<br>Look at surroundings<br>Listen to victim<br>Ask observers<br>Smell odors | Burns on mouth | Caustic poisoning |
| | | Nausea | Drug overdose; ingested poison; poison inhaled in gas form; poison or drug injected; plant poisoning |
| **LEVEL OF CONSCIOUSNESS** | General observation | Brief periods of unconsciousness | Simple fainting; concussion |
| | Ask victim questions | Confusion, disorientation | Slight blow to head; psychiatric disorder; concussion; hysteria; alcohol or drug overdose; cerebral oxygen insufficiency; emotional disturbance |
| | | Stupor | Cerebral oxygen deficiency; alcohol intoxication |
| | | Deep coma | Concussion; brain damage; skull fracture; severe blow to head; diabetic shock; hysteria; poisoning |
| | | Convulsions | Insulin shock; epilepsy |

**Table 2-1 (Continued)**

| CHECK | OBSERVE | SIGNS | POSSIBLE PROBLEMS/CAUSES |
|---|---|---|---|
| **PUPIL REACTION** | Lift victim's eyelids and check pupil response to light | Dilated | Shock; unconsciousness; cardiac arrest; brain damage; drug use or overuse; disorder of the central nervous system |
| | | Constricted | Head injury; stroke |
| | | Unequal | Head injury |
| | | No response to light, eyes rolled back in head | Death; coma; false eye; cataracts |
| **SKIN COLOR** | Check extremities and fingernails; check inside of lips on dark-skinned victim | Red skin | High blood pressure; carbon monoxide poisoning; heart attack; skin burn |
| | | White skin | Fright; shock; heart attack |
| | | Blue skin (cyanosis) | Asphyxia; anoxia; heart attack; electrocution; poisoning |
| **SKIN TEMPERATURE** | Take temperature with thermometer, orally or rectally; feel with back of hand | Cool, clammy skin | Trauma; hemorrhage; shock; heat exhaustion; nervous stimulation; bleeding |
| | | Cool, dry skin | Exposure to excessive cold |
| | | Hot, dry skin | Fever (in illness); exposure to excessive heat (sun stroke) |
| **REACTION TO PAIN** | Touch victim in various spots | Numbness or tingling in extremities | Injury to spinal cord |
| | | Severe pain and no pulse in extremity | Occlusion of main artery to that extremity |
| | | No feeling of pain or sensation with obvious injury | Hysteria; violent shock; excessive alcohol or drug usage; spinal cord injury |
| | | General pain with injury | Body injury; probably no spinal damage |
| | | Local pain in extremity | Fracture |
| **ABILITY TO MOVE** | Ask victim to move extremities; use hand pressure test | Limited use of any or all extremities | Injury to spinal cord in neck |
| | | Paralysis on one side | Injury to spinal cord in lower back; stroke |
| | | Inability to move arms and hands | Pressure on spinal cord or in brain |
| | | Inability to move legs and feet | Stroke; head injury with brain damage or hemorrhage |

## Work Exercises

Priorities of proper emergency care need to be evaluated, planned, and given. In order to do this properly, what must you, the First Aider, do as you approach and enter the accident scene?

What is a very important consideration as you introduce yourself to the victim and bystanders?

### Primary Victim Survey

Certain conditions are life-threatening and require immediate discovery and care. They are:

1.

2.

3.

4.

An effective First Aider uses well-trained senses to quickly evaluate the condition of each victim and the possible care needed. The senses used by a First Aider are

1. ____________________

2. ____________________

3. ____________________

4. ____________________

You are now looking for signs and symptoms to tell you the proper emergency care to give. It is important to distinguish between signs and symptoms.

(Please complete):

A SIGN is: ____________________

A SYMPTOM is: ____________________

As you approach a conscious victim, you should (complete):

1. Position yourself close to the victim and make eye contact.
2. 
3. 
4. Begin the victim survey.

## Vital Signs

Vital signs tell the victim's condition and are included in the primary and secondary evaluation. Complete the following table by providing the probable causes.

### OBSERVATION OF VITAL SIGNS AND THEIR PROBABLE CAUSES

| Diagnostic Area | Normal Observation | Signs and Symptoms | Probable Cause |
|---|---|---|---|
| State of consciousness | Alert: | Well aware of what is going on, reacts appropriately to factors in the environment; he may ask for water or may tell you that he is in pain. | |
| | Réstless: | Extremely sensitive to the environment; exaggerates environmental factors; wants constant attention; thrashes around. | |
| | Stuporous: | Quiet; seems to be sleeping; can be awakened but returns quickly to sleeplike condition; may involuntarily urinate or defecate; can be awakened by voice or by tapping on body. | |
| | Comatose: | Appears to be sleeping; cannot be awakened. | |
| Respiration or breathing rate | Adults = ________ respirations per minute<br>Child = ________ respirations per minute<br>Depth of breathing also important. | Rapid and shallow<br>Irregular snoring or blowing<br>Deep, labored, gasping<br>Has to sit up to breathe<br>Tendency to hold breathing back<br>Bright red frothy blood from mouth with each exhalation. | |

**OBSERVATION OF VITAL SIGNS AND THEIR PROBABLE CAUSES (Continued)**

| Diagnostic Area | Normal Observation | Signs and Symptoms | Probable Cause |
|---|---|---|---|
| Pulse (indication of heart action) | Adults = ______ beats per minute<br>Child = ______ beats per minute | Rapid and Weak<br>Rapid and Bounding<br>Slowing and Weak<br>Absent | |
| Body and skin temperature | Normal = ______ | Cool and clammy, cold and moist<br>Cool and dry, chills<br>Hot and dry | |
| Skin color | No standard for comparison. Natural skin tone. | Red<br>White<br>Blue | |

A MEDIC ALERT TAG, bracelet or necklace is for what purpose?

REMEMBER — A visual and physical sweep of the body right after you take the pulse is essential.

## Primary and Secondary Surveys

Below are important measures to perform in the primary and secondary survey. They are not listed in order of priority.

- ★ Check the head for laceration.
- ★ Check arms and legs for fractures.
- ★ Check the neck and back for fractures.
- ★ Check for an open airway.
- ★ Check for adequate breathing.
- ★ Check the clavicle and chest for movement on both sides and for fractures.
- ★ Check for a pulse.
- ★ Check the skull for depressions.
- ★ Check the pelvis for fractures.
- ★ Check for any severely bleeding injuries.
- ★ Check for paralysis of extremities.
- ★ Check the abdomen for tenderness and spasms or rigidity.

Place yourself in the following accident situation: A young boy falls out of a tree onto a rock pile below. You are the first person to get to the boy, who is unconscious. In what order would you give this boy a victim survey?

(Rearrange the list from the preceding page in priority order as you imagine yourself performing a primary and secondary survey on the injured boy.)

---

**The Primary Survey**

1. __________
2. __________
3. __________
4. __________

**The Secondary Survey**

5. __________
6. __________
7. __________
8. __________
9. __________
10. __________
11. __________
12. __________

## SELF-TEST

### Part I: True and False

If you believe the statement is true, circle the T. If you believe the statement is false, circle F.

T F 1. Serious injuries are usually very obvious to the First Aider.

T F 2. It is important for a First Aider to know how an accident took place.

T F 3. A spinal injury in the lower back will usually cause paralysis in the victim's arms.

T F 4. The "B" in the "A-B'C's" of first aid stands for "broken bones."

T F 5. The number one treatment priority is an open airway.

T F 6. In a victim survey you begin at the head and usually work down the body.

T F 7. The victim's story about his injuries cannot usually be trusted.

T F 8. The normal breathing rate in the average adult is about 20-25 breaths per minute.

T F 9. The normal pulse rate in adults is 80-100 beats per minute.

T F 10. A rapid and weak pulse is an indication of shock.

T F 11. Constricted pupils are a sign of cardiac arrest.

T F 12. Unequal pupils are a sign of head injury.

T F 13. Paralysis limited to one side of the body is an indication of stroke.

T F 14. Cold and dry skin is an indication of shock.

T F 15. The First Aider should look for a card or bracelet on the victim that gives emergency medical identification.

### Part II: Multiple Choice

For each question, circle the answer that best reflects an accurate statement.

1. In the order of priorities, which of the following are the three primary first aid measures?
   a. maintain breathing, stop bleeding, manage shock
   b. stop bleeding, maintain breathing, reduce shock
   c. prevent shock, stop bleeding, maintain breathing
   d. stop bleeding, prevent shock, avoid infection

2. If you find an unconscious person whose face is red, you should:
   a. raise his/her hips and legs
   b. raise his/her head and shoulders
   c. place him/her on his/her abdomen
   d. do nothing until the doctor arrives

3. A grayish-blue color in the tongue, lips, nail beds, and skin is a sign that the brain is getting too little oxygen. This sign is called:
   a. silicosis
   b. halitosis
   c. cyanosis
   d. symbiosis

4. What should be looked for while conducting the body survey?
   a. blood in the hair
   b. abdominal spasms and tenderness
   c. paralysis of the extremities
   d. all of the above

5. What does loss of fluid or bleeding from the ears and nose indicate?
   a. spinal injury
   b. shock
   c. eye damage
   d. skull fracture

6. During the course of the secondary survey, what should be done if a spinal injury is suspected?
   a. stop the survey and call for more assistance
   b. stabilize the head
   c. continue the survey to find other problems
   d. stop the survey altogether

7. What may constricted pupils indicate?
   a. drug addiction
   b. shock
   c. stroke; head injury
   d. concussion

8. How long should the First Aider spend on the secondary body survey?
   a. 10 to 12 minutes
   b. 5 to 10 minutes
   c. 2 to 3 minutes
   d. less than one minute

9. Medic Alert tags are worn:
   a. to identify allergies
   b. to warn of hidden medical conditions such as diabetes
   c. to provide pertinent information about a victim's special medical needs if he is unable to communicate due to an accident or illness
   d. all of the above

10. Which step in emergency care should be taken first?
    a. treat for shock
    b. remove victims from life-threatening situations
    c. summon police authorities to control bystanders and traffic
    d. determine the mechanism of injury

11. The primary survey, a search for immediate life-threatening problems, is conducted according to the following order:
    a. check for bleeding, breathing, and pulse
    b. check for breathing, pulse, and bleeding
    c. check for pulse, breathing, and bleeding
    d. check for pulse, bleeding, and breathing

Corresponds with:
**American Red Cross**
**Standard First Aid & Personal Safety**
Chapter 5, pages 66-94
and
**Advanced First Aid & Emergency Care**
Chapter 5, pages 65-83

# 3 Respiratory Emergencies

## HOW RESPIRATION WORKS

Oxygen is essential to human life; all living tissue depends on the oxygen carried by the blood. Oxygen enters the body through respiration, the breathing process. Any interference with breathing produces oxygen depletion (anoxia) throughout the entire body. Knowledge of the respiratory system and the organs concerned with respiration will greatly aid in understanding artificial respiration.

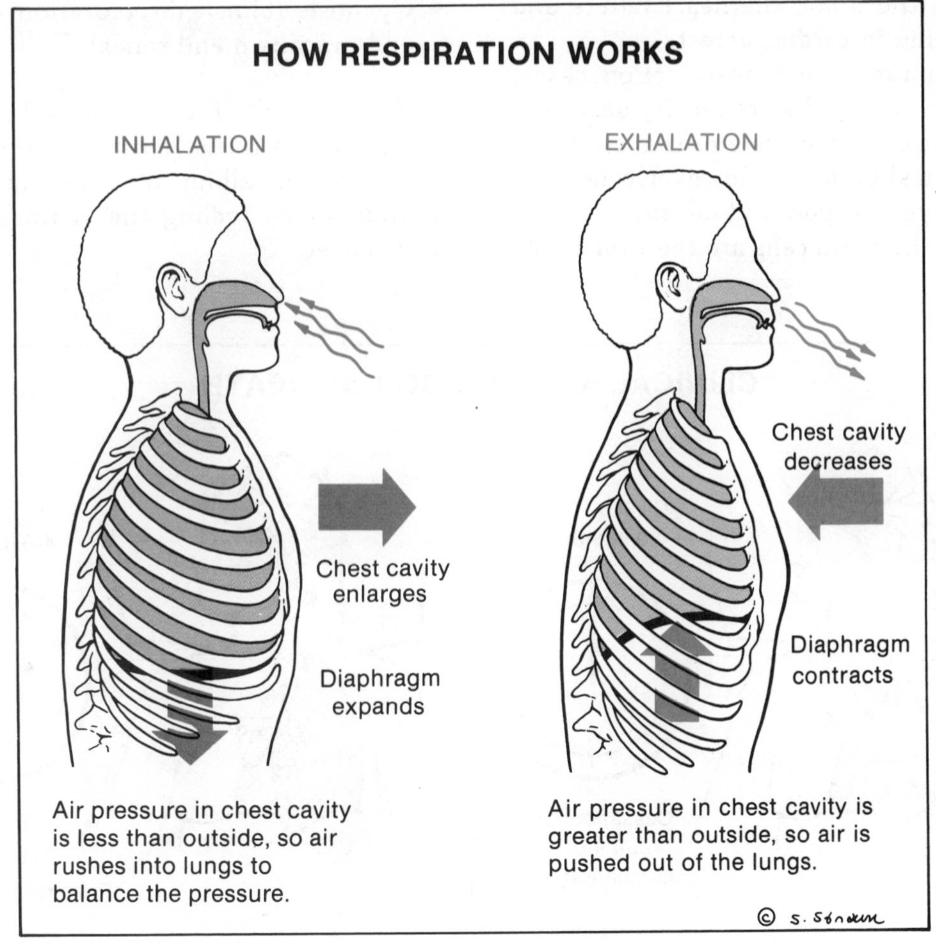

## CAUSES OF RESPIRATORY ARREST

Breathing may stop as a result of a variety of serious accidents. The most common causes of **respiratory arrest** are electric shock, drowning, suffocation, inhalation of poisonous gases, head injuries, and heart problems.

## THE NEED FOR OXYGEN

Without oxygen, cells cannot produce energy and therefore die. If the respiratory system fails to place oxygen in the blood, or if the circulatory system fails to carry oxygen to the cells, then cells, tissue, organs, and finally the system (the victim) dies. Time is critical.

Many victims die from failure of the respiratory and/or circulatory systems. When oxygen is cut off to the lungs, hence to the brain and heart, the heart will continue to pump, gradually becoming weaker as the brain cells that send signals to the heart begin to die from lack of oxygen. When it does not receive signals from the brain, the heart falters and stops, resulting in **cardiac arrest**.

When respiration and heart action cease, the victim is classified as **clinically dead**, because the two essential systems that continue life have been shut down. However, cells have a residual oxygen supply and can survive for a short time. The brain cells are the first to die — usually four to six minutes after being deprived of **oxygenated blood**. Irreversible brain damage occurs, and the system dies. This is called **biological death**. The period between clinical and biological death is short, which means that the First Aider must act quickly to reoxygenate the blood and get it to flow to the brain.

## SIGNS OF RESPIRATORY DISTRESS

Look for the signs of respiratory distress, which include:

- Nasal flaring: the nostrils open wide during inhalation.
- Tracheal tugging: the Adam's apple is pulled upward during inhalation.
- Retraction of **intercostal muscles** (those between the ribs) during inhalation.
- Use of the diaphragm and neck muscles to assist in inhalation.
- Use of the abdominal muscles during exhalation.
- Cyanosis (bluish discoloration of the skin and mucous membranes).

You can tell if a victim is breathing by looking to see if the victim's chest or abdomen is rising and falling, by listening for breath sounds, or by feeling the victim's breath on your cheek.

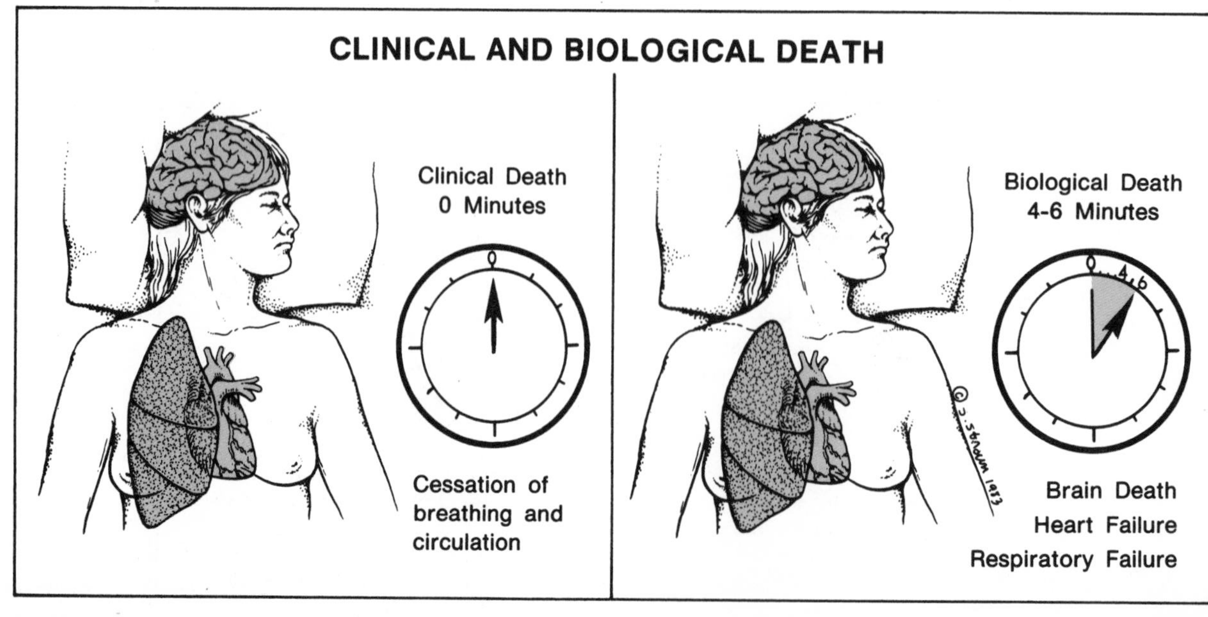

## BASIC LIFE SUPPORT

It has been estimated that many deaths due to cardiac arrests and other injuries that cause breathing to stop could be prevented if the steps of basic life support were started immediately. Briefly, these are:

1. **Assess and open the airway.** Even if the victim has not completely stopped breathing, you need to clear any debris out of his/her mouth and throat. This can include broken teeth, **vomitus,** broken dentures, mucous, or foreign matter that got into the mouth as a result of injury.
2. **Restore breathing.** Once you have cleared out and opened the airway, you have to restore the breathing of a victim who has stopped breathing (no exhaled air can be felt/heard). If the victim is still breathing, stay alert and watch him/her carefully in case he/she does stop breathing.
3. **Restore circulation.** If the victim's heart has stopped beating (neck pulse [carotid] cannot be felt), start **cardiopulmonary resuscitation** to artificially ventilate and circulate the patient.

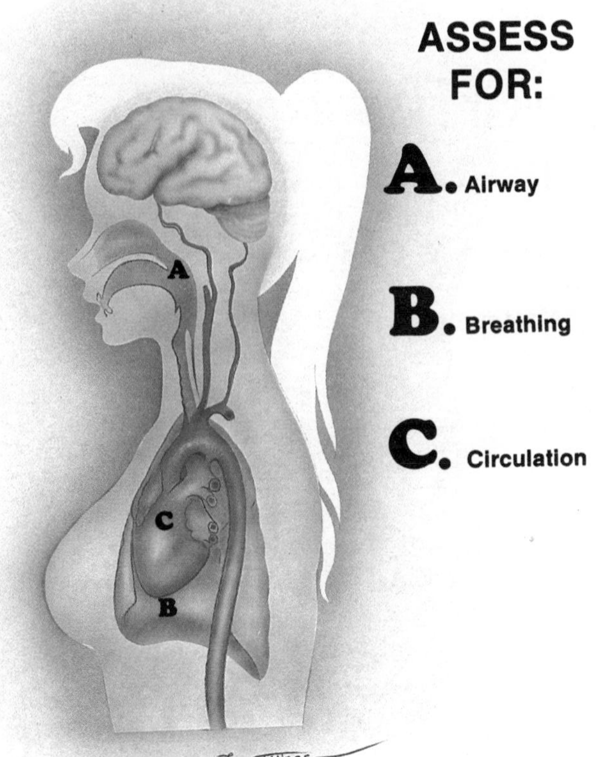


A,B,Cs OF BASIC LIFE SUPPORT

## HOW TO DETERMINE IF A VICTIM IS BREATHING

### 1. Find out if the victim is conscious.

Gently try to arouse him/her by shaking a shoulder, leg, or foot. Speak loudly. If he/she does not respond, lightly scratch the palm of the hand with a pin or needle, or rub the sternum with your knuckles. If he/she does not respond to pain, the victim is unconscious.

### 2. Position the victim on his/her back

Do this only if cervical or spinal injury can be ruled out and if the victim is not already lying on his/her back. If you suspect spinal injury, determine respirations and heartbeat if possible, then find help and roll the victim as a unit (head and neck in alignment) onto his/her back.

### 3. Open the airway.

#### Head Tilt-Chin Lift

This is the most important step in opening the airway.

- Place the palm of one hand on the patient's forehead.
- Apply firm, backward pressure, tipping the victim's head backward.
- Additional assistance is gained by placing the fingers of the other hand under the bony part of the lower jaw near the chin and lift to bring the chin forward and line teeth almost to occlusion.

#### Jaw Thrust

The jaw thrust maneuver is accomplished by displacing the lower jaw forward while tilting the head backward.

**If a neck injury is suspected, the safest, first approach is to perform the jaw thrust without head tilt. After the mandible is displaced forward, support the head carefully without tilting it backward or turning it from side to side.**

### 4. Examine the victim's mouth.

The mouth and throat must be examined for debris that may be obstructing breathing.

**When performing the Head Tilt-Chin Lift Maneuver, the thumb should not be used for lifting the chin and the fingers must not press deeply into the soft tissue under the chin, which might obstruct the airway. Care must also be exercised not to close the mouth completely.**

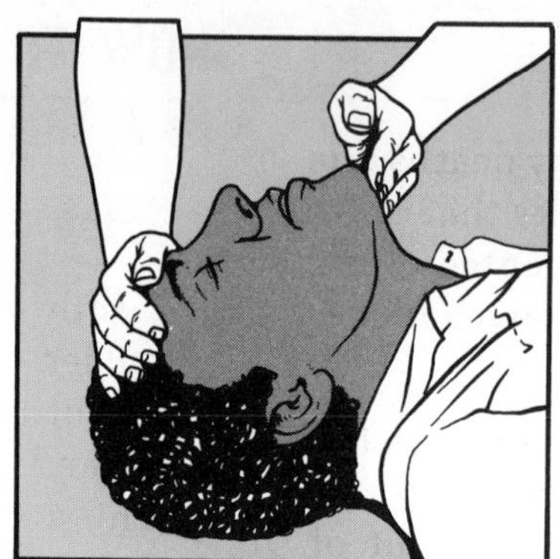

HEAD TILT-CHIN LIFT MANEUVER (Preferred Method)

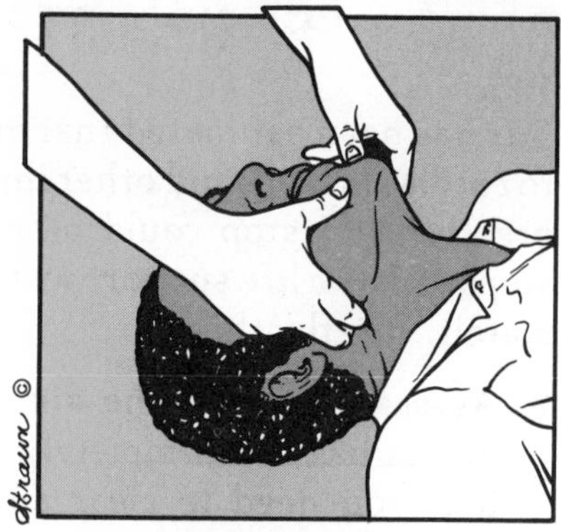

JAW-THRUST MANEUVER

Look for pieces of food, vomitus, broken teeth or dentures, or debris from an automobile or boating accident.

## 5. Establish breathlessness.

Kneel beside the victim and put your ear near his/her mouth and nose, looking toward the chest and stomach. Watch closely to see if the abdomen or chest is rising and falling with breathing. With your cheek next to the victim's nose and mouth, listen for breathing sounds. If the victim is breathing adequately, you should be able to feel him/her exhale against your cheek.

Once you have determined that the victim is not breathing, you must start basic life support within seconds. Give two initial full ventilations at 1-1.5 seconds per ventilation, allowing for deflation between breaths. Vital brain tissue can die within four to six minutes if it is deprived of oxygen. Remember that for any trauma victim, check for and immobilize spinal injury. If the initial attempt to ventilate is unsuccessful, reposition the victim's head and repeat rescue breathing.

## RESTORING BREATHING WITH ARTIFICIAL VENTILATION

The atmosphere that we breathe in contains about 21 percent oxygen. Of this 21 percent, only 5 percent is used by the body, and the remaining 16 percent is exhaled. Because the exhaled breath contains about 16 percent oxygen, a victim can be ventilated using only the First Aider's breath.

The following sequence of photographs shows the procedure for rescue breathing.

Guard against the common mistakes in administering ventilation:

- Not keeping the head tilted.
- Not pinching the nose closed.
- Not making a good enough seal with your mouth.
- Not giving two initial breaths.
- Not giving full breaths during the first two breaths.
- Giving too many or too few breaths.
- Remember not to tilt a child's head too far, and not to breathe too hard.

## AIRWAY OBSTRUCTION

An estimated 3,100 people per year die suddenly while eating; an unknown proportion of these people choke on food stuck in their throats.

An important part of emergency care is educating people to prevent accidents. The following suggestions will help to avoid airway obstructions.

1. Avoid excessive intake of alcohol before and during meals.
2. Cut food into small pieces. Denture wearers especially should chew slowly and thoroughly.
3. Avoid talking and laughing during chewing and swallowing.
4. Teach children not to put foreign objects in their mouths.
5. Do not allow children to run about when they are eating.

## RESCUE BREATHING

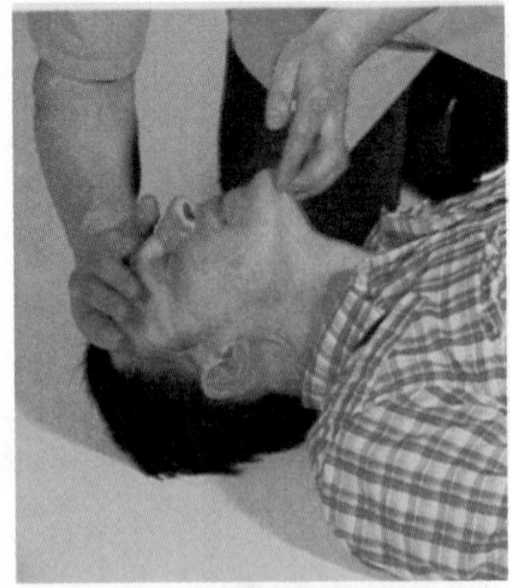

1
Opening the airway by the head tilt-chin lift maneuver (preferred).

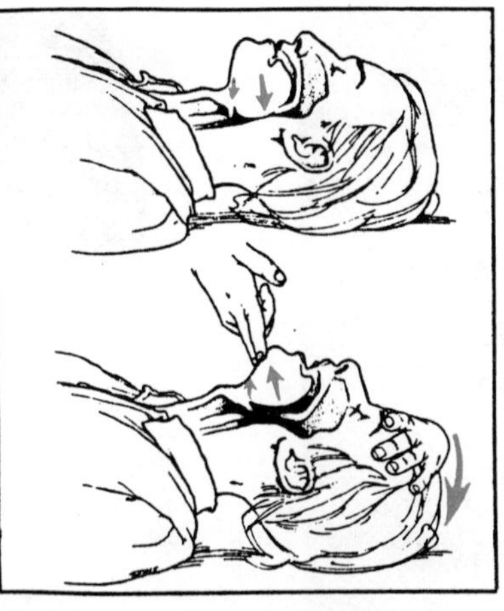

2
Opening the airway. Top, airway obstruction produced by tongue and epiglottis; bottom, relief by head-tilt/chin-lift.

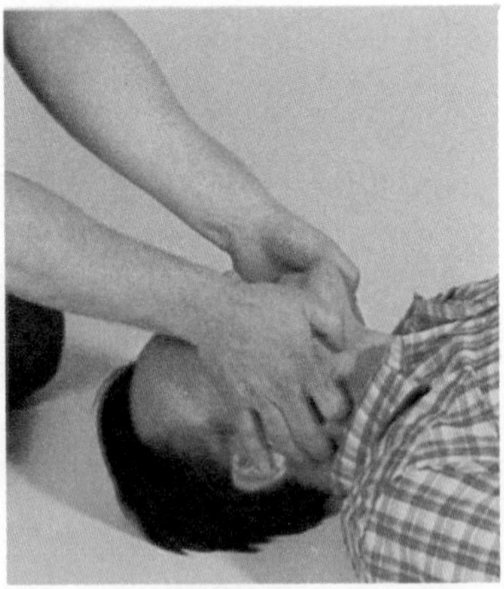

3
Opening the airway by the modified jaw thrust.

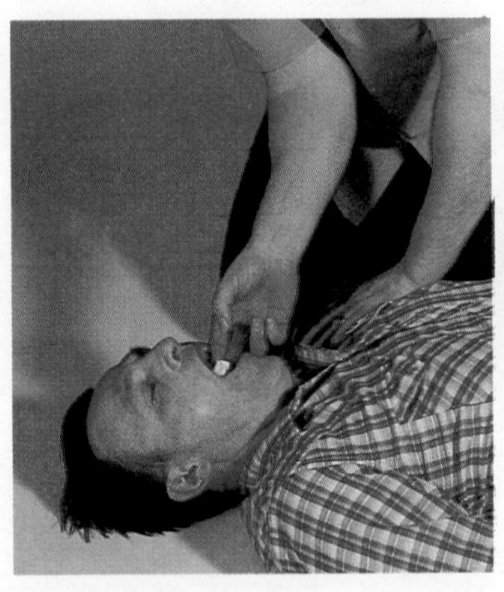

4
Remove any obstructions from the mouth if they are visible.

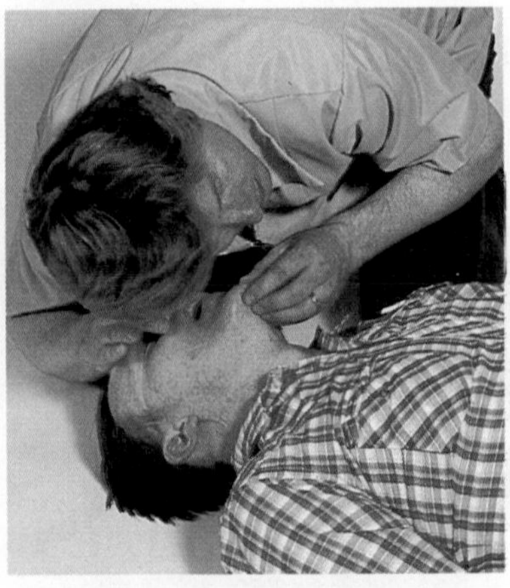

5
Establishing breathlessness with the Look-Listen-Feel method.

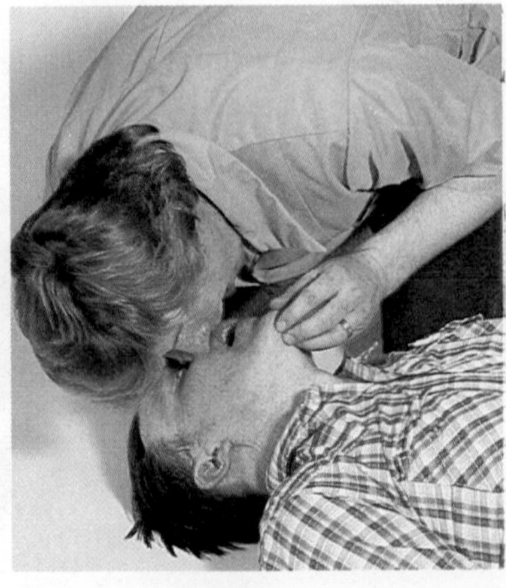

6
Mouth-to-mouth resuscitation. Give two full breaths of air, allowing for deflation between ventilations.

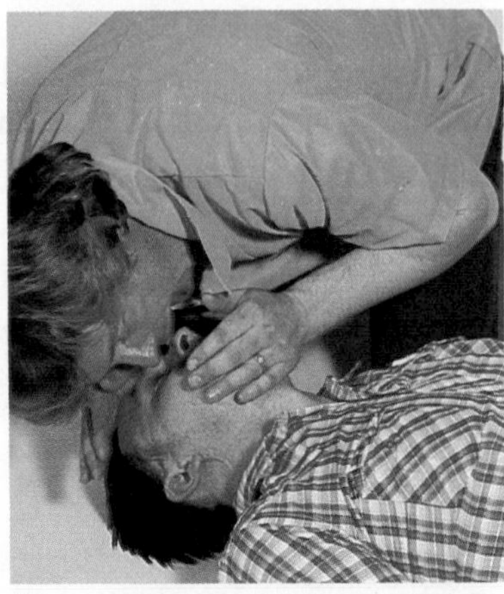

7
Mouth-to-nose ventilation.

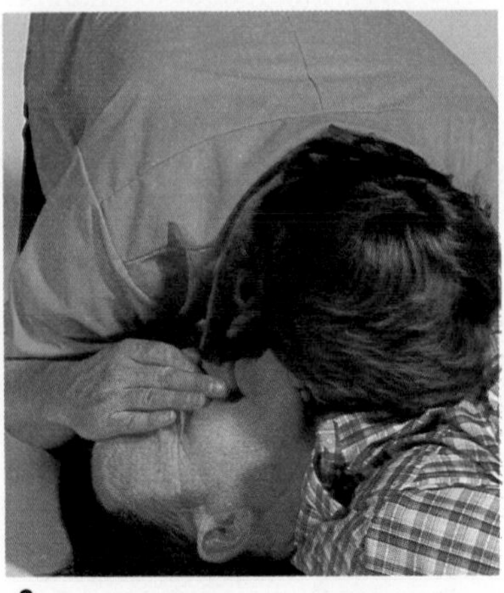

8
Mouth-to-stoma ventilation.

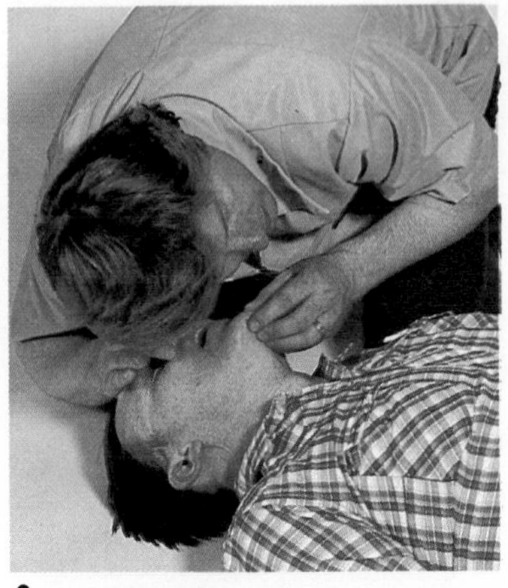

9
Passive exhaling of the victim.

## INFANT VENTILATION

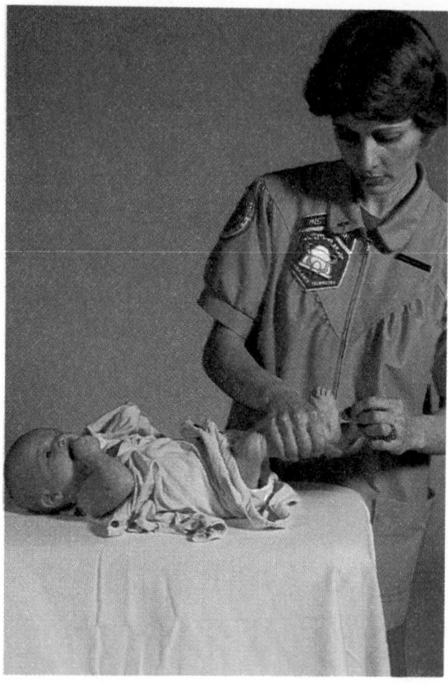

1
Flick the soles of the feet to arouse the baby.

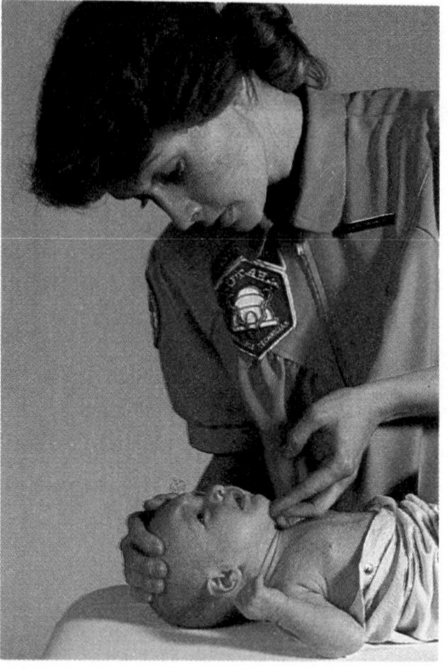

2
Gently open the baby's airway with the head tilt-chin lift method. Do **NOT** exaggerate the head tilt.

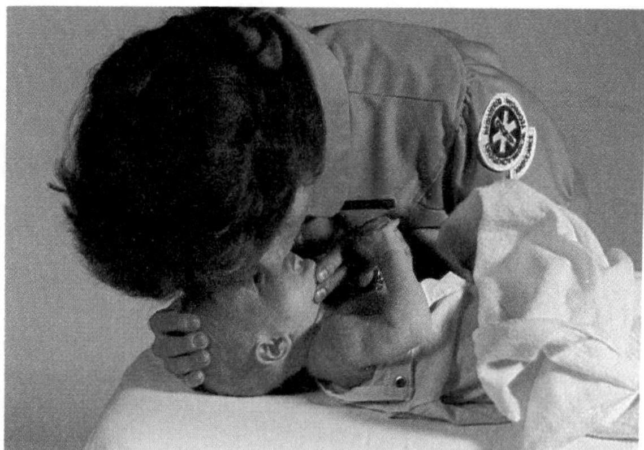

3
Ventilating the baby with mouth-to-mouth and nose resuscitation, using a tight seal and small puffs every 3-4 seconds.

## GASTRIC DISTENTION

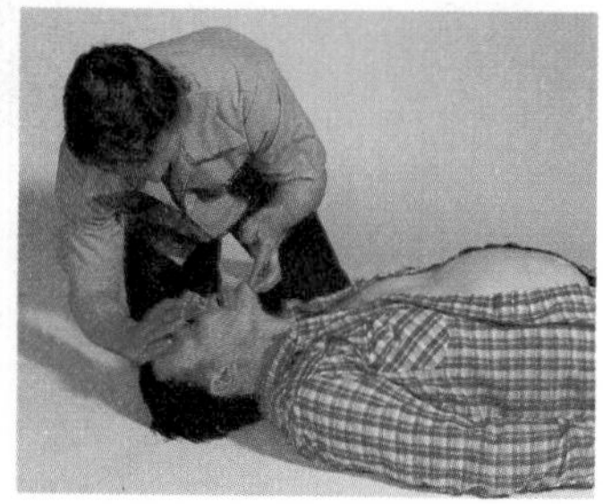

1
When gastric distention occurs, first reposition the airway.

2
To relieve **severe** gastric distention, exert moderate pressure on the abdomen.

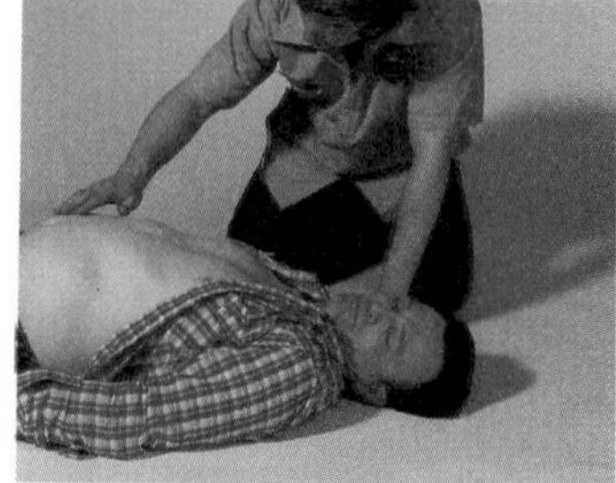

# WHEN BREATHING STOPS

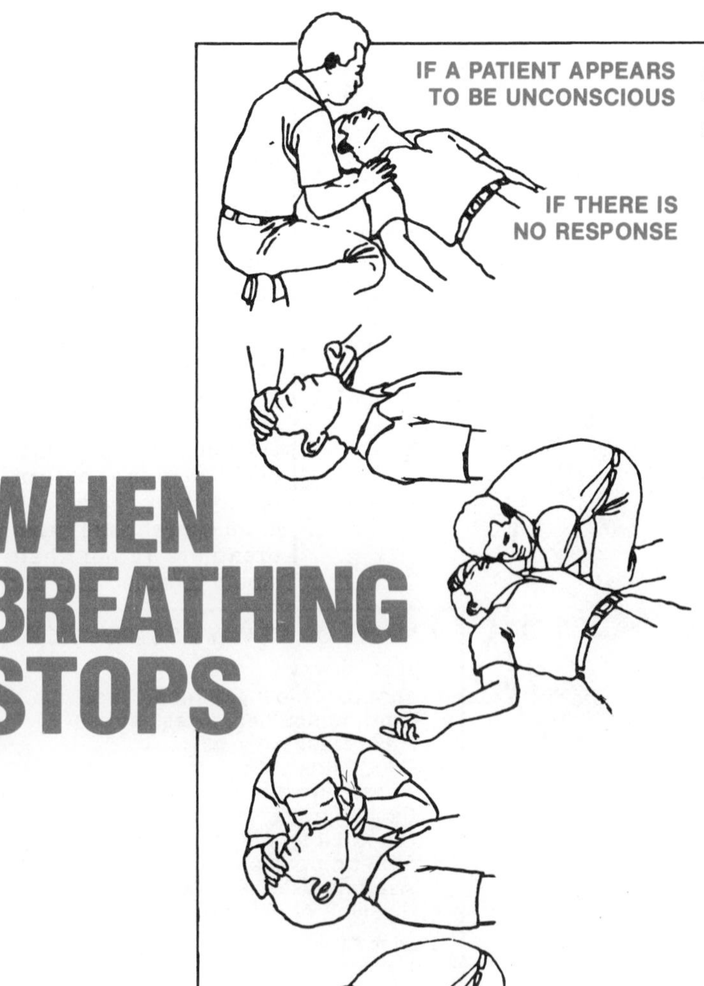

**IF A PATIENT APPEARS TO BE UNCONSCIOUS**

Establish unresponsiveness by:

TAPPING PATIENT ON THE SHOULDER AND SHOUTING, "ARE YOU OKAY?"

**IF THERE IS NO RESPONSE**

CALL for HELP.

**ASSESS** for and OPEN the AIRWAY.

OPEN THE AIRWAY WITH THE HEAD TILT-CHIN LIFT MANEUVER. Tilt the head back by pushing on the forehead with the heel of one hand while pushing the jaw upward with the fingers of the other hand. This will move the tongue away from the back of the throat to open the airway.

**BREATHE** — IMMEDIATELY LOOK, LISTEN, AND FEEL FOR AIR.

While maintaining the backward head tilt position, place your cheek and ear close to the patient's mouth and nose. Look for the chest to rise and fall while you listen and feel for the return of air. Check for about 5 seconds.

GIVE TWO FULL BREATHS.
Maintain the backward head tilt, pinch the patient's nose with the hand that is on the patient's forehead to prevent leakage of air, open your mouth wide, take a deep breath, seal your mouth around the patient's mouth, and blow into the patient's mouth with two full breaths, allowing for deflation. **For an infant,** give gentle puffs and blow through the mouth *and* nose and do not tilt the head back as far as for an adult.

If you do not get an air exchange when you blow, it may help to reposition the head and try again.

AGAIN, LOOK, LISTEN, AND FEEL FOR AIR EXCHANGE.

**IF THE PATIENT IS NOT BREATHING BUT DOES HAVE A PULSE**

**CIRCULATE** — check the pulse. If there is a pulse: continue ventilations.

**IF THERE IS STILL NO BREATHING**

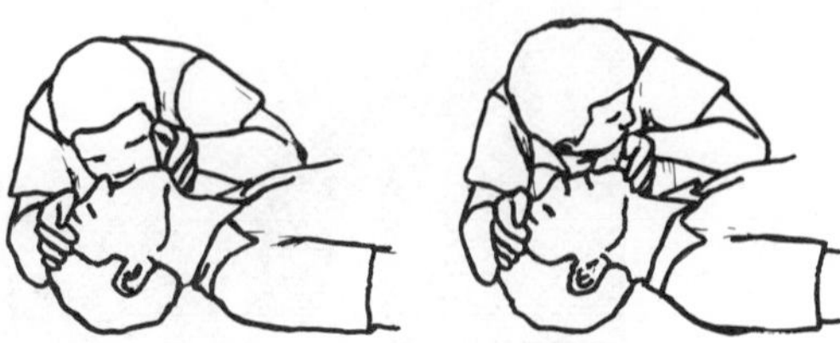

CHANGE RATE TO ONE BREATH EVERY 5 SECONDS **FOR AN ADULT.**

**FOR AN INFANT,** GIVE ONE GENTLE PUFF EVERY 3 SECONDS.

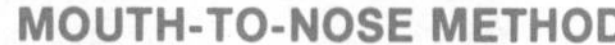

**MOUTH-TO-NOSE METHOD**

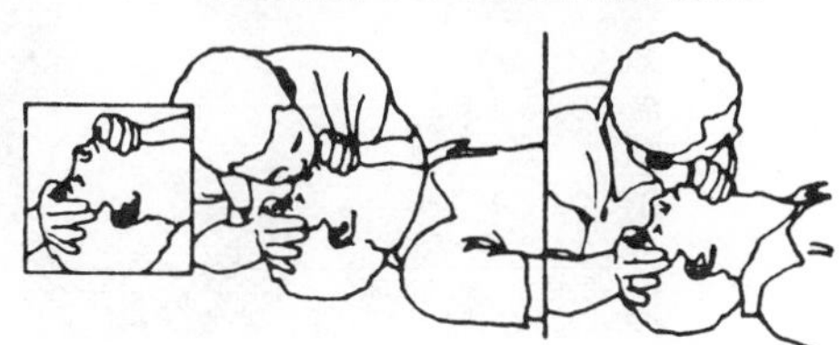

The mouth-to-nose method can be used with the sequence described above instead of the mouth-to-mouth method. Maintain the backward head-tilt position with the hand on the victim's forehead. With the other hand close the victim's mouth. Blow into the victim's nose. Open the victim's mouth for the look, listen, and feel step.

Adapted from American Red Cross.

## AIRWAY ANATOMY

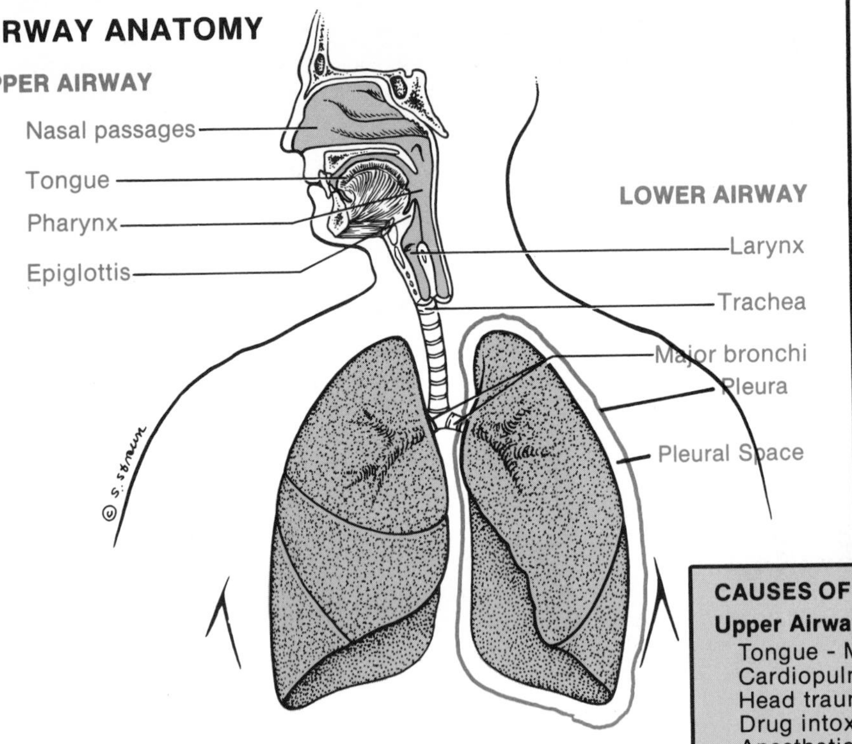

**UPPER AIRWAY**

Nasal passages
Tongue
Pharynx
Epiglottis

**LOWER AIRWAY**

Larynx
Trachea
Major bronchi
Pleura
Pleural Space

© S. Strawn

The structure most commonly responsible for upper airway obstruction is the tongue. The type of foreign object that most frequently causes upper airway obstruction is food. Another common cause of obstruction is acute epiglottitis, which is more frequently seen in children than in adults. Do not overlook nasal obstruction as a cause of upper airway obstruction in infants who are nasal breathers rather than mouth breathers.

**CAUSES OF AIRWAY OBSTRUCTION**

**Upper Airway**
- Tongue - Most common cause
- Cardiopulmonary arrest, stroke
- Head trauma
- Drug intoxication
- Anesthetic drugs
- Facial trauma
- Blood clots: trauma or surgery
- Foreign bodies
- Aspirated stomach contents
- Swelling of epiglottis

**Lower Airway**
- Foreign bodies:
  - Ranging from peanuts to toys

## Emergency Care

The performance sheets on pages 37-40 will guide you through the proper procedures for emergency care for obstruction by a foreign object. Also see photos on pages 35 and 36.

## CHOKING INFANTS AND CHILDREN

In the case of an infant who is choking, you should "straddle" the infant over one arm with the face down and the head lower than the trunk. With the other hand, deliver the four back blows rapidly and forcefully between the shoulder blades — but remember this is an infant. See performance sheets on pages 39 and 40.

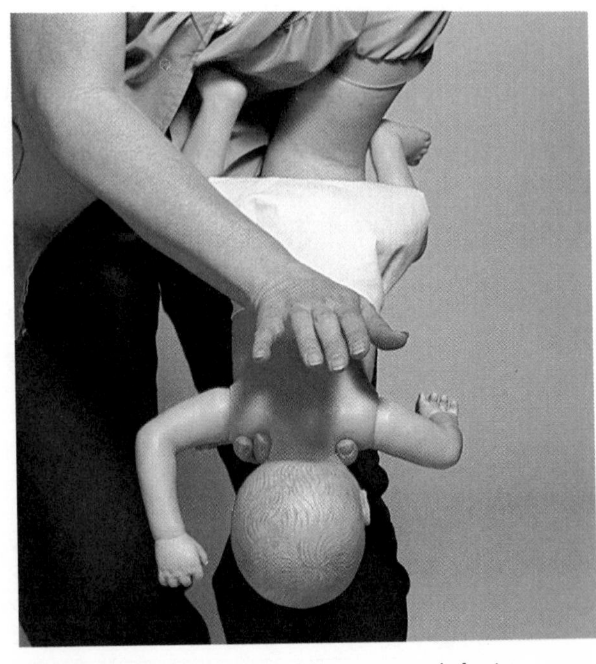

Performing back blows on an infant.

## EMERGENCY CARE FOR OBSTRUCTION BY A FOREIGN OBJECT

**NOTE: Each new thrust should be a separate and distinct movement**

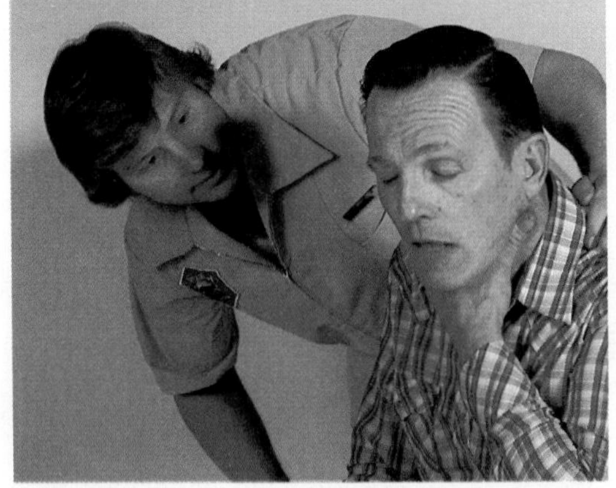

1
The universal sign of choking. Ask the victim "Are You Choking?"

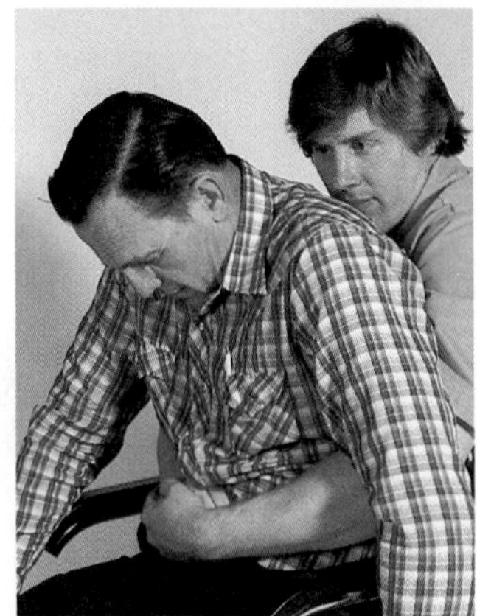

2
Administering the abdominal thrust (Heimlich maneuver) to a sitting victim.

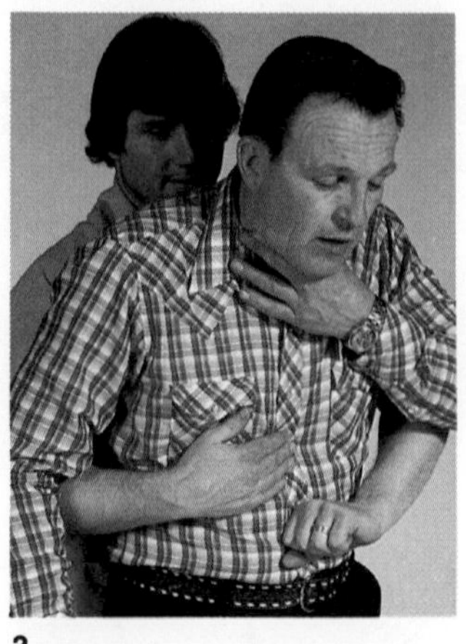

3
Positioning of the fist, thumb side in, for the abdominal thrust.

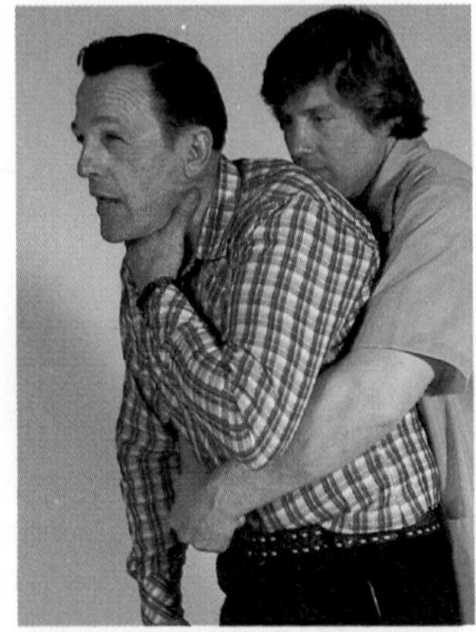

4
Administering the abdominal thrust on a standing victim.

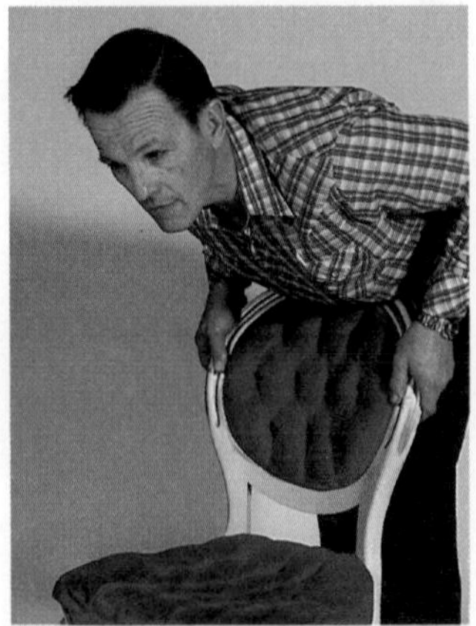

5
The choking victim performing an abdominal thrust on self.

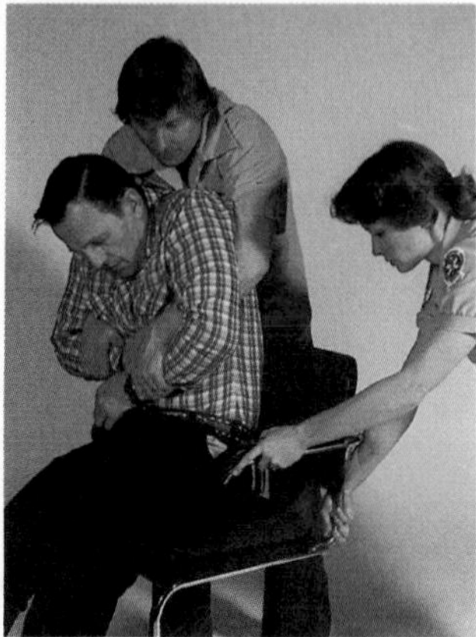

6
Remove an unconscious, sitting victim from the chair and lie him face-up on the floor.

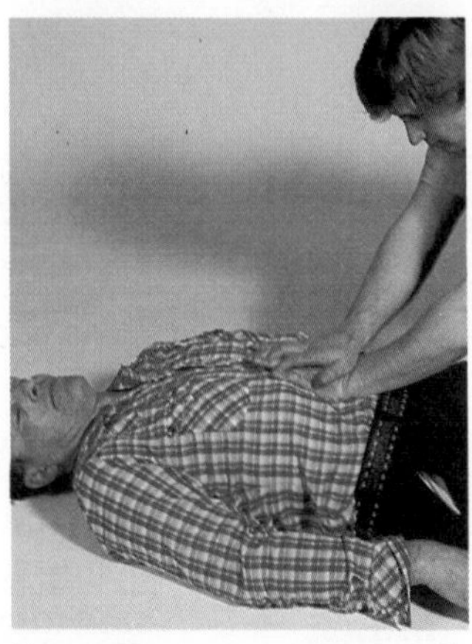

7
Performing abdominal thrusts on an unconscious victim.

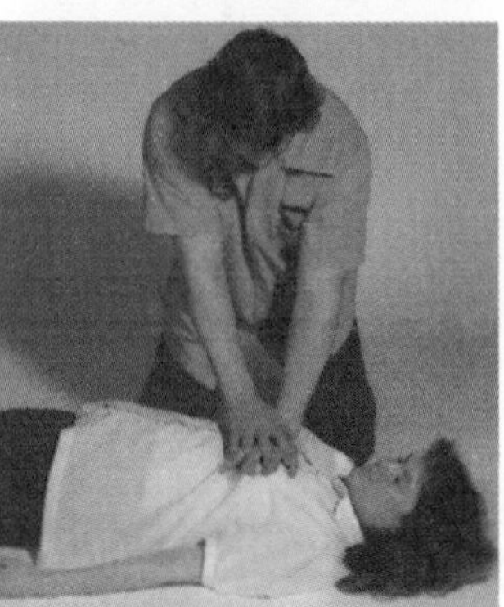

8
Performing chest thrusts on unconscious advanced pregnancy or markedly obese victim — lying down. Chest thrusts can also be performed on a pregnant or obese standing victim.

## FOREIGN OBJECT OBSTRUCTION — MANEUVERS FOR CHILDREN

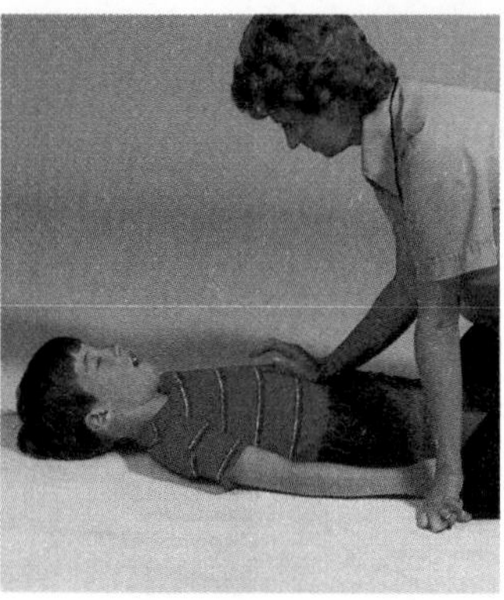

Performing abdominal thrusts on a child lying down. For a larger child, place other hand on top of first hand as in adult.

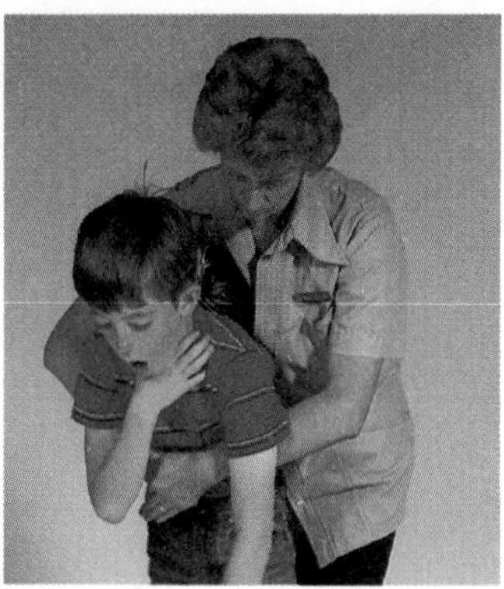

Performing abdominal thrust on a child standing up.

## CHEST THRUSTS

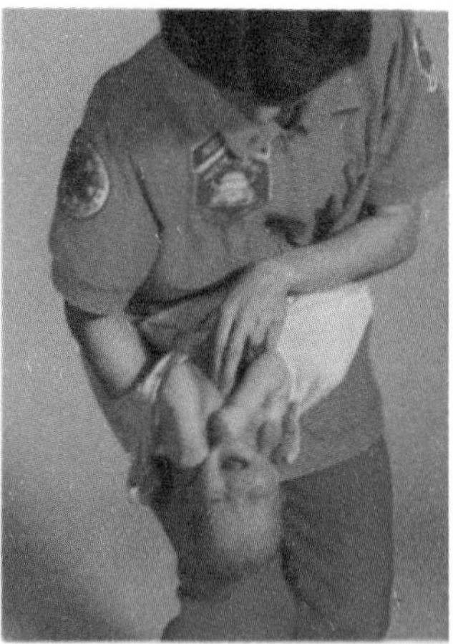

Performing chest thrusts on an infant.

## Chest Thrust — For an Infant (Under One Year)

- Position the infant face-up over your forearm with the infant's head lower than the rest of his body.
- Open the airway. Place the flat part of your index finger on the intermammary line (an imaginary line between the nipples). Use the flat part of your next two fingers below the line to compress the infant's sternum one-half to one inch.

Note: When practicing these maneuvers, do not follow through with the action or you may seriously injure someone.

# Obstructed Airway: Conscious Adult

| Step | Activity | Critical Performance |
|---|---|---|
| **1. Assessment** | Determine airway obstruction. | Ask "Are you choking?" |
| | | Determine if victim can cough or speak. |
| **2. Heimlich Maneuver** | Perform abdominal thrusts. | Stand behind the victim. |
| | | Wrap arms around victim's waist. |
| | | Make a fist with one hand and place the thumb side against victim's abdomen in the midline slightly above the navel and well below the tip of the xiphoid. |
| | | Grasp fist with the other hand. |
| | | Press into the victim's abdomen with quick upward thrusts. |
| | | Each thrust should be distinct and delivered with the intent of relieving the airway. |
| | | Repeat thrusts until either the foreign body is expelled or the victim becomes unconscious (see below). |

## Victim with Obstructed Airway Becomes Unconscious

| Step | Activity | Critical Performance |
|---|---|---|
| **3. Additional Assessment** | Position the victim. | Turn on back as unit. |
| | | Place face up, arms by side. |
| | Call for help. | Call out "Help!" or, if others respond, activate EMS system. |
| **4. Foreign Body Check** | Perform finger sweep.** | Keep victim's face up. |
| | | Use tongue-jaw lift to open mouth. |
| | | Sweep deeply into mouth to remove foreign body. |
| **5. Breathing Attempt** | Attempt ventilation (airway is obstructed). | Open airway with head-tilt/chin-lift. |
| | | Seal mouth and nose properly. |
| | | Attempt to ventilate. |
| **6. Heimlich Maneuver** | Perform abdominal thrusts. | Kneel astride victim's thighs. |
| | | Place heel of one hand against victim's abdomen, in the midline slightly above the navel and well below the tip of the xiphoid. |
| | | Place second hand directly on top of first hand. |
| | | Press into the abdomen with quick upward thrusts. |
| | | Perform 6-10 abdominal thrusts. |
| **7. Foreign Body Check** | Perform finger sweep.** | Keep victim's face up. |
| | | Use tongue-jaw lift to open mouth. |
| | | Sweep deeply into mouth to remove foreign body. |
| **8. Breathing Attempt** | Reattempt ventilation. | Open airway with head-tilt/chin-lift. |
| | | Seal mouth and nose properly. |
| | | Attempt to ventilate. |
| **9. Sequencing** | Repeat sequence. | Repeat Steps 6-8 until successful.† |

** During practice and testing, simulate finger sweeps.

† After airway obstruction is removed, check for pulse and breathing. (a) If pulse is absent, ventilate a second time and start cycles of compressions and ventilations. (b) If pulse is present: Open airway and check for spontaneous breathing. (c) If breathing is present, monitor breathing and pulse closely, maintain open airway. (d) If breathing is absent, perform rescue breathing at 12 times/min. and monitor pulse.

**Source: American Heart Association**

# Obstructed Airway: Unconscious Adult

| Step | Activity | Critical Performance |
|---|---|---|
| **1. Assessment/Airway** | Determine unresponsiveness. | Tap or gently shake shoulder. Shout "Are you OK?" |
| | Call for help. | Call out "Help!" |
| | Position the victim. | Turn on back as unit, if necessary, supporting head and neck (4-10 sec.). |
| | Open the airway. | Use head-tilt/chin-lift maneuver. |
| | Determine breathlessness. | Maintain open airway. |
| | | Ear over mouth, observe chest: look, listen, feel for breathing (3-5 sec.). |
| **2. Breathing Attempt** | Attempt ventilation (airway is obstructed). | Maintain open airway. |
| | | Seal mouth and nose properly. |
| | | Attempt to ventilate. |
| | Reattempt ventilation (airway remains blocked). | Reposition victim's head. |
| | | Seal mouth and nose properly. |
| | | Reattempt to ventilate. |
| | Activate EMS system. | If someone responded to call for help, send him/her to activate EMS system. |
| **3. Heimlich Maneuver** | Perform abdominal thrusts. | Kneel astride victim's thighs. |
| | | Place heel of one hand against victim's abdomen in the midline slightly above the navel and well below the tip of the xiphoid. |
| | | Place second hand directly on top of first hand. |
| | | Press into the abdomen with quick upward thrusts. |
| | | Each thrust should be distinct and delivered with the intent of relieving the airway. |
| | | Perform 6-10 abdominal thrusts. |
| **4. Foreign Body Check** | Perform finger sweep.** | Keep victim's face up. |
| | | Use tongue-jaw lift to open mouth. |
| | | Sweep deeply into mouth to remove foreign body. |
| **5. Breathing Attempt** | Reattempt ventilation. | Open airway with head-tilt/chin-lift maneuver. |
| | | Seal mouth and nose properly. |
| | | Attempt to ventilate. |
| **6. Sequencing** | Repeat sequence. | Repeat Steps 3-5 until successful.† |

** During practice and testing, simulate finger sweeps.

† After airway obstruction is removed, check again for pulse and breathing. (a) If pulse is absent, ventilate a second time and start cycles of compressions and ventilations. (b) If pulse is present, open airway and check for spontaneous breathing. (c) If breathing is present, monitor breathing and pulse closely, maintain open airway. (d) If breathing is absent, perform rescue breathing at 12 times/min. and monitor pulse.

Source: American Heart Association

# Obstructed Airway: Conscious Child

| Step | Activity | Critical Performance |
|---|---|---|
| **1. Assessment** | Determine airway obstruction. | Ask "Are you choking?" |
| | | Determine if victim can cough or speak. |
| **2. Heimlich Maneuver** | Perform abdominal thrusts (only if victim's cough is ineffective and there is increasing respiratory difficulty). | Stand behind the victim. |
| | | Wrap arms around victim's waist. |
| | | Make a fist with one hand and place the thumb side against victim's abdomen, in the midline slightly above the navel and well below the tip of the xiphoid. |
| | | Grasp fist with the other hand. |
| | | Press into the victim's abdomen with quick upward thrusts. |
| | | Each thrust should be distinct and delivered with the intent of relieving the airway. |
| | | Repeat thrusts until either the foreign body is expelled or the victim becomes unconscious. |

## Obstructed Airway: Unconscious Child

| Step | Activity | Critical Performance |
|---|---|---|
| **1. Assessment/Airway** | Determine unresponsiveness. | Tap or gently shake shoulder. |
| | | Shout "Are you OK?" |
| | Call for help. | Call out, "Help!" |
| | Position the victim. | Turn on back as unit, if necessary, supporting head and neck (4-10 sec.). |
| | Open the airway. | Use head-tilt/chin-lift maneuver. |
| | Determine breathlessness. | Maintain open airway. |
| | | Ear over mouth, observe chest: look, listen, feel for breathing (3-5 sec.). |
| **2. Breathing Attempt** | Attempt ventilation (airway is obstructed). | Maintain open airway. |
| | | Seal mouth and nose properly. |
| | | Attempt to ventilate (1-1.5 sec./ventilation). |
| | Reattempt ventilation (airway remains blocked). | Reposition victim's head. |
| | | Seal mouth and nose properly. |
| | | Reattempt to ventilate (1-1.5 sec./ventilation). |
| | | Total time, Steps 1 and 2: 15-35 sec. |
| | Activate EMS system. | If someone responded to call for help, send him/her to activate EMS system. |
| **3. Heimlich Maneuver** | Perform abdominal thrusts. | Kneel at victim's feet if on the floor, or stand at victim's feet if on a table. |
| | | Place heel of one hand against victim's abdomen in the midline slightly above navel and well below tip of xiphoid. |
| | | Place second hand directly on top of first hand. |
| | | Press into the abdomen with quick upward thrusts. |
| | | Each thrust should be distinct and delivered with the intent of relieving the airway. |
| | | Perform 6-10 abdominal thrusts. |
| **4. Foreign Body Check** | Perform tongue-jaw lift. Do not perform blind finger sweep; remove foreign body only IF VISUALIZED. | Keep victim's face up. |
| | | Use tongue-jaw lift to open mouth. |
| | | Look into mouth and remove foreign body IF VISUALIZED. |
| **5. Breathing Attempt** | Reattempt ventilation. | Open airway with head-tilt/chin-lift maneuver. |
| | | Seal mouth and nose properly. |
| | | Attempt to ventilate (1-1.5 sec./ventilation). |
| **6. Sequencing** | Repeat sequence. | Repeat Steps 3-5 until successful.** |

** After airway obstruction is removed, check again for pulse and breathing. (a) If pulse is absent: Ventilate a second time and start cycles of compressions and ventilations. (b) If pulse is present: Open airway and check for spontaneous breathing. If breathing is present, monitor breathing and pulse closely, maintain open airway. If breathing is absent, perform rescue breathing at 15 times/min. and monitor pulse.

Source: American Heart Association

# Obstructed Airway: Conscious Infant*

| Step | Activity | Critical Performance |
|---|---|---|
| **1. Assessment** | Determine airway obstruction.* | Observe breathing difficulties.* |
| **2. Back Blows** | Deliver 4 back blows. | Supporting head with one hand, straddle infant face down, head lower than trunk, over your forearm supported on your thigh. |
| | | Deliver 4 back blows, forcefully, between the shoulder blades with the heel of the hand (3-5 sec.). |
| **3. Chest Thrusts** | Deliver 4 chest thrusts. | While supporting the head, sandwich infant between your hands and turn on back, with head lower than trunk. |
| | | Deliver 4 thrusts in the midsternal region in the same manner as external chest compressions, but at a slower rate (3-5 sec.). |
| **4. Sequencing** | Repeat sequence. | Repeat Steps 2 and 3 until either the foreign body is expelled or the infant becomes unconscious. |

## Obstructed Airway: Unconscious Infant

| Step | Activity | Critical Performance |
|---|---|---|
| **1. Assessment/Airway** | Determine unresponsiveness. | Tap or gently shake shoulder. |
| | Call for help. | Call out, "Help!" |
| | Position the infant. | Turn on back as unit, if necessary, supporting head. |
| | | Place on firm, hard surface. |
| | Open the airway. | Use head-tilt/chin-lift maneuver to sniffing or neutral position. |
| | | Do not overextend the head. |
| | Determine breathlessness. | Maintain open airway. |
| | | Ear over mouth, observe chest: look, listen, feel for breathing (3-5 sec.). |
| **2. Breathing Attempt** | Attempt ventilation (airway is obstructed). | Maintain open airway. |
| | | Make tight seal on mouth and nose of infant with rescuer's mouth. |
| | | Attempt to ventilate (1-1.5 sec./ventilation). |
| | Reattempt ventilation (airway remains blocked). | Reposition infant's head. |
| | | Seal mouth and nose properly. |
| | | Reattempt to ventilate (1-1.5 sec./ventilation). |
| **3. EMS** | Activate EMS system. | If someone responded to call for help, send him/her to activate EMS system. |
| | | Total time, Steps 1-3: 10-25 sec. |
| **4. Back Blows** | Deliver 4 back blows. | Supporting head with one hand, straddle infant face down, head lower than trunk, over your forearm supported on your thigh. |
| | | Deliver 4 back blows, forcefully, between the shoulder blades with the heel of the hand (3-5 sec.). |
| **5. Chest Thrusts** | Deliver 4 chest thrusts. | While supporting the head, sandwich infant between your hands and turn on back, with head lower than trunk. |
| | | Deliver 4 thrusts in the midsternal region in the same manner as external chest compressions, but at a slower rate (3-5 sec.). |
| **6. Foreign Body Check** | Perform tongue-jaw lift. Do not perform blind finger sweep; remove foreign body only IF VISUALIZED. | Do tongue-jaw lift by placing thumb in infant's mouth over tongue. Lift tongue and jaw forward with fingers wrapped around lower jaw. |
| | | Remove foreign body IF VISUALIZED. |
| **7. Breathing Attempt** | Reattempt ventilation. | Open airway with head-tilt/chin-lift. |
| | | Seal mouth and nose properly. |
| | | Attempt to ventilate (1-1.5 sec./ventilation). |
| **8. Sequencing** | Repeat sequence. | Repeat Steps 4-7 until successful.** |

** After airway obstruction is removed, check again for pulse and breathing. (a) If pulse is absent: Ventilate a second time and start cycles of compressions and ventilations. (b) If pulse is present: Open airway and check for spontaneous breathing. If breathing is present, monitor breathing and pulse closely, maintain open airway. If breathing is absent, perform rescue breathing at 15 times/min. and monitor pulse.

Source: American Heart Association

## Work Exercises

### Normal Breath Sounds

List the three major ways you can recognize adequate breathing:

Seeing Chest & Abdomen Rise & Fall

Hearing For Breath

Feeling Feeling breath on your cheek

### Causes of Respiratory Distress and Arrest

List below six major causes of respiratory arrest:

1. Electric shock
2. Drowning
3. Suffocation
4. Inhalation of poisonous gases
5. Head Injuries
6. Heart problems

2. A respiratory emergency occurs when a victim stops breathing and is signalled by various signs and symptoms; list those that affect each of the following:

A. Consciousness: Unconcious

B. Pupils: Dilated

C. Tongue:

D. Lips: Discolored Blue

E. Fingernail beds:

3. Identify below four major symptoms of suffocation in an unconscious person.

1. Nasal Flaring
2. Tracheal Tugging
3. Cyanosis - Blue Discoloration
4. Use of Abdominal Muscles in exhalation

3.

4.

4. As a trained First Aider, you may be called upon to teach groups basic emergency care. What precautions could you explain to a neighborhood gathering to prevent suffocation?

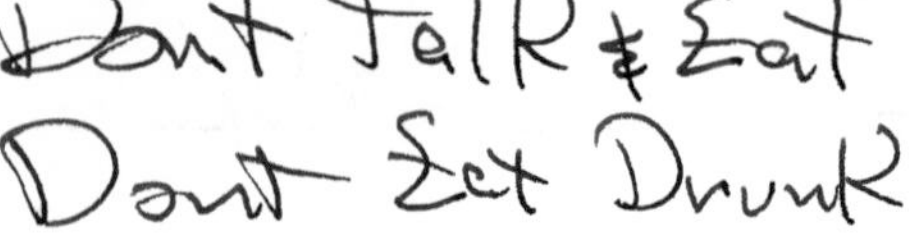


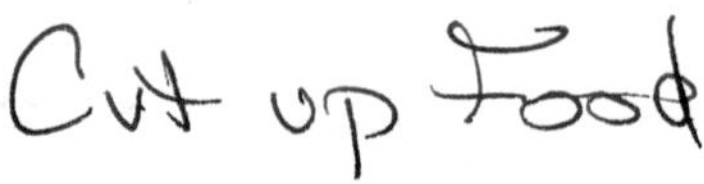


5. Basic Life Support is a systematic approach to saving the life of a victim who is not breathing and may not have a heart beat. The three major steps of Basic Life Support are:

1. A. = Airway Open
2. B. = Restore Breathing
3. C. = Restore Circulation

Select the proper technique for each of the following ways the airway may be opened.

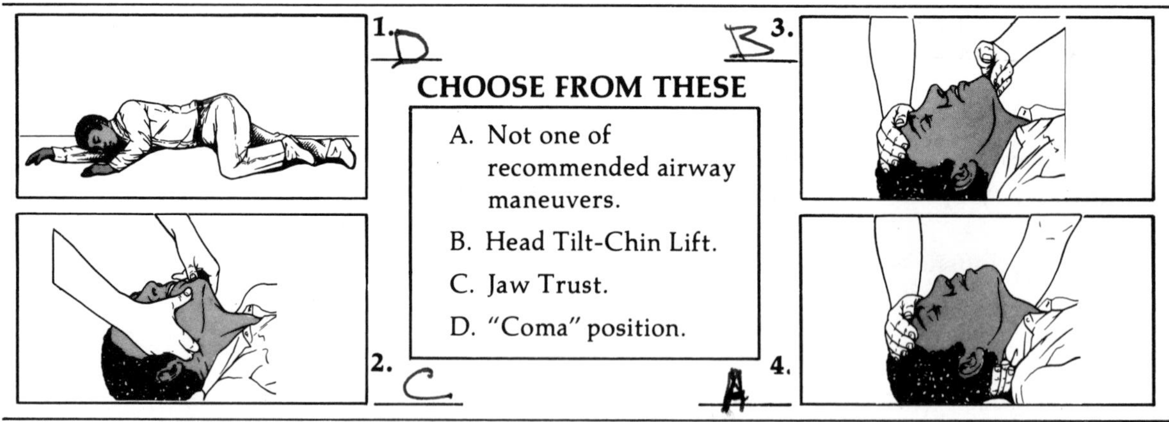


## Artificial Ventilation

Oxygen is essential for the normal functioning of body cells. When the oxygen supply is cut off, the first cells to die are the brain cells. These oxygen deprived brain cells may die within 4 to 6 minutes.

The most effective type of artificial ventilation is ______________ resuscitation.

Fill in the following chart.

# LIFE SUPPORT DECISION CHART

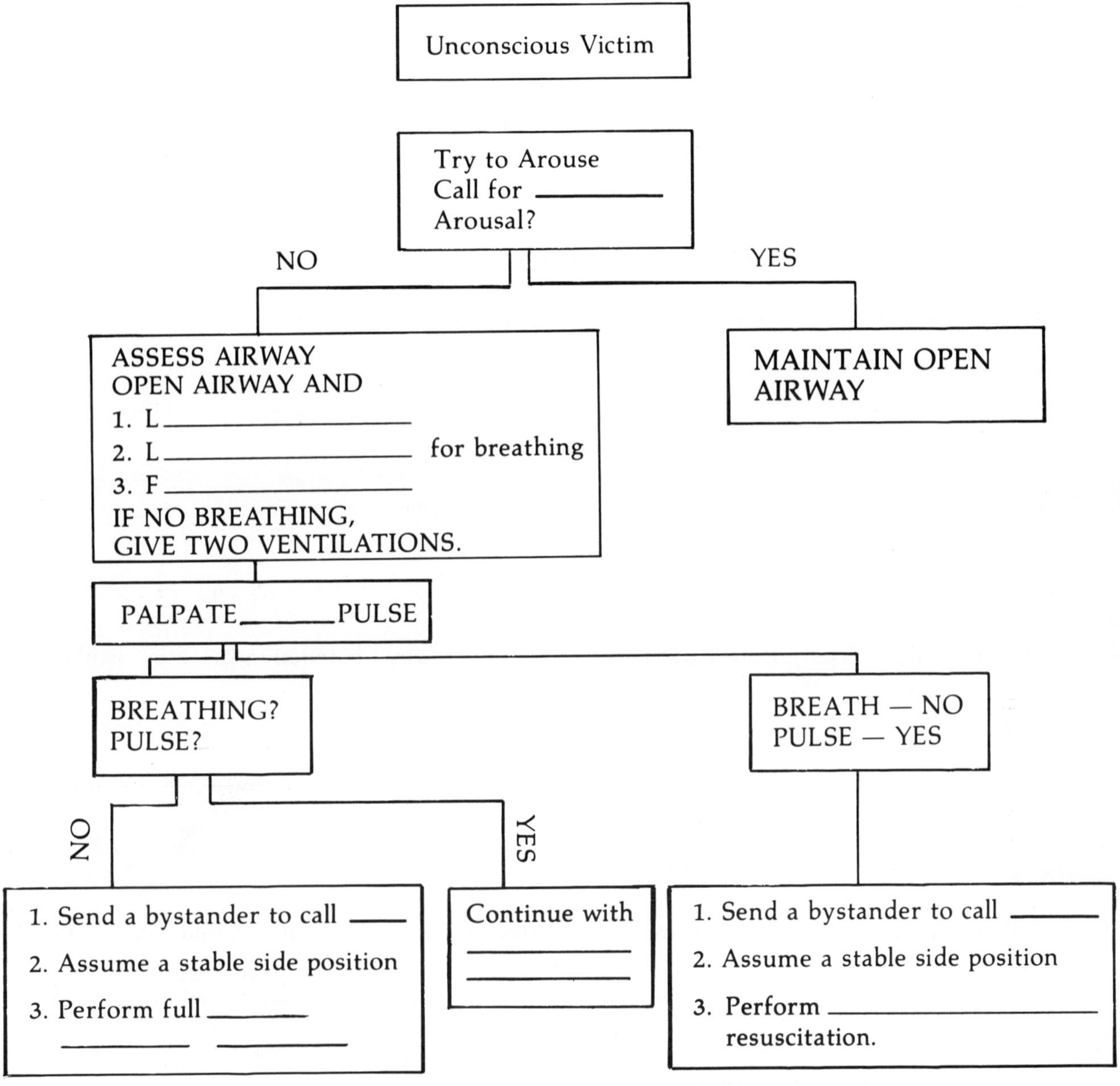


## Infant Resuscitation

Describe the differences between infant and adult mouth-to-mouth resuscitation.

1. 1 Breath every 3 sec Infant (5 sec Adult)
2. Seal Nose as well as mouth - Infant

## Airway Obstruction

A significant ventilation problem is airway obstruction. Who is one of the most common victims of airway obstructions? ______________________.

Airway obstruction causes hypoxemia or ______________________.

The brain cannot sustain more than ________ to ________ minutes of hypoxemia.

The most common source of upper airway obstruction is Tongue.

List four signs and symptoms shown by a victim of airway obstruction.

1.

2.

3.

4.

When a victim experiences a partial or complete airway obstruction, he may display the universal distress signal for choking, which is ______________________

______________________

## Emergency Care For Airway Obstruction

When you recognize partial or incomplete airway obstruction you should ask the victim

______________________

### EMERGENCY CARE FOR AIRWAY OBSTRUCTION

Outline below the most effective method used to overcome an airway obstruction and the number of times this method should be applied.

| Method | Number of Times |
|---|---|
| 1. | |
| For Infants | |
| 1. | Four |
| 2. | |

## SELF-TEST

### Part I: True and False

If you believe the statement is true, circle the T. If you believe the statement is false, circle F.

T F 1. The most common respiratory emergency is blockage of the air passage by a solid foreign object lodged in the throat.

T F 2. If a choking person is unable to speak, you should assume the emergency is life-threatening.

T F 3. Adults have a faster rate of respiration than children, so require more rapid artificial ventilation.

T F 4. In mouth-to-mouth respiration it is important to tilt the victim's head back with his chin pointing up so his tongue won't block his airway.

T F 5. When resuscitating infants or small children, use more frequent, less powerful puffs of air into both the nose and mouth simultaneously.

T F 6. To check effectiveness of artificial respiration, you should watch to make sure that the stomach is bulging.

T F 7. If you suspect that the heart has stopped beating, you should not attempt artificial respiration.

T F 8. In cardiopulmonary resuscitation (CPR), you can perform external heart compression without artificial ventilation if the victim seems to be breathing normally.

T F 9. An adult victim should be provided with one breath every 8 to 9 seconds.

T F 10. Blue fingernail beds and dilated pupils are signs of a respiratory emergency.

T F 11. The average person may die in six minutes or less if his oxygen supply is cut off.

T F 12. Recovery is usually very slow when you perform artificial ventilation.

T F 13. You should only do artificial ventilation for thirty minutes; longer than that will do no good if the victim has not already responded.

T F 14. The victim of a respiratory emergency should always be treated for shock and should always see a doctor.

T F 15. Use only small puffs when giving artificial resuscitation to a baby.

T F 16. If the victim's stomach begins to bulge during artificial ventilation, just ignore it and continue your first aid efforts.

T F 17. The best way to see if a person has stopped breathing is to check the rising of the chest.

T F 18. The brain can survive for approximately ten to twelve minutes before permanent brain damage occurs due to oxygen deprivation.

T F 19. Mouth-to-mouth is the most effective method of artificial respiration.

T F 20. When giving mouth-to-nose resuscitation, you keep the mouth tightly closed through the *complete* process.

T F 21. The *first* step in clearing a blocked airway is to check for breathing obstructions.

### Part II: Multiple Choice

For each question, circle the answer that best reflects an accurate statement.

1. The purpose of artificial ventilation is to:

a. prevent the tongue from being swallowed
b. provide a method of air exchange
c. clear an upper air passage obstruction
d. clear a lower air passage obstruction

2. You should always continue giving artificial ventilation until:
   a. the victim is dead beyond any doubt
   b. the victim starts breathing on his own
   c. the victim is pronounced dead by a doctor
   d. all of the above

3. A respiratory emergency can result from:
   a. drowning
   b. alcohol overdose
   c. electrocution
   d. vomiting
   e. burns to the face
   f. all of the above

4. As compared to mouth-to-mouth ventilation, in mouth-to-stoma respiration you should:
   a. blow the air at a slower rate
   b. blow the air at the same rate
   c. blow the air at a faster rate

5. A major sign of a respiratory emergency is:
   a. bluish discoloration of the tongue, lips, and/or nailbeds
   b. distended abdomen
   c. hot, flushed skin
   d. constricted pupils
   e. all of the above

6. Artificial respiration should be started as soon as possible — once the oxygen supply is cut off completely, the average person may die within:
   a. 2 minutes
   b. 6 minutes
   c. 10 minutes

7. The first priority in an emergency is:
   a. call the police
   b. check for a pulse
   c. establish and maintain an airway
   d. get consent to treat

8. Which one is not a part of the respiratory system?
   a. larynx
   b. trachea
   c. esophagus
   d. pharynx

9. A healthy adult breathes approximately:
   a. 8-10 times a minute
   b. 12-15 times a minute
   c. 17-20 times a minute
   d. 22-25 times a minute

10. Clinical death occurs:
    a. after biological death
    b. when respiration and heart action cease
    c. when brain cells are irreversibly damaged
    d. 4-6 minutes after respiration ceases

11. Brain cells die after ________________ without oxygen:
    a. 1-2 minutes
    b. 4-6 minutes
    c. 6-8 minutes
    d. after 10 minutes

12. The preferable method of opening the airway is the:
    a. jaw thrust
    b. neck lift-jaw thrust
    c. head tilt-jaw thrust
    d. head tilt-chin lift

13. The three facets of Basic Life Support are:
    a. primary survey, secondary survey, transport
    b. assess the airway, breathe, circulate
    c. maintain life, prevent injury, get medical attention
    d. treatment for ABC's, shock, bleeding

14. You can tell that you are performing mouth-to-mouth ventilation correctly if you can:
    a. see the victim's chest rise and fall
    b. feel resistance as you blow air in
    c. feel air escaping from the victim's mouth as he exhales
    d. all of the above

15. When you are giving mouth-to-mouth resuscitation, you should:
    a. hold the victim's nostrils closed while breathing into his mouth
    b. avoid touching the nostrils unless cardiopulmonary resuscitation is being given at the same time
    c. pinch the nostrils as you lift your mouth from his mouth
    d. keep nostrils pinched all the time

16. When ventilating nonbreathing adult victims by the mouth-to-mouth method, the First Aider should provide breaths approximately:

    a. every 60 seconds, or about 60 times a minute
    b. every two seconds, or about 30 times a minute
    c. every five seconds, or about 12 times a minute
    d. every 10 seconds, or six times a minute

17. The artificial ventilation rate for an infant is:

    a. once every three seconds
    b. once every second
    c. once every five seconds
    d. about ten breaths per minute

18. The most common source of upper airway obstruction is:

    a. fluid-mucous
    b. food
    c. tongue
    d. swollen trachea

19. To avoid airway obstruction,

    a. cut food into small pieces
    b. avoid talking and laughing during chewing and swallowing
    c. don't allow children to run about where they are eating
    d. all of the above are correct

20. The universal distress sign of choking is:

    a. cyanosis
    b. pointing at the throat with a finger
    c. inability to speak
    d. clutching the throat with the thumb on one side and fingers on the other

21. The most reliable indication of a blocked airway in a conscious person is:

    a. the inability to speak
    b. a compression accident
    c. partially digested food in mouth
    d. cherry red skin color

Corresponds with:
**American Red Cross**
**Standard First Aid & Personal Safety**
Chapter 5, page 88
and
**Advanced First Aid & Emergency Care**
Chapter 5, page 83

# 4 Cardiopulmonary Resuscitation

Cardiopulmonary resuscitation (CPR) involves the use of artificial ventilation (mouth-to-mouth breathing) and external heart compression (rhythmic pressure on the breastbone). These techniques can only be learned through training and supervised practice. Incorrect application of external heart compressions may result in complications such as damage to internal organs, fracture of ribs or sternum, or separation of cartilage from ribs. (Rib fractures may occur when compressions are being correctly performed but this is not an indication to stop compression.) Application of cardiopulmonary resuscitation when not required could result in cardiac arrest. It should be emphasized that when CPR is properly applied, the likelihood of complications is minimal and acceptable in comparison with the alternative — death.

## SUDDEN DEATH

Sudden death is the immediate and unexpected cessation of respiration and functional circulation. The term "sudden death" is synonymous with cardiopulmonary arrest or heart-lung arrest. In the definition, the phrase "sudden and unexpected" is extremely important. A person who dies gradually of an organic disease such as cancer, or is under treatment for a chronic heart condition and has gradual but progressive loss of heart function, cannot be correctly classified as "sudden death." Cardiac arrest, when the heart stops pumping blood, may occur suddenly and unexpectedly in younger, healthy people for any one of a number of reasons:

- Heart attack
- Electric shock
- Asphyxiation
- Suffocation
- Drowning
- Allergic reaction
- Choking
- Secondary to severe injury.

The moment the heart stops beating and breathing ceases, the person is considered **clinically dead.** However, the vital centers of the central nervous system within the brain may remain viable for four to six minutes more. Indeed, much of the body remains "biologically alive" for much longer. The tissue most sensitive to oxygen deprivation is the brain. Irreversible death probably begins to occur to human brain cells somewhere between four and six minutes after oxygen has been excluded. This condition is referred to as **biological death.** Resuscitation in the treatment of sudden death depends upon this grace period of four to six minutes. After that period, even though the heart might yet be restarted, the chance of return to a normal functional existence is lessened. In sudden death, CPR should be started even though the four-to-six minute mark has been passed. The urgency of re-establishing the oxygenation system of the body, that is, ventilation and circulation, within this four- to six-minute grace period cannot be overemphasized.

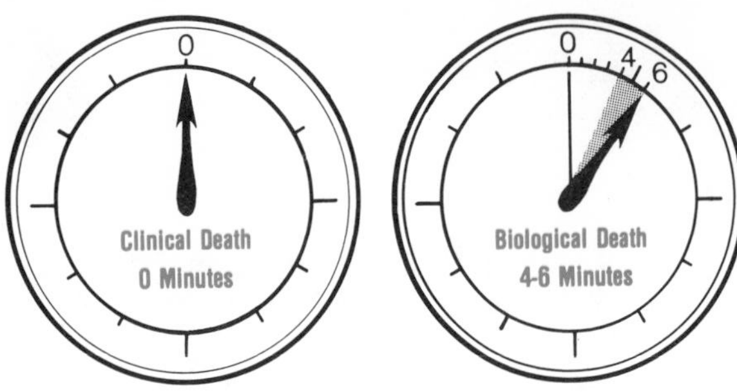


Time — clinical and biological death.

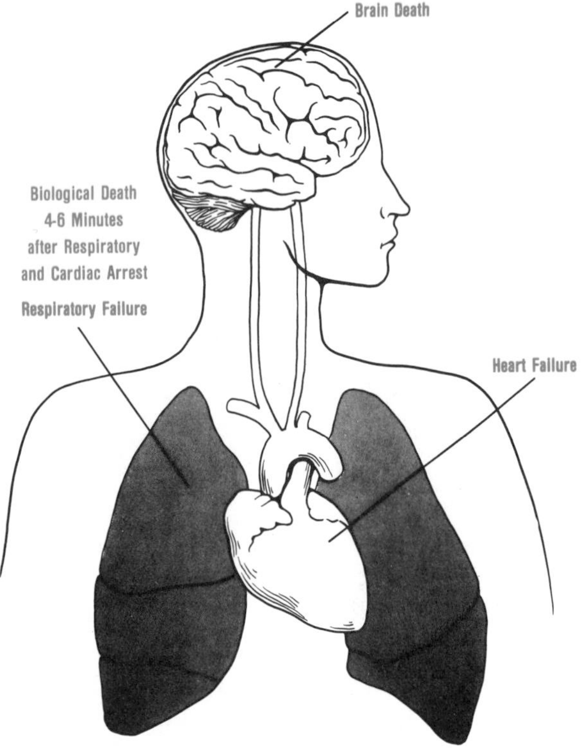


Biological death.

## Early Warning Signs

Recognition of the early warning signs of heart attack is extremely important. The following are the early warning signs of an impending heart attack:

- Uncomfortable pressure, squeezing, fullness, tightness, or dull pain in the center of the chest.
- Pain may radiate into the shoulders, arm, neck or jaws.
- Sweating.
- Nausea.
- Shortness of breath.
- Feeling of weakness.
- Pale and sick look.

A person need not exhibit all these symptoms to have a heart attack. The symptoms of a heart attack may come and go. Also, quite often the victim attributes these symptoms to another cause such as indigestion or flu.

## A CONSCIOUS HEART ATTACK VICTIM

When a victim of heart attack is conscious, give the following emergency care:

1. Place the victim in a semi-reclining position..
2. Loosen any tight clothing.
3. Give calming reassurance, trying to help the victim relax as much as possible.
4. Call an ambulance as soon as possible.
5. Constantly check breathing and heart beat.

## UNCONSCIOUS HEART ATTACK VICTIM

A victim who is unconscious will not be able to tell you how he/she feels; in a person who has lost consciousness, look for these signs:

1. An absence of a pulse in either the neck or the groin.
2. An absence of breathing. (This sign is a result of a temporary halt of brain activity, causing the brain to stop sending impulses that control respiration.)
3. Dilated pupils. (Brain impulses that control dilation and constriction of pupils cease.)
4. Limpness.
5. Flaccidity or weakness of the muscles.
6. A bluish color of the skin, the lips, or the beds of the fingernails. (This bluish or purplish color, called cyanosis, results from deficient oxygenation in the blood.)
7. Lack of a heartbeat.

## Checklist of Heart Attack Early Signals

None of the symptoms below is conclusive proof of a heart attack. But the more of them present, the more likely it is that the patient *is* undergoing a heart attack.

| | |
|---|---|
| DIFFICULTY BREATHING | COLD SWEAT |
| PALPITATIONS | PALENESS |
| NAUSEA | WEAKNESS |
| VOMITING | ANXIETY |

## How to Help a Possible Heart Attack Victim

You can best help — possibly save a life — if you know in advance: 1) The nearest hospital equipped to handle heart attack emergencies. 2) How to do Cardiopulmonary Resuscitation (CPR).* 3) How quickly to call a doctor, the hospital and/or an ambulance. 4) The fastest route to the hospital. Knowing these things, you should:

**1** Help victim to least painful position — usually sitting with legs up and bent at knees. Loosen clothing around neck and midriff. Be calm, reassuring.

**2** Quickly call ambulance to get victim to hospital via local rescue squad, police, fire or other available service. Once the ambulance is on the way, notify family physician, if you have one.

**3** If ambulance is coming, comfort victim while waiting. Otherwise, help victim to car, trying to keep victim's exertion to minimum. If possible, take another CPR-trained person with you. Victim should sit up.

**4** Drive cautiously to hospital. Watch victim closely (or have other passenger do so). If he or she loses consciousness, check for breathing, and feel for neck pulse under side angle of lower jaw to check for circulation. If no pulse, start CPR. Continue CPR until trained help arrives to take over.

**5** If victim retains consciousness to hospital, make sure he or she is carried, not walked, to emergency room.

*Get in touch with local Heart Association or Red Cross.

Courtesy Metropolitan Life Insurance Company ©

## RECOGNIZE THE PROBLEM

The person who initiates emergency heart-lung resuscitation has two responsibilities:

- To apply emergency measures to prevent irreversible changes to the vital centers of the body.
- To be sure the victim receives definitive medical care; this requires hospitalization.

When sudden death occurs, the First Aider must act immediately upon recognition of heart failure. In order to prevent biological death, the First Aider must be able to do the following:

- Recognize rapidly the apparent stoppage of heart action and respiration.
- Provide artificial ventilation to the lungs.
- Provide artificial circulation of the blood.

In addition to performing CPR, the First Aider must summon help in order that an ambulance and/or a physician may be called to the scene.

## STEPS PRECEDING CPR

A victim of cardiac arrest will be unconscious, have no pulse in the large arteries, have absence of breathing, and have a death-like appearance (grayish-blue skin, heavy perspiration, dilated pupils). The major factor, however, is an **absent pulse.** For a victim of cardiac arrest, take these steps before beginning CPR:

1. **Establish unresponsiveness.** Establish that the victim is unconscious.
   - Try to rouse the victim by tapping him/her gently on the shoulder and loudly asking, "Are you okay? Are you okay?"

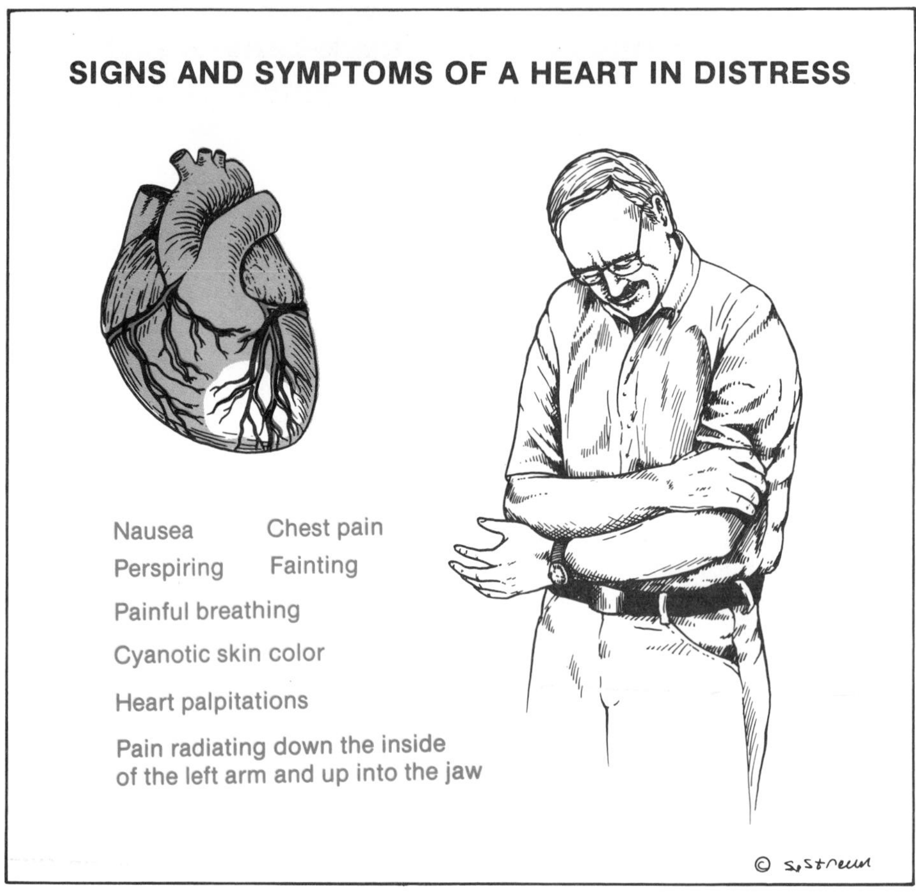


- If the victim does not gain consciousness, you may rub his/her sternum with your knuckles.

If the victim does not respond to touch, your voice, or pain, he/she is unconscious. This evaluation should take no more than ten seconds.

2. **Call for help.** You may have to send someone later to call for the ambulance and/or to help you do CPR.
3. **The victim needs to be positioned on his back on a hard, flat surface** (floor, sidewalk, etc.). A victim with a suspected neck injury who is lying on his stomach needs the neck stabilized during the roll onto the back. This necessitates at least two rescuers. The First Aider applying gentle traction on the victim's head gives the commands to roll as he keeps the head and neck in alignment.
4. **AIRWAY: Assess for an open airway.** Properly open the airway, if needed, by the head tilt-chin lift (preferred), or jaw thrust technique.
5. **BREATHE: Check the victim for breathing by using the LOOK, LISTEN, FEEL approach.** If breathless, give two full ventilations, allowing for deflation between ventilations. If the initial attempt to ventilate is unsuccessful, reposition the victim's head and repeat rescue breathing.
6. **CIRCULATE:** Establish pulselessness. Feel the victim's neck to find the carotid pulse. Keep your thumb out of the way, and *do not* rest your hand across the trachea. This step should take five to ten seconds.
7. **ADMINISTER the proper emergency care:**
   - **Activate the Emergency Medical Service (EMS) system. The EMS system is activated by calling the local emergency telephone number (911, if available).** The person who calls the EMS system should be prepared to give the following information as calmly as possible: (1) where the emergency is (with names of cross streets or roads, if possible); (2) the telephone number from which the call is made; (3) what happened — heart attack, auto accident, etc; (4) how many persons need help; (5) condition of the victim(s); (6) what aid is being given to the victim(s); (7) any other information requested.
   - **Take a stable side position by the victim.**

- **If the victim is breathless, give two full breaths in succession.** If the victim has a pulse, continue on with mouth-to-mouth resuscitation. Continue good airway maintenance.
- **If the victim has no pulse, perform full C.P.R.**
- **Clear an obstructed airway.** If the victim's chest does not rise and fall with the ventilations, give care for an obstructed airway. Open the mouth and check for foreign matter in the mouth and throat; if you see nothing, perform abdominal thrusts (see Chapter 3).

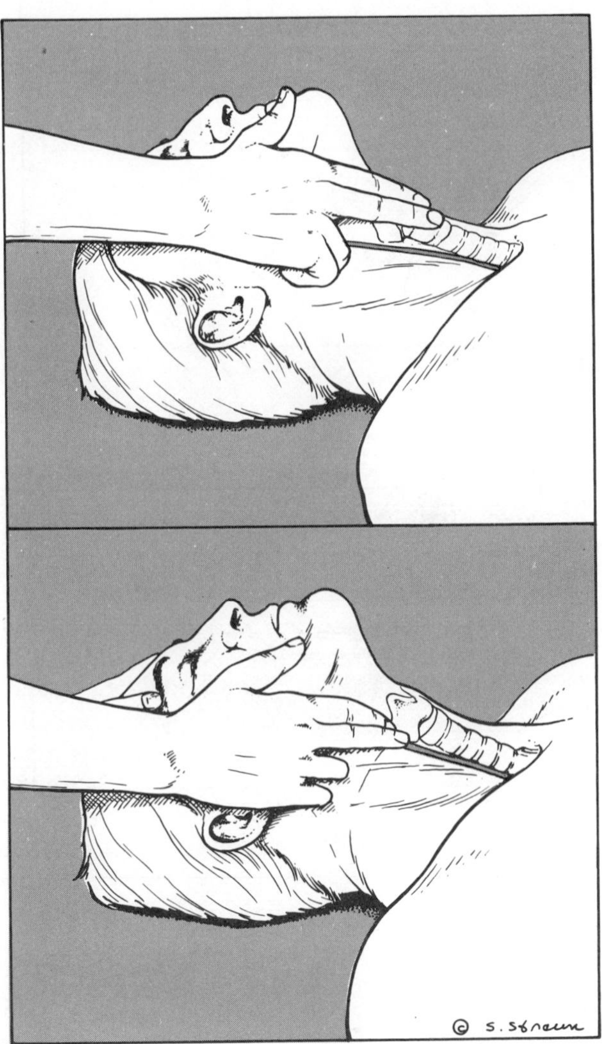

After you have checked breathing, check the carotid pulse. Palpate the thyroid cartilage in the midline with your index and middle fingers. Slide your fingers laterally to the groove between the trachea and the sterno-cleidomastoid muscle, and gently feel for the carotid pulse. If you do not feel a pulse, administer the proper emergency care.

8. If the victim's heart is not beating, begin cardiac compressions. Effective CPR is essential if the victim is to survive.

# CPR TECHNIQUE

## Administering Cardiac Compressions

1. The victim should be positioned horizontally on the back, with the legs elevated, on a firm surface, preferably the ground, the floor, or a **spineboard**.
2. If the victim's chest is covered, uncover it. (Do not waste time taking off a shirt — rip it open or pull it up.) In the case of a female victim, the brassiere will need to be removed or cut in two to expose the sternal area, or possibly slipped up to the neck.
3. Kneel on the firm surface **close** to the side of the victim's shoulder.
4. Locate the lower tip (**xiphoid process**) of the victim's breastbone (sternum) by feeling the lower margin of the rib cage on the side nearest you with the middle and index fingers of your hand closest to the victim's feet. Then run your fingers along the victim's rib cage to the notch where the ribs meet the breastbone in the center of the lower chest.
5. Place one finger on that notch, and put your other finger on the lower end of the victim's sternum.
6. Now place the heel of your other hand **above** the two fingers. When you apply pressure at that point with the heel of your hand, the sternum is flexible enough to be compressed. (If you do not position your hand properly, compression can fracture the breastbone or the ribs, lacerating the heart, the lungs, and/or the liver.)

   Another way of providing hand placement that does not require location of the xiphoid process and that is becoming widely accepted uses the following method:

   - With the index and middle fingers of your hand closest to the victim's feet,

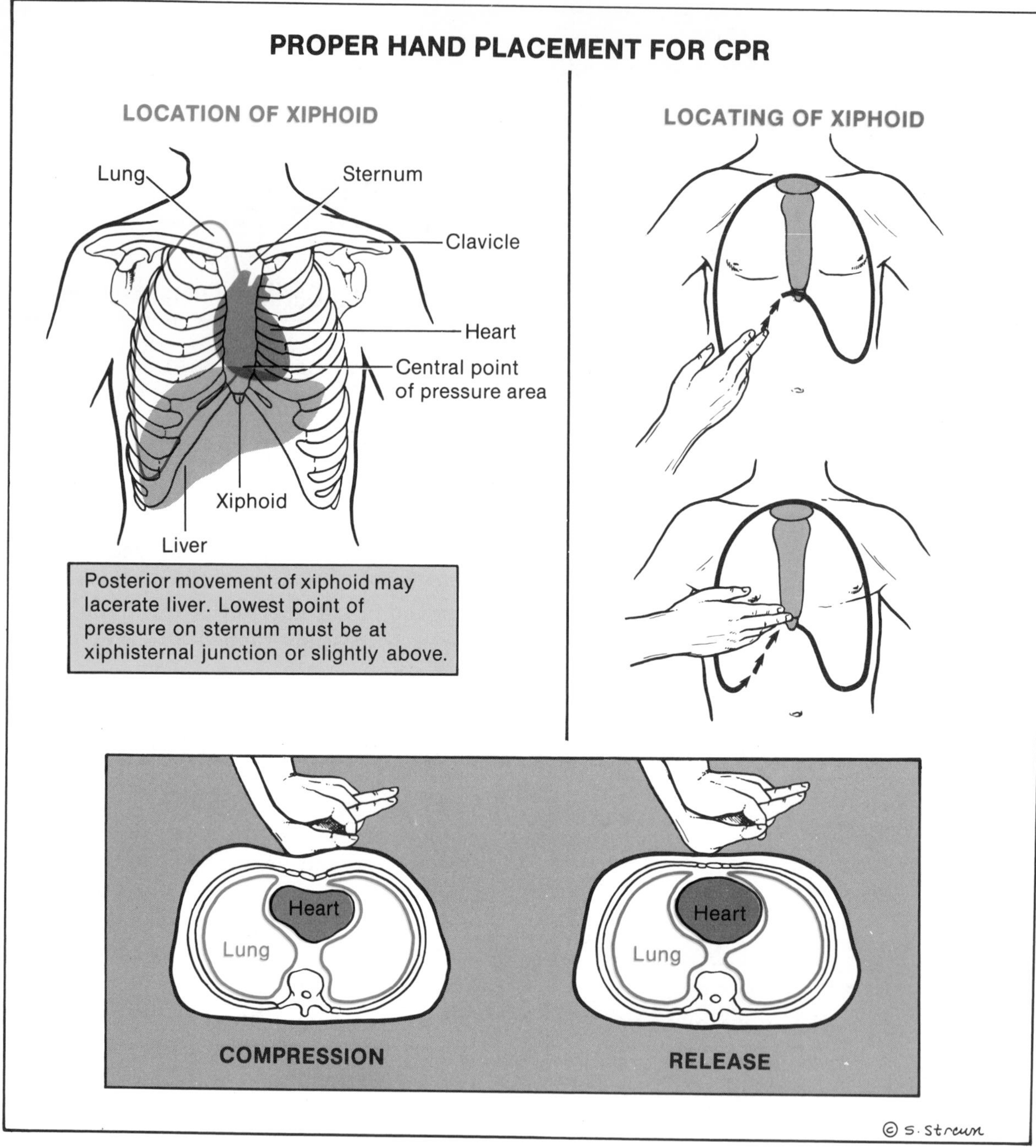


locate the lower border of the rib cage closest to you.

- Put your fingers along the rib cage until you find the **substernal notch** (where the ribs meet the sternum).
- Keep your index finger on the lower end of the sternum and your middle finger on the notch.
- Now move your free hand to the midline of the sternum and place the thumb side against the index finger of your lower hand, making sure that the heel of your free hand is on the midline of the sternum.

7. Place your second hand on top of your first, bringing your shoulders directly over the victim's sternum.

## ONE-RESCUER CPR

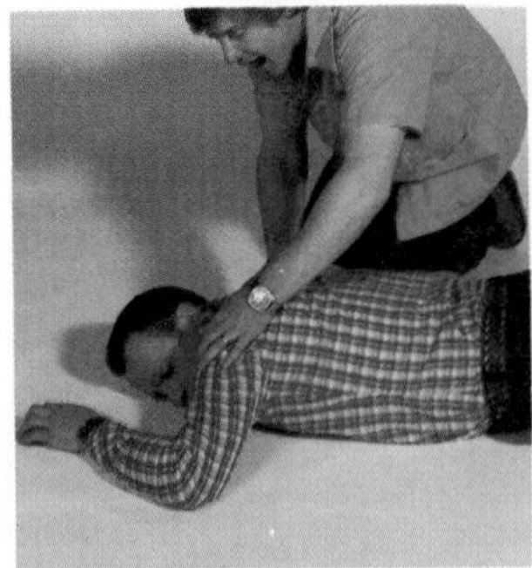

1
Establish unresponsiveness by the "gently shake and shout" method.

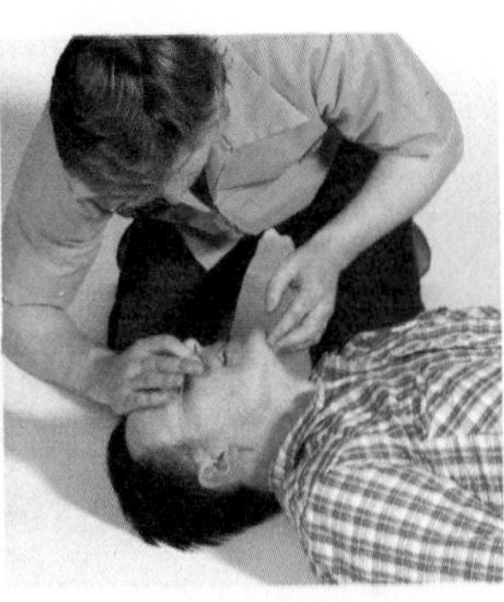

2
If necessary, roll the victim as a unit onto his back, then open his airway.

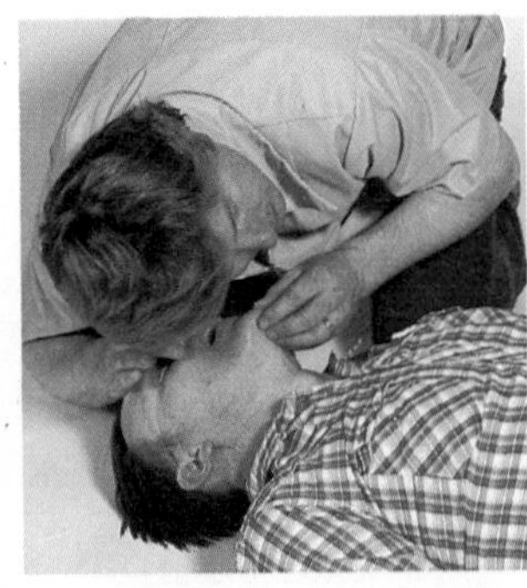

3
Establish breathlessness with the Look-Listen-Feel method.

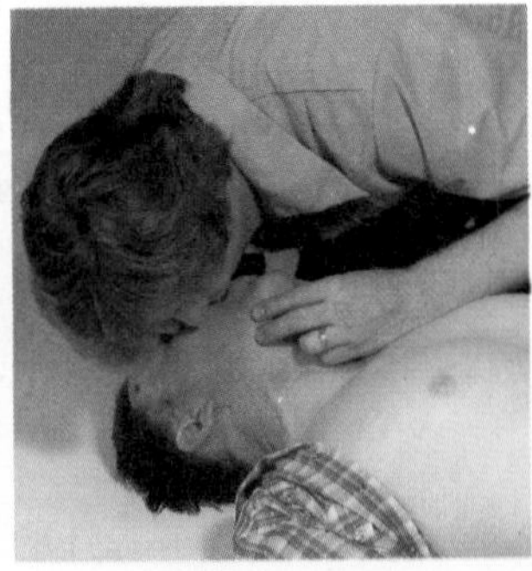

4
If breathing is absent, give two breaths of air, allowing for deflations between ventilations.

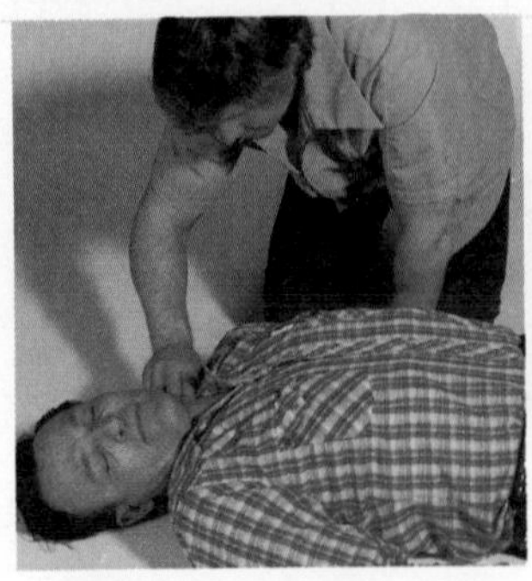

5
Establish pulselessness by checking the carotid artery in the neck.

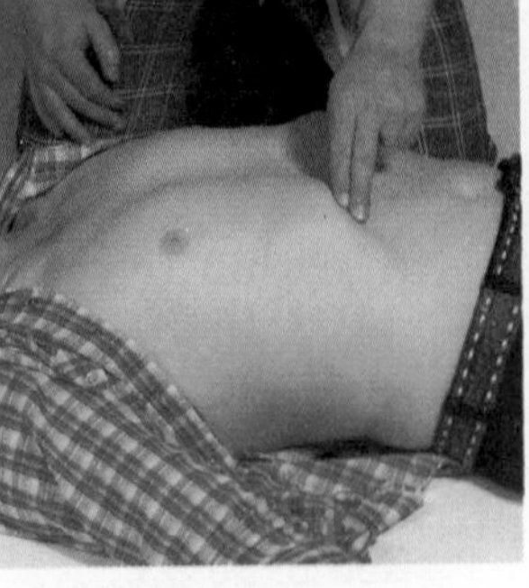

6
If you detect no pulse, run two fingers up the rib cage to locate the xiphoid process or sternal notch.

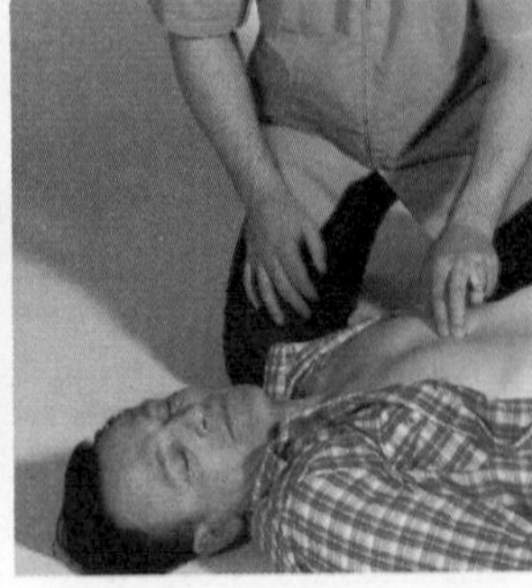

7
Locate the correct chest compression site by finding the xiphoid process or sternal notch, and measure two finger widths above the xiphoid process.

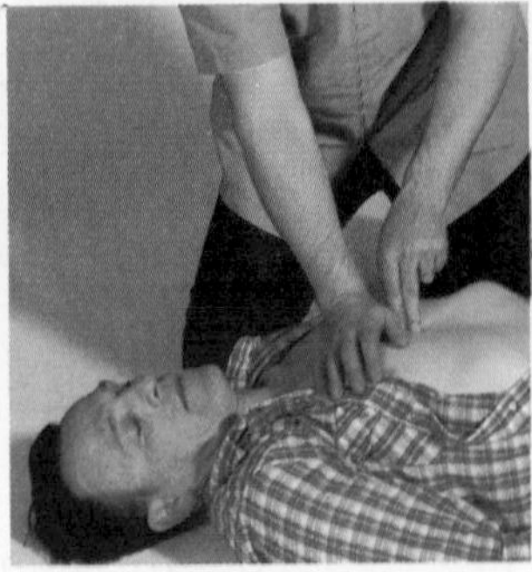

8
Place the heel of your other hand on the lower half of the sternum, next to the fingers of your first hand.

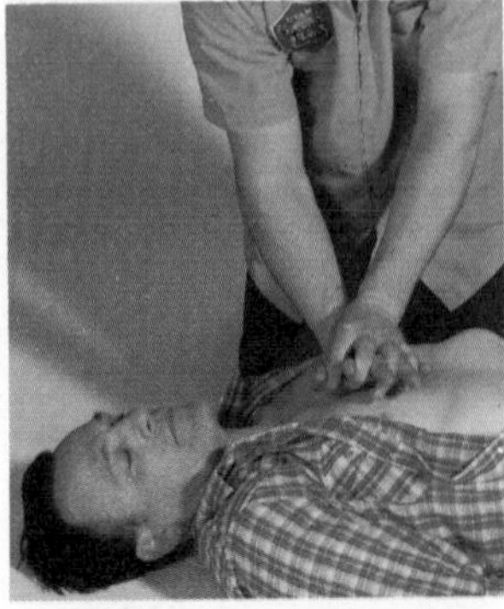

9
Proper hand and body placement for chest compressions.

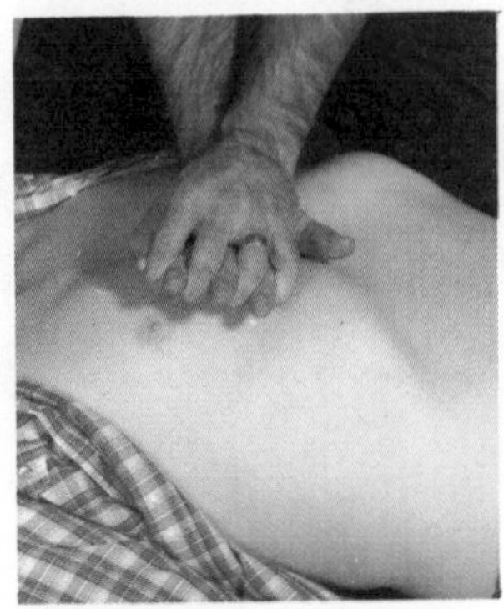

10
Compress 1½ to 2 inches on an adult, at the rate of 80-100 per minute.

**NOTE: The American Heart Association recommends that lay persons only learn one rescuer CPR.**

8. Pull your fingers up from the chest by interlacing them. If your fingers stay on the chest, the pressure from your compressions will dissipate and may fracture the victim's ribs.
9. Keeping your arms straight and your elbows locked, apply firm, heavy pressure so that you depress the sternum about one and one-half to two inches (four to five centimeters). Use the weight of your upper body as you lean down over the victim to deliver the compressions. If necessary, add additional weight with your shoulders, but never with your arms — the force is too great, and you will fracture the sternum.

   An acceptable alternative for those who have hand or wrist problems is to grasp the wrist of the hand lying on the chest with the hand that has been locating the lower end of the breastbone.
10. After each compression, completely relax the pressure so that the sternum returns to its normal position, but **never** move your hands off the victim's chest **at any time,** or you will lose the proper positioning. Keep the heel of your bottom hand touching the chest even during relaxation.
11. Your compressions should be regular, smooth, and uninterrupted, with compression and relaxation time being about equal. Make sure that you administer pressure directly from above, not from the side. If the victim is not breathing, deliver compressions at the rate of about eighty to one hundred per minute for an adult or child, and at least one hundred per minute for an infant.

## One-Man CPR

1. If the victim still is not breathing, administer artificial ventilation while you continue cardiac compressions.
   - If you are alone, continue cardiac compressions at the rate of eighty to one hundred per minute for an adult, and give two full lung inflations after each fifteen compressions, allowing for deflation between ventilations.
   - To maintain proper rate and rhythm, use an audible count such as "one-and, two-and," with the downstroke on the number and the upstroke on the "and."
   - You must give the two lung inflations within five seconds.
2. After the first minute of CPR, and then periodically, feel the carotid pulse to check for the return of a spontaneous, effective heartbeat. Do this pulse check regularly. See page 65.
3. Relieving a fatigued rescuer, the following steps are recommended for entry of the

### HAND POSITIONING FOR CHEST COMPRESSIONS

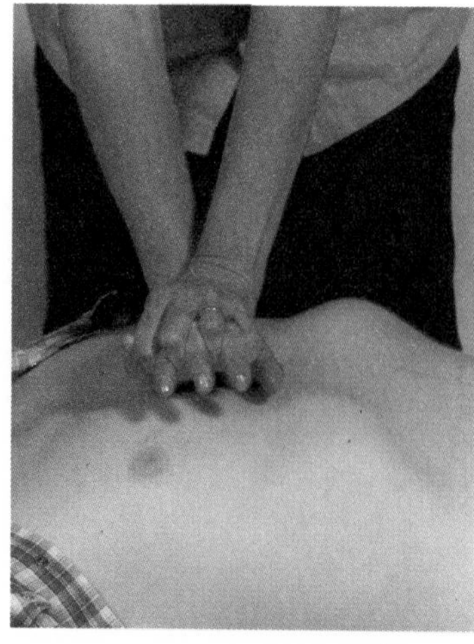

Preferred hand position.

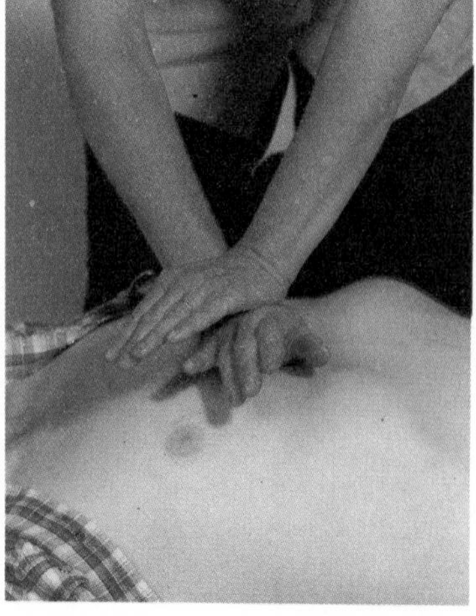

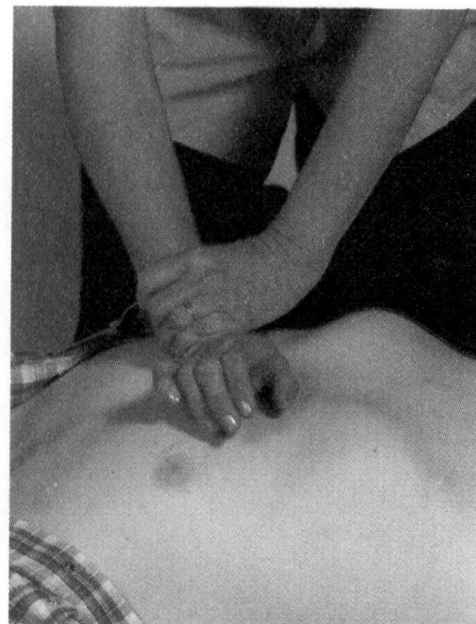

Acceptable alternatives, if necessary.

second rescuer. The second person should identify himself or herself as a qualified rescuer who is willing to help. If the first rescuer is fatigued and has requested help, the logical sequence is as follows: (1) The first rescuer stops CPR after two ventilations. (2) The second rescuer kneels down and checks for pulse for 5 seconds. (3) If there is no pulse, the second rescuer gives two breaths. (4) The second rescuer commences external chest compressions at the recommended rate and ratio for one-person CPR. (5) The first rescuer assesses the adequacy of the second rescuer's ventilations and compressions. This can be done by watching the chest rise during rescue breathing and by checking the pulse during the chest compressions.

## Two-Man CPR

1. If there are two First Aiders, one should kneel at the victim's side and perform cardiac compression while the other kneels (at the opposite side, if possible) near the victim's head and delivers artificial ventilation.
2. In this case, a ventilation should be delivered during a pause after every fifth cardiac compression so that ventilation is at the rate of twelve per minute.
3. The First Aider performing ventilations should ventilate after each fifth compression during a pause of compressions. The compression rate is 80-100 per minute. Use an audible count of "one-and-two-and-three-and," etc.
4. The compression First Aider counts aloud the sequence "one-and-two-and-three-and-four-and-five" - pause. Compressions occur on each number (one, two, etc.)
5. The ventilation First Aider takes a deep breath on "three-and," positions himself to ventilate on "four-and," and begins blowing into the victim after "five." See page 66.

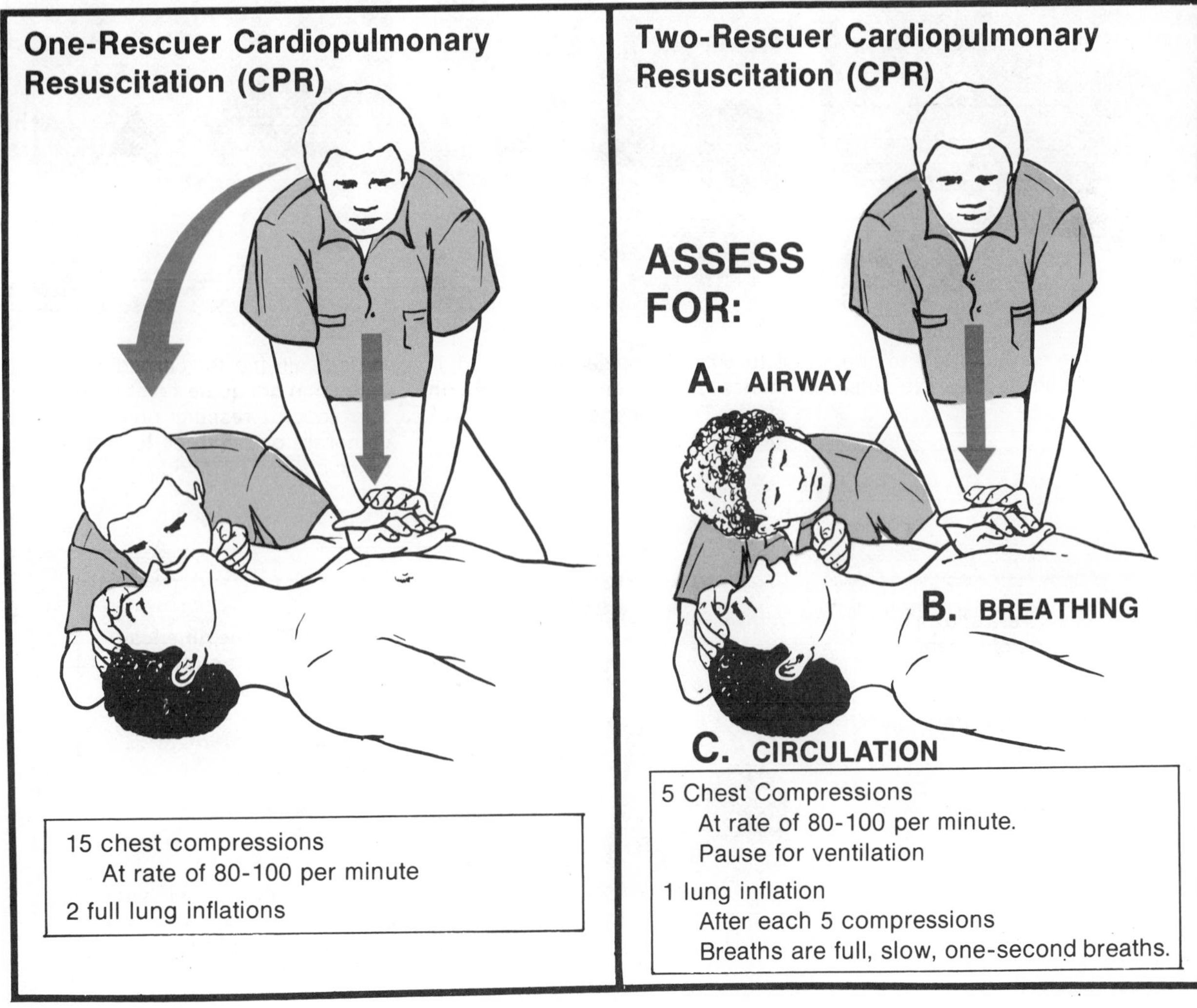

## TWO-RESCUER CPR

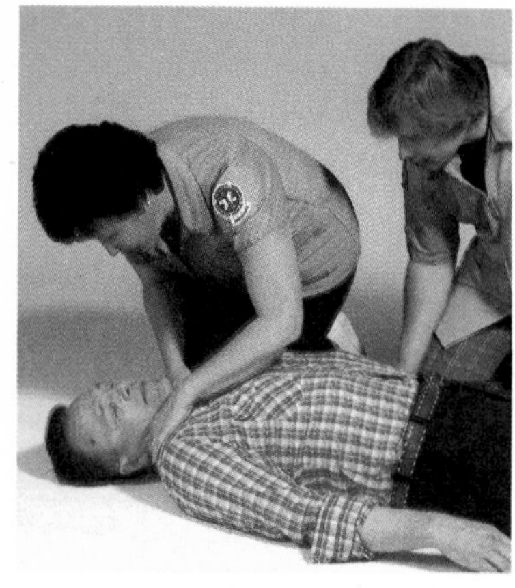

1
Establish unresponsiveness.

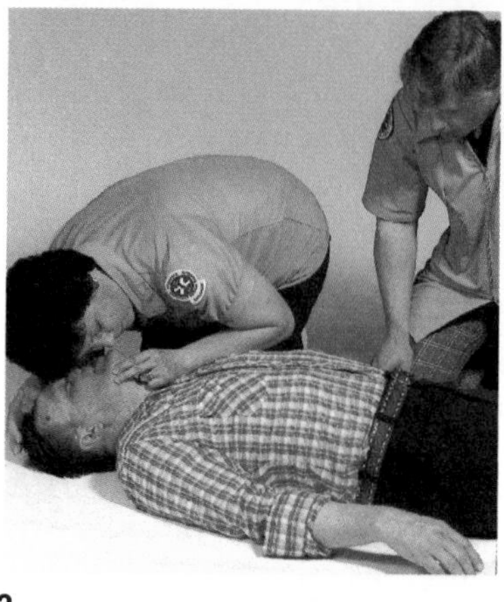

2
Open the airway, then look, listen, and feel for breathlessness, and say, "No breathing."

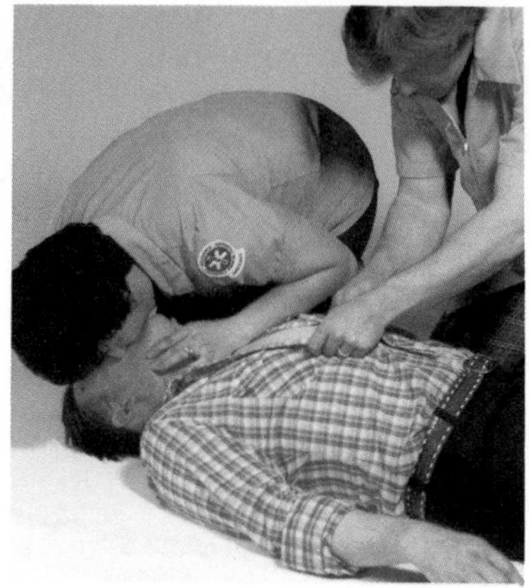

3
Give two full breaths of air within four to five seconds while the second rescuer bares the chest.

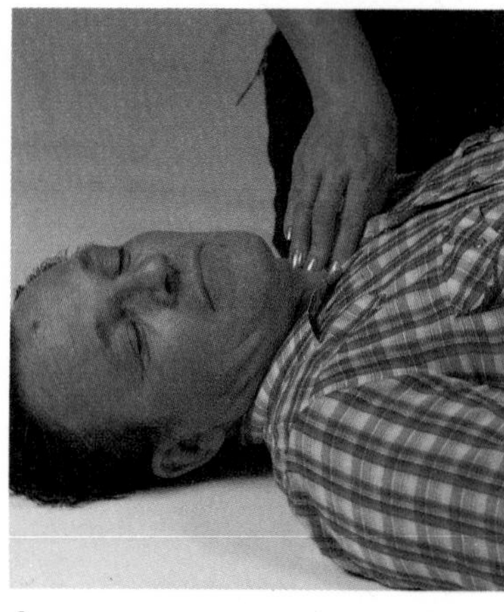

4
Palpate the carotid artery to check for pulselessness. Say, "No pulse."

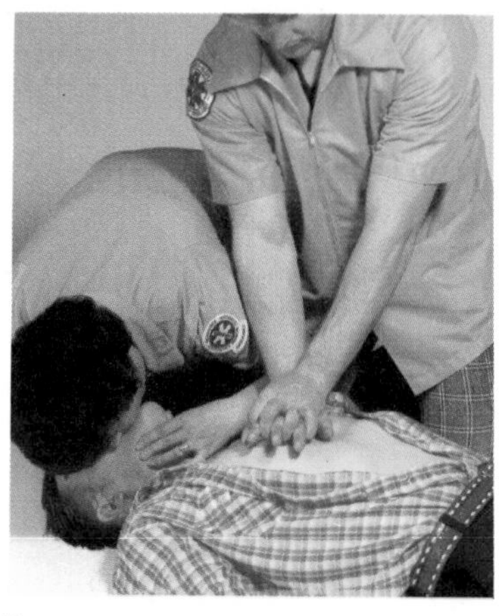

5
If the patient is pulseless, say "Commence CPR," then give one breath of air. The second rescuer commences chest compressions.

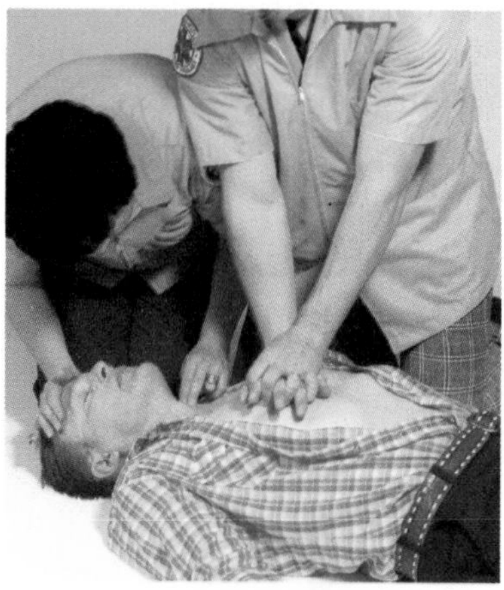

6
Periodically feel the carotid pulse to determine adequate compressions. The second rescuer delivers five compressions in three to four seconds, counting out loud.

Rescuers are shown on same side of patient for photo clarity. However, when possible, it is best to have Rescuers on opposite sides.

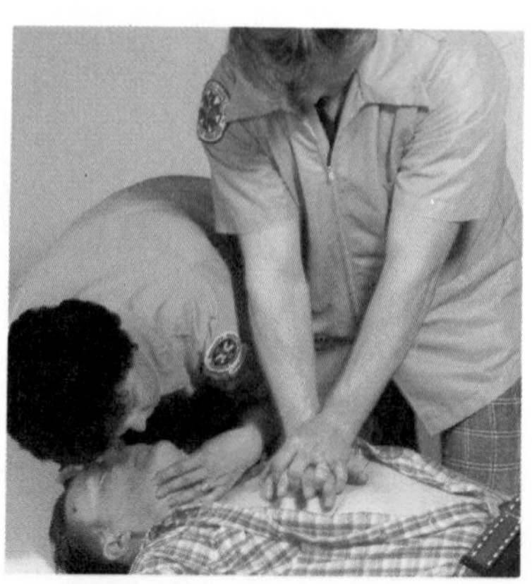

**NOTE: The American Heart Association recommends that lay persons learn only one-rescuer CPR.**

7
After each fifth compression, the compressor pauses while the ventilator gives a full ventilation.

When the First Aider performing cardiac compressions gets tired, he should switch with the one who is performing ventilations. To do this, use the following method:

1. **The First Aider doing compressions requests a switch at the end of a compression cycle. The First Aider who is performing compressions calls for the change by substituting "change and" for "one-and" The audible count remains the same for the remaining four compressions. (Any mnemonic that satisfactorily accomplishes the change is acceptable. Another popular technique uses as the count, "Change, on, the, next, breath.")**
2. **During the fifth compression, the First Aider performing the ventilations breathes after "five"-pause, then moves to the chest and gets into position.**
3. **The First Aider performing the compressions moves quickly to the victim's head after the fifth compression and checks the carotid pulse and breathing for a maximum of five seconds.**
4. **If no pulse is found, the First Aider at the head announces, "No pulse;' commence CPR," and administers a ventilation.**
5. **The First Aider at the chest is in position and begins compressions.**

**Note:** The switch may require seven seconds to complete, which is acceptable.

If one First Aider is performing CPR and a second First Responder or other rescuer becomes available, follow this procedure:

1. **He should identify himself as qualified in CPR and as a First Aider.**
2. **The first rescuer nods as compressions are continued, and he completes the cycle of fifteen compressions and two ventilations, while the second rescuer kneels on the opposite side and checks the pulse. A pulse should be felt with each compression.**
3. **At the end of the cycle (15-2), the second First Aider checks the carotid pulse for five seconds, while the first rescuer discontinues compressions.**
4. **If he finds no pulse, he says, "No pulse," gives one ventilation, and CPR is continued.**
5. **Compressions are then resumed. A ventilation should be given during a pause after each fifth chest compression.**

## Signs of Successful CPR

1. Each time that the sternum is compressed, a pulse will be perceptible (it will feel like a flutter).
2. Lung expansion will occur with each breath.
3. The pupils will react to light or will appear normal.
4. A normal heartbeat will return.
5. A spontaneous gasp of breathing will occur.
6. The victim's skin color will improve or return to normal.
7. The victim will move arms or legs on his own.

Continue administering CPR until the victim is breathing and the heart is beating on its own, until other trained personnel can relieve you, or until you are too exhausted to continue.

## CPR for Infants and Children

Infants (up to one year) and children (one to eight years) require slightly different procedures for evaluation and performance of CPR. (See pages 67-68.)

### Establishing Unresponsiveness or Respiratory Difficulty

Evaluating for cardiorespiratory arrest is based on any of the following:

- No obtainable blood pressure.
- Brachial pulse is absent.
- Chest is not moving.
- No audible heart sounds.
- Child appears blue or pale.
- Child is unresponsive when shaken or gently tapped.
- Gasps, muscle contractions, and seizure-like, convulsive activity.

If in doubt about the assessment of cardiorespiratory arrest, assume that an arrest has occurred, and begin resuscitative procedures immediately. It is better to start unnecessary resuscitation than to waste time during an actual arrest.

### Assess For An Open Airway

All other measures will fail if the airway is inadequate. Follow these steps in establishing and maintaining an airway:

1. **As soon as unconsciousness or breathing difficulty is established, open the airway using the head tilt-chin lift. (Head tilt-neck lift maneuver may also be used.)**
2. **An infant or child who shows breathing difficulty but whose color is not blue probably has an adequate airway and should be immediately transported to a medical facility.**
3. **If necessary, clear the mouth and throat of all secretions.**
4. **Open the airway, but make sure that the mouth is open and that your fingers are not causing undue pressure on the soft tissue underneath the jaw. Be gentle!**
5. **Do not overextend the neck — a neutral position is best. An overextended neck may kink the trachea.**

### Breathing

1. **Establish breathlessness.** Use the same method as for the adult. Often, the infant will resume breathing when the airway is open. If the child gasps or struggles to catch his breath after the airway is open, decide whether to apply emergency breathing. Your key here is the child's lips. If they are pink, enough oxygen is reaching the blood, so do not perform emergency breathing. If the lips are blue (cyanotic), apply emergency breathing. If patient is not breathing, begin ventilations by giving two gentle breaths at 1-1.5 seconds per ventilation, allowing for deflation between breaths.
2. **Establish pulselessness. Check the carotid pulse in a child, but check the brachial pulse in the infant.** Use your index and middle fingers to feel for the pulse.
3. **Activate the EMS system.**
4. **Begin ventilations at twenty breaths per minute for infants (once every three seconds) and fifteen breaths per minute for children (once every four seconds).** Cover the mouth and nose of the infant, and use the mouth seal and nose pinch on the child. Give two gentle breaths, allowing for deflation between ventilations.

   Force and volume used should be that of a deep sigh. Do not overinflate. Ventilation is limited to the amount of air needed to cause the chest to rise. Your blowing pressure will probably have to be greater than imagined, however.

   Watch the motion of the chest wall with each breath to assess the adequacy of ventilation.

## Administering CPR

1. **Begin CPR, if necessary, in the following manner:**
   - Make sure the patient is lying on a firm surface.
   - If an *Infant,* place the flat part of your index finger just below the intermammary line (an imaginary line between the nipples).

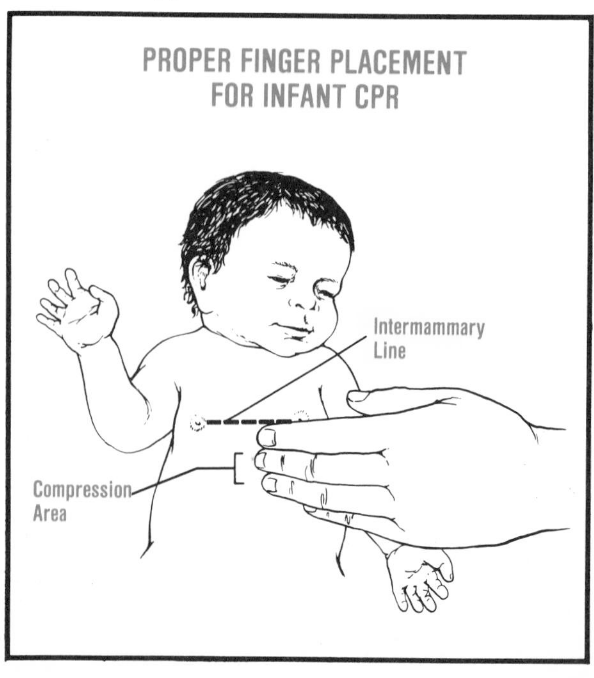

## INFANT AND CHILD CPR

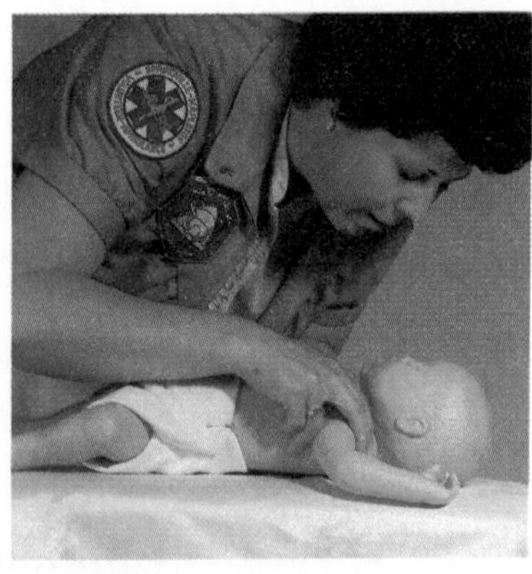

1
Determine unresponsiveness in the infant by a gentle "shake and shout" method.

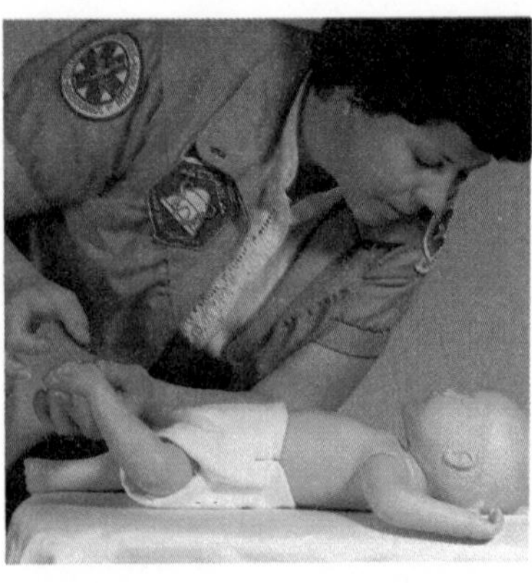

2
You may also try flicking the soles of the baby's feet.

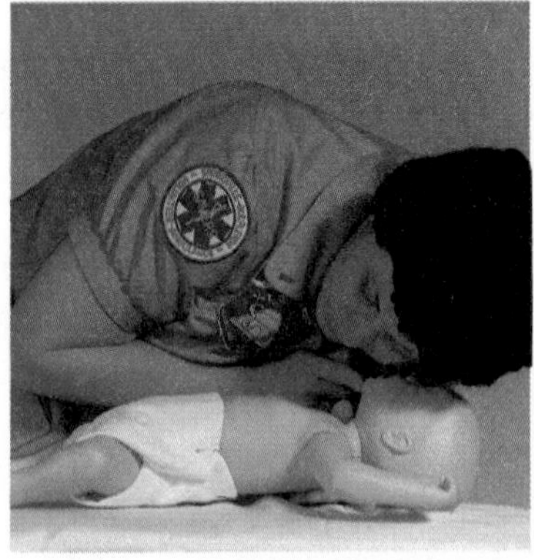

3
Establish breathlessness by the Look-Listen-Feel method.

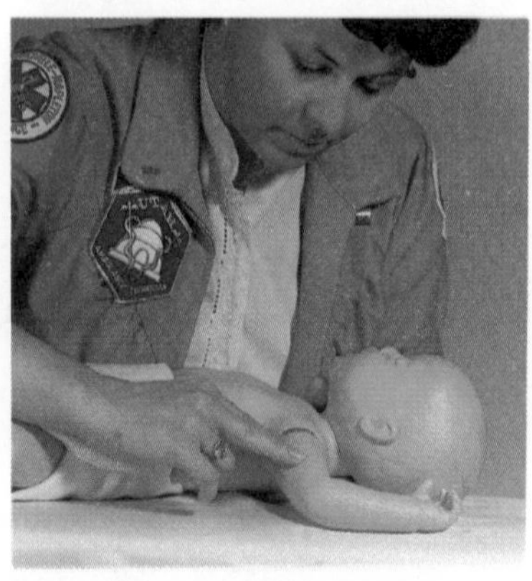

4
Infant mouth-to-mouth and nose resuscitation. The rescuer gently opens the airway, covers the baby's mouth and nose with a good seal, then gives two ventilations.

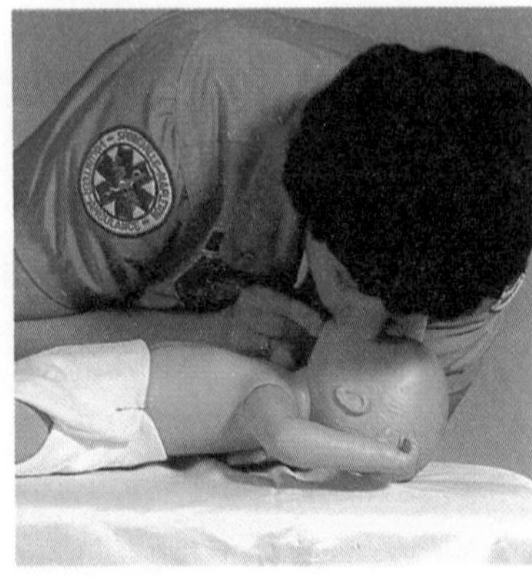

5
Check the infant for pulselessness by gently palpating the brachial artery.

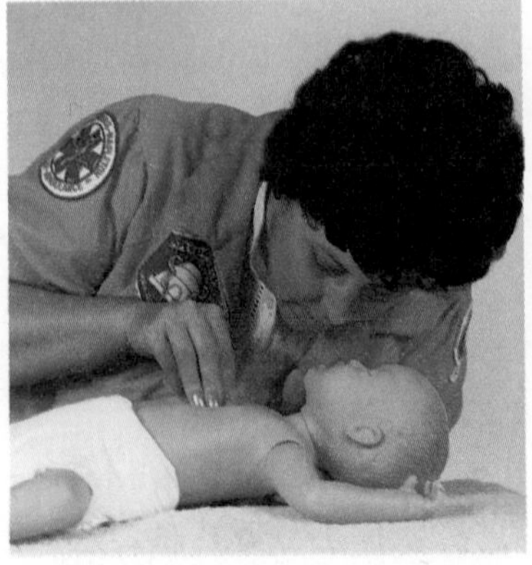

6
Single-rescuer infant CPR: Chin lift method. Landmark by placing index finger just below intermammary line. Use middle and ring fingers for compressions.

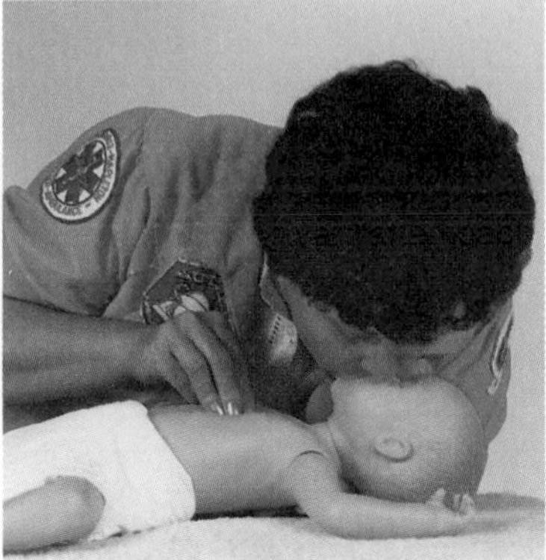

7
A ventilation is given after each fifth compression.

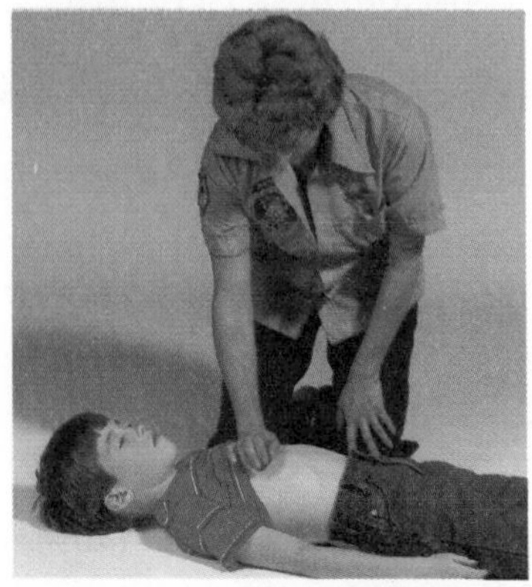

8
Performing chest compressions on a child.

- Use the flat part of your second and third fingers to compress the infant's sternum one-half to one inch (see page 61). For a larger child, you may need to compress the sternum to one and one-half inches with the heel of one of your hands.
- The compression rate for infants is at least 100 per minute; for children, it is 80-100 compressions per minute.
- The ratio of compressions to respirations is five to one for infants and children.
- The single rescuer breathes once for the patient after each fifth compression.
- With two-man CPR, the breath is given during a pause after each fifth compression. The compressions are counted by the First Responders in the following manner:

  Infant — one, two, three, four, five, breathe.

  Child — one and two and three and four and five and breathe.

### Checking for Successful CPR

The methods of checking for successful CPR in infants or children are almost the same as for adults.

- Check the infant's brachial pulse periodically.
- Check the dilated pupils to see if they regain activity or constrict.
- Watch for a spontaneous heartbeat to be reestablished, spontaneous breathing to be resumed, and consciousness to return.

## MISTAKES IN THE PERFORMANCE OF CPR

Following are the most common mistakes made by First Aiders using CPR procedures.

Some common resuscitation mistakes:

1. Failing to tip the head back far enough, thereby not giving adequate ventilations.
2. Failing to maintain an adequate head tilt.
3. Failing to pinch the nose or maintain the pinched nose during ventilations.
4. Not giving full breaths.
5. Completing a cycle in less than five seconds.
6. Failing to watch and listen for exhalation.
7. Failing to maintain an adequate seal around the victim's mouth, nose, or both during ventilation. (The seal should be released when the victim exhales.)

Some common chest compression mistakes:

1. Elbows bent instead of straight.
2. Shoulders not directly above sternum of the victim.
3. Heel of bottom hand not in line with the sternum, or too low; not depressing the chest (sternum) one-half to two inches.
4. Fingers touching the victim's chest.
5. Pivoting at knees instead of at hips.
6. Compression rate incorrect.
7. Compressions given in jerks rather than smoothly.
8. Hand not remaining on victim's chest between compressions.
9. Bobbing of First Aider's head instead of compressing victim's chest.

## IMPORTANT POINTS TO REMEMBER ABOUT CPR

When CPR is performed improperly or inadequately, artificial ventilation and artificial circulation may be ineffective in providing basic life support. Important points to remember in performing external cardiac compression and artificial ventilation include the following:

1. Do not interrupt CPR for more than seven seconds for any reason, except when transporting on stairs. When moving a victim up or down a stairway, it is difficult to continue effective CPR. Under these circumstances, it is best to perform effective CPR at the head or foot of the stairs, then interrupt CPR at a given signal and move quickly to the next level, where effective CPR is resumed. Such interruptions usually should not be longer than thirty seconds.

2. Do not move the victim to a more convenient site until he has been stabilized

and is ready for transportation, or until arrangements have been made for uninterrupted CPR during movement.

3. Never compress over the xiphoid process at the tip of the sternum. The xiphoid extends downward over the abdomen. Pressure on it may cause laceration of the liver, which can lead to severe internal bleeding.
4. Between compressions, the heel of the hand must release its pressure completely but should remain in constant contact with the chest wall over the lower one-half of the sternum.
5. The First Aider's fingers should not rest on the victim's ribs during compression. Interlocking the fingers of the two hands may help to avoid this. Finger pressure on the ribs or lateral pressure increases the possibility of rib fractures and rib-joint separation.
6. Sudden or jerking movements should be avoided when compressing the chest. The compression should be smooth, regular, and uninterrupted (50 percent of the cycle should be compression, and 50 percent should be relaxation). Quick jabs increase the possibility of injury and produce quick jets of flow; they do not enhance the amount of blood pumped from the heart.
7. Do not maintain continuous pressure on the abdomen (to decompress the stomach) while performing external cardiac compression. This may cause the liver to rupture.
8. The shoulders of the First Aider should be directly over the victim's sternum. The elbows should be straight. Pressure is applied vertically downward on the lower sternum. This provides a maximally effective thrust, minimal fatigue for the First Aider and reduced hazard of complications for the victim. When the victim is on the ground or floor, the First Aider can kneel or stand at his/her side. When the victim is on a bed, the First Aider must be on a step or chair or be kneeling on the bed.
9. The lower sternum of an adult must be depressed one and one-half to two inches by external cardiac compression. Lesser amounts of compression are ineffectual, since even well-performed cardiac compression provides only about one-quarter to one-third of the normal blood flow.

## WHEN TO TERMINATE CPR

First Aiders, as they recognize cardiac arrest, should administer CPR to the best of their ability and knowledge and should not be held liable for failure to initiate CPR if that decision is consistent with current American Red Cross or Heart Association standards. They should continue resuscitation efforts until one of the following occurs:

1. Effective, spontaneous ventilation and circulation have been restored.
2. Another responsible or professional person assumes responsibility for life support.
3. A physician, physician-directed individual, or physician-directed team assumes responsibility for life support.
4. The victim is transferred to an appropriate emergency medical service facility.
5. The First Aider is exhausted and unable to continue life support.

# One-Rescuer CPR: Adult

| Step | Activity | Critical Performance |
|---|---|---|
| **1. Assessment/Airway** | Determine unresponsiveness. | Tap or gently shake shoulder. |
| | | Shout "Are you OK?" |
| | Call for help. | Call out, "Help!" |
| | Position the victim. | Turn on back as unit, if necessary, supporting head and neck (4-10 sec.). |
| | Open the airway. | Use head-tilt/chin-lift maneuver. |
| | Determine breathlessness. | Maintain open airway. |
| | | Ear over mouth, observe chest: look, listen, feel for breathing (3-5 sec.). |
| **2. Breathing** | Ventilate twice. | Maintain open airway. |
| | | Seal mouth and nose properly. |
| | | Ventilate 2 times at 1-1.5 sec./ventilation. |
| | | Observe chest rise (adequate ventilation volume?) |
| | | Allow deflation between breaths. |
| **3. Circulation** | Determine pulselessness. | Palpate carotid pulse on near side of manikin. |
| | | Maintain head-tilt with other hand (5-10 sec.). |
| | Activate EMS system. | If someone responded to call for help, send him/her to activate EMS system.I |
| | Begin chest compressions. | Rescuer's knees by victim's shoulders. |
| | | Landmark check prior to hand placement. |
| | | Proper hand position throughout. |
| | | Rescuer's shoulders over victim's sternum. |
| | | Equal compression-relaxation. |
| | | Compress 1½ to 2 inches. |
| | | Keep hands on sternum during upstroke. |
| | | Complete chest relaxation on upstroke. |
| | | Say any helpful mnemonic. |
| | | Compression rate: 80-100/min (15 per 9-11 sec.). |
| **4. Compression/ventilation Cycles** | Do 4 cycles of 15 compressions and 2 ventilations. | Proper compression/ventilation ratio: 15 compressions to 2 ventilations per cycle. |
| | | Observe chest rise: 1-1.5 sec./ventilation; 4 cycles/52-73 sec. |
| **5. Reassessment** | Recheck pulse. (If no pulse: Step 6. If pulse felt: **. If 2nd rescuer arrives: †.) | Palpate carotid pulse (5 sec.) |
| **6. Continue CPR** | Ventilate twice. | Ventilate 2 times. |
| | | Observe chest rise; 1-1.5 sec./ventilation. |
| | Resume compression/ ventilation cycles. | Resume Step 4. |

**If pulse is present, open airway and check for spontaneous breathing. If breathing is present, monitor breathing and pulse closely, maintain open airway. If breathing is absent, perform rescue breathing at 12 times/min. and monitor pulse.

† 2nd rescuer arrives to replace rescuer: (a) 2nd rescuer identifies self by saying "I know CPR. Can I help?" (b) 2nd rescuer then does pulse check in Step 5 and continues with Step 6. (During practice and testing only one rescuer actually ventilates the manikin. The other rescuer simulates ventilation.) (c) 1st rescuer assesses the adequacy of 2nd rescuer's CPR by observing chest rise during ventilations and by checking the pulse during chest compressions.

**Source: American Heart Association**

# Two-Rescuer CPR: Adult*

| Step | Activity | Critical Performance |
|---|---|---|
| **1. Assessment/Airway** | One rescuer (ventilator): | |
| | Determine unresponsiveness. | Tap or gently shake shoulder. |
| | | Shout "Are you OK?" |
| | Positions the victim. | Turn on back if necessary (4-10 sec.) |
| | Opens the airway. | Use a proper technique to open airway. |
| | Determines breathlessness. | Look, listen and feel (3-5 sec.).<br>Say "No breathing." |
| **2. Breathing** | Ventilator ventilates twice. | Observe chest rise: 1-1.5 sec./ventilation. |
| **3. Circulation** | Determines pulselessness. | Palpate carotid pulse (5-10 sec.). |
| | States assessment results. | Say "No pulse." |
| | Other rescuer (compressor) simultaneously: | |
| | Locates landmark notch. | Landmark check. |
| | Gets into position for compressions. | Hands, shoulders in correct position? |
| **4. Compression/ventilation cycles.** | Compressor begins chest | Correct ratio compressions/ventilations: 5/1. |
| | | Compression rate: 80-100/min (5 compressions/3-4 sec.). |
| | | Say any helpful mnemonic. |
| | | Stop compressing for each ventilation. |
| | Ventilator ventilates after every 5th compression and checks compression effectiveness. | Ventilate 1 time (1-1.5 sec.).<br>Check pulse to assess compressions. |
| | (Minimum of 10 cycles.) | Time for 10 cycles: 40-53 sec. |
| **5. Call for Switch** | Compressor calls for switch when fatigued. | Give clear signal to change. |
| | | Compressor completes 5th compression. |
| | | Ventilator completes ventilation after 5th compression. |
| **6. Switch** | Simultaneously switch: | |
| | Ventilator moves to chest. | Move to chest. |
| | | Become compressor. |
| | | Locate landmark notch. |
| | | Get into position for compressions. |
| | Compressor moves to head. | Move to head. |
| | | Become ventilator. |
| | | Check carotid pulse (5 sec.). |
| | | Say "No pulse." |
| | | Ventilate once.† |
| **7. Continue CPR** | Resume compression/ventilation cycles. | Resume Step 3. |

* If CPR is already in progress with one rescuer, the switch to the two new rescuers occurs after the completion of one rescuer's cycle of 15 compressions and 2 ventilations. The two new rescuers start with Step 6. The EMS should be activated before this sequence is used.

† During practice and testing only one rescuer actually ventilates the manikin. The other rescuer simulates ventilation.

**Source: American Heart Association**

# One-Rescuer CPR: Child

| Step | Activity | Critical Performance |
|---|---|---|
| **1. Assessment/Airway** | Determine unresponsiveness. | Tap or gently shake shoulder. |
| | | Shout "Are you OK?" |
| | Call for help. | Call out, "Help!" |
| | Position the victim. | Turn on back as unit, if necessary, supporting head and neck (4-10 sec.). |
| | Open the airway. | Use head-tilt/chin-lift maneuver. |
| | Determine breathlessness. | Maintain open airway. |
| | | Ear over mouth, observe chest: look, listen, feel for breathing (3-5 sec.). |
| **2. Breathing** | Ventilate twice. | Maintain open airway. |
| | | Seal mouth and nose properly. |
| | | Ventilate 2 times at 1-1.5 sec./ventilation. |
| | | Observe chest rise (adequate ventilation volume?) |
| | | Allow deflation between breaths. |
| **3. Circulation** | Determine pulselessness. | Palpate carotid pulse on near side of manikin. |
| | | Maintain head-tilt with other hand (5-10 sec.). |
| | Activate EMS system. | If someone responded to call for help, send him/her to activate EMS system. |
| | Begin chest compressions. | Rescuer's knees by victim's shoulders. |
| | | Landmark check prior to hand placement. |
| | | Proper hand position throughout. |
| | | Rescuer's shoulders over victim's sternum. |
| | | Equal compression-relaxation. |
| | | Compress 1 to 1½ inches. |
| | | Keep hands on sternum during upstroke. |
| | | Complete chest relaxation on upstroke. |
| | | Say any helpful mnemonic. |
| | | Compression rate: 80-100/min. |
| **4. Compression/Ventilation Cycles** | Do 10 cycles of 5 compressions and 1 ventilation | Proper compression/ventilation ratio: 5 compressions to 1 slow ventilation per cycle. |
| | | Observe chest rise: 1-1.5 sec./ventilation |
| **5. Reassessment** | Recheck pulse. (If no pulse: Step 6. If pulse felt: †. If 2nd rescuer arrives: ‡.) | Palpate carotid pulse (5 sec.) |
| **6. Continue CPR** | Ventilate once. | Ventilate one time. |
| | | Observe chest rise; 1-1.5 sec./ventilation. |
| | Resume compression/ ventilation cycles. | Resume Step 4. |

* If child is above age of approximately 8 years, the method for adults should be used.

† If pulse is present, open airway and check for spontaneous breathing. (a) If breathing is present, monitor breathing and pulse closely, maintain open airway. (b) If breathing is absent, perform rescue breathing at 12 times/min. and monitor pulse.

‡ 2nd rescuer arrives to replace 1st rescuer: (a) 2nd rescuer identifies self by saying "I know CPR. Can I help?" (b) 2nd rescuer then does pulse check in Step 5 and continues with Step 6. (During practice and testing only one rescuer actually ventilates the manikin. The other rescuer simulates ventilation.) (c) 1st rescuer assesses the adequacy of 2nd rescuer's CPR by observing chest rise during ventilations and by checking the pulse during chest compressions.

Source: American Heart Association

# Two-Rescuer CPR: Child

| Step | Activity | Critical Performance |
|---|---|---|
| **1. Assessment/Airway** | One rescuer (ventilator): | |
| | Determines unresponsiveness. | Tap or gently shake shoulder. |
| | | Shout "Are you OK?" |
| | Positions the victim. | Turn on back if necessary (4-10 sec.) |
| | Opens the airway. | Use a proper technique to open airway. |
| | Determines breathlessness. | Look, listen and feel (3-5 sec.).<br>Say "No breathing." |
| **2. Breathing** | Ventilator ventilates twice. | Observe chest rise: 1-1.5 sec./ventilation. |
| **3. Circulation** | Determines pulselessness. | Palpate carotid pulse (5-10 sec.). |
| | States assessment results. | Say "No pulse." |
| | Other rescuer (compressor) simultaneously: | |
| | Locates landmark notch. | Landmark check. |
| | Gets into position for compressions. | Hands, shoulders in correct position? |
| **4. Compression/ventilation cycles.** | Compressor begins chest compressions. | Correct ratio compressions/ventilations: 5/1. |
| | | Compression rate: 80-100/min (5 compressions/3-4 sec.). |
| | | Say any helpful mnemonic. |
| | | Stop compressing for each ventilation. |
| | Ventilator ventilates after every 5th compression and checks compression effectiveness. | Ventilate 1 time (1-1.5 sec.).<br>Check pulse to assess compressions. |
| | (Minimum of 10 cycles.) | Time for 10 cycles: 40-53 sec. |
| **5. Call for Switch** | Compressor calls for switch when fatigued. | Give clear signal to change. |
| | | Compressor completes 5th compression. |
| | | Ventilator completes ventilation after 5th compression. |
| **6. Switch** | Simultaneously switch: | |
| | Ventilator moves to chest. | Move to chest. |
| | | Become compressor. |
| | | Locate landmark notch. |
| | | Get into position for compressions. |
| | Compressor moves to head. | Move to head. |
| | | Become ventilator. |
| | | Check carotid pulse (5 sec.). |
| | | Say "No pulse." |
| | | Ventilate once.† |
| **7. Continue CPR** | Resume compression/ventilation cycles. | Resume Step 3. |

* If CPR is already in progress with one rescuer, the switch to the two new rescuers occurs after the completion of one rescuer's cycle of 15 compressions and 2 ventilations. The two new rescuers start with Step 6. The EMS should be activated before this sequence is used.

† During practice and testing only one rescuer actually ventilates the manikin. The other rescuer simulates ventilation.

**Source: American Heart Association**

# One-Rescuer CPR: Infant

| Step | Activity | Critical Performance |
|---|---|---|
| **1. Assessment/Airway** | Determine unresponsiveness. | Tap or gently shake shoulder. |
| | Call for help. | Call out "Help!" |
| | Position the infant. | Turn on back as unit, supporting head and neck. |
| | Open the airway. | Use head-tilt/chin-lift maneuver to sniffing or neutral position. |
| | | Do not overextend the head. |
| | Determine breathlessness. | Maintain open airway. |
| | | Ear over mouth, observe chest: look, listen, feel for breathing (3-5 sec.). |
| **2. Breathing** | Ventilate twice. | Maintain open airway. |
| | | Make tight seal on infant's mouth and nose with rescuer's mouth. |
| | | Ventilate 2 times at 1-1.5 sec./ventilation. |
| | | Observe chest rise (adequate ventilation volume?) |
| | | Allow deflation between breaths. |
| **3. Circulation** | Determine pulselessness. | Palpate brachial pulse. |
| | | Maintain head-tilt with other hand (5-10 sec.). |
| | Activate EMS system. | If someone responded to call for help, send him/her to activate EMS system. |
| | Begin chest compressions. | Draw imaginary line between nipples. |
| | | Place 2-3 fingers on sternum, 1 finger's width below imaginary line. |
| | | Equal compression-relaxation. |
| | | Compress vertically, ½ to 1 inch. |
| | | Keep fingers on sternum during upstroke. |
| | | Complete chest relaxation on upstroke. |
| | | Say any helpful mnemonic. |
| | | Compression rate: at least 100/min. (5 compressions/3 sec. or less.) |
| **4. Compression/Ventilation Cycles** | Do 10 cycles of 5 compressions and 1 ventilation. | Proper compression/ventilation ratio: 5 compressions to 1 slow ventilation per cycle. |
| | | Pause for ventilation. |
| | | Observe chest rise: 1-1.5 sec./ventilation; 10 cycles/45 sec. or less. |
| **5. Reassessment** | Recheck pulse. (If no pulse: Step 8. If pulse felt: **.) | Palpate brachial pulse (5 sec.). |
| **6. Continue CPR** | Ventilate. | Ventilate 1 time. |
| | | Observe chest rise; 1-1.5 sec./ventilation. |
| | Resume compression/ ventilation cycles. | Resume Step 3. |

**If pulse is present, open airway and check for spontaneous breathing. (a) If breathing is present, monitor breathing and pulse closely, maintain open airway. (b) If breathing is absent, perform rescue breathing at 20 times/min. and monitor pulse.

Source: American Heart Association

## Work Exercises

### Clinical and Biological Death

Quick action is needed before the victim experiences clinical, then biological death. Identify those two terms by completing the following table:

| Lapsed Time | Type of Death (Clinical or Biological) | Possibility of Brain Damage |
|---|---|---|
| 0-4 minutes | | Small, but brain cells are being weakened by lack of fuel. |
| 4-6 minutes | | Brain cells are rapidly dying. |
| 6-10 minutes | | Extensive irreversible brain damage has occurred and death is imminent. |
| over 10 minutes | | Too many brain cells have usually been destroyed for life to continue. |

### CPR — Cardiopulmonary Resuscitation

Identify 6 signs and symptoms of a heart attack.

1. — No Pulse
2. — No Breathing
3. — Dilated Pupils
4. — Bluish Coloration (Skin, Lips, Fingernails)
5. — Tightness in chest
6. — Pain Left Arm up to neck } Concious

Nausea
Profuse Sweating
Fainting

In order to avert biological death in a heart attack victim, immediately begin CPR, which means caring for the ABC's.

The ABC's of CPR are:

A = Airway

B = Breathing

C = Circulation

## A — Airway

Match the following diagrams with their appropriate names.

A. Not one of the recommended techniques B. Head Tilt-Chin Lift C. Jaw Thrust

1. B 2. A 3. C

## B — Breathing

To recognize breathing cessation; tilt the victim's head backward and check for breathing;

1. LOOK for Chest Rise & Fall
2. LISTEN for Breath
3. FEEL for Breath

- **LOOK**
- **LISTEN**
- **FEEL**

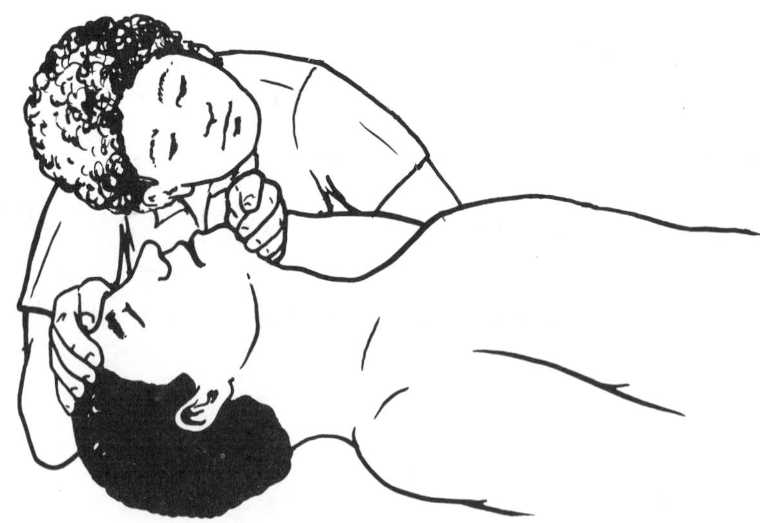

Remember: Airway obstruction is usually found by blowing in and finding ventilation difficult to impossible to perform on the victim.

CYANOSIS is a condition characterized by a blue or grey color in the tongue, lips, nail beds and skin. It is a dependable sign that No $O_2$ in blood

## C — Circulation

You can identify whether the heart is beating by trying to locate a pulse. Match the two types of pulses with the proper diagram.

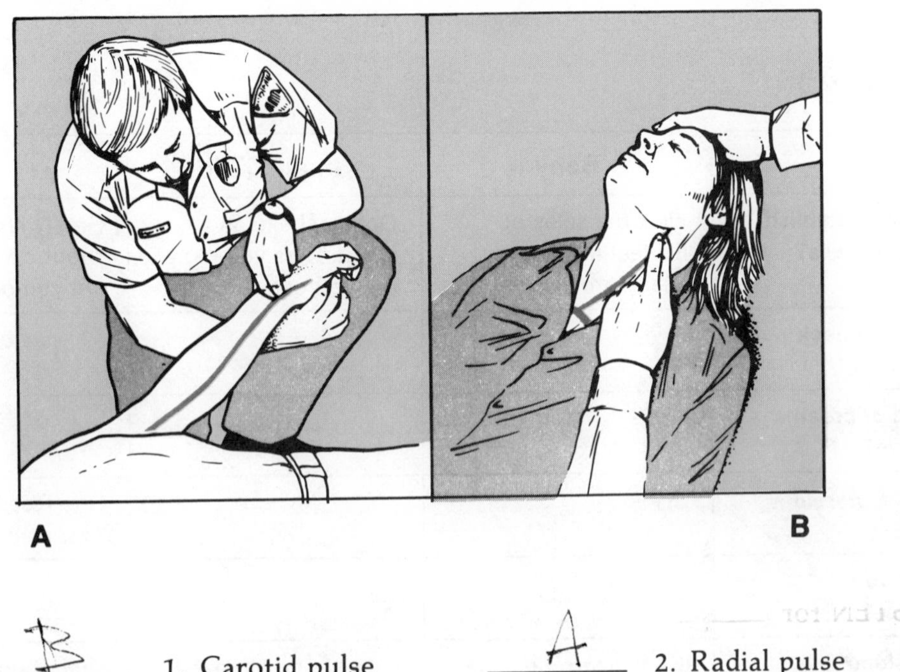


B 1. Carotid pulse A 2. Radial pulse

## Cardiopulmonary Resuscitation

When do you begin CPR?

## Proper Positioning

Describe the proper positioning of the First Aider who is performing cardiac compressions.

Why is the proper hand placement on the chest so important?

## CPR Review

Effective CPR is learned and maintained through proper knowledge and constant practice. Fill in the following table to test your CPR knowledge.

### CPR REVIEW

| | Baby | Small Child | Adult |
|---|---|---|---|
| **How do you establish unresponsiveness?** | Flick the soles of his feet and shout "Baby are you okay?" | Gently shake and shout, "Are you okay, are you okay?" | Gently shake and and shout, "Are you okay, are you okay?" |
| **How do you check breathing?** | | | |
| **What kind of breaths do you give?** | | | |
| **Ratio of compressions to breaths** | | | One rescuer:<br>Two rescuers: |
| **Where do you check pulse?** | | | |
| **Compressions: hand position?** | two fingers, one finger width below the intermammary line | heel of one hand, middle of sternum | heel of one hand, other hand on top, 1" to 1½" from xiphoid |
| **Compressions: how far:** | Gently<br>______ to ______ | Moderately<br>______ to ______ | Firmly<br>______ to ______ |
| **Compression rate** | ______ per min. | ______ per min. | One rescuer:<br>______ per min.<br>Two rescuers:<br>______ per min. |
| **Pause to check pulse** | ______ seconds | ______ seconds | ______ seconds |
| **Pause to move patient** | ______ seconds | ______ seconds | ______ seconds |

Adapted from American Red Cross

## SELF-TEST

### Part I: True and False

If you believe the statement is true, circle the T. If you believe the statement is false, circle F.

T F 1. During a heart attack pain may radiate from the chest to the shoulder of the victim.

T F 2. The carotid pulse is at the wrist. Radial

T F 3. Cardiac compressions on a male adult should depress the sternum four to five inches. 1½-2

T F 4. Cardiac arrest means the lungs have stopped working effectively. Heart

T F 5. If a person stops breathing, his/her heart could keep beating for awhile.

T F 6. The best way to find out if a person has stopped breathing is to check the carotid pulse. LLF

T F 7. The xiphoid process is found at the lower end of the sternum.

T F 8. Even though a person's heart stops beating, he/she may keep breathing for awhile.

T F 9. The moment the heart stops beating and breathing ceases, the person is considered biologically dead. Clinically

T F 10. The pain from a heart attack may radiate into the neck, shoulders, and jaw.

T F 11. You should begin CPR immediately after you find the victim is not breathing. has No Pulse

T F 12. For adult CPR, proper hand placement on the chest is two finger widths above the xiphoid process.

T F 13. One rescuer should give compressions at the rate of 60 per minute. 80-100

T F 14. It is possible to change positions during two-rescuer CPR.

T F 15. Successful CPR should cause the victim's pupils to appear normal.

T F 16. An infant should be given twenty breaths per minute.

T F 17. Heartbeat in an infant should be checked by palpating the carotid pulse. Bracial

T F 18. A First Aider should terminate CPR if the victim doesn't respond within fifteen minutes.

### Part II: Multiple Choice

Circle the answer that best reflects an accurate statement.

1. In artificial circulation, the First Aider should place his hands on the victim's sternum and should:
   a. fold his fingers under, making a fist
   b. allow his fingers to curve into the victim's chest
   c. hold his fingers outward and as high off the victim's chest as possible
   d. it does not matter how the fingers are held

2. The First Aider should assume that the victim is in cardiac arrest if:
   a. there are no signs of respiration
   b. there is no pulse
   c. the pupils of the eyes are dilated
   d. all of the above signs are present

3. The pulse that is most easily felt in an adult is the:
   a. radial pulse
   b. brachial pulse
   c. carotid pulse
   d. femoral pulse

4. Once the victim remains in clinical death, the brain cells begin to die after:
   a. 2-4 minutes
   b. 4-6 minutes
   c. 5-7 minutes
   d. 10 minutes or more

5. To check the pulse on an infant use:
   a. the brachial artery
   b. the carotid artery
   c. the pedal pulse
   d. the radial pulse

6. The correct hand position for administering CPR to an infant is:
   a. two fingers above the sternal notch
   b. at the base of the sternum
   c. in the lower 1/3 of the sternum
   d. two fingers, one finger width below the intermammary line

7. To establish an airway, the First Aider should do all of the following *except:*
   a. the head tilt-chin lift
   b. the head tilt-jaw thrust
   c. the jaw thrust
   d. the neck lift-jaw thrust

8. When performing external cardiac compressions on an adult, the sternum should be depressed:
   a. ½ to 1 inch
   b. 1 inch to 1½ inches
   c. 1½ to 2 inches
   d. 2 to 2½ inches

9. After each chest compression during CPR, your hands should:
   a. come completely off the chest
   b. apply small amount of pressure on the chest
   c. rest on the chest in normal CPR position
   d. none of the above

10. If you are alone and performing CPR, you will be giving:
    a. 60-80 compressions per minute
    b. 80-100 compressions per minute
    c. 100-120 compressions per minute
    d. 70-90 compressions per minute

11. If you are alone, giving CPR, you should give ________ inflations after each ________ compressions.
    a. 2, 15
    b. 15, 2
    c. 1, 2
    d. 1, 4

12. If there are two rescuers in CPR, the second should give ventilations:
    a. on the upstroke of each fifth compression
    b. during a pause after each fifth compression
    c. before the fifth compression
    d. on the downstroke of the sixth compression

13. The compression rate for two-man CPR is:
    a. 40-60 per minute
    b. 50-70 per minute
    c. 60-80 per minute
    d. 80-100 per minute

14. Correct hand placement for CPR is:
    a. in the middle of the sternum
    b. two fingers below the sternal notch
    c. at the apex of the rib cage
    d. two fingers above the sternal notch

15. Cardiac arrest can be caused by:
    a. electrocution
    b. suffocation
    c. trauma accidents
    d. all of the above

16. Basic Life Support consists of:
    a. recognition of cardiac arrest and providing artificial ventilation and circulation
    b. checking for breathing and applying rescue breathing
    c. checking for heart beat and applying artificial circulation
    d. checking for heart beat and applying rescue breathing

17. CPR must begin when a need for it is recognized and continue until *all but one* of the following occurs:
    a. the patient is declared dead by the First Aiders
    b. the patient is resuscitated
    c. the rescuer can no longer go on
    d. a qualified medical person takes over

18. To check for a carotid pulse and circulation:
    a. use your thumb
    b. take the pulse on the opposite side of the trachea so that you can feel air exchange in the trachea
    c. check the pulse with your fingertips after you give two full breaths
    d. none of the above

Corresponds with:
**American Red Cross**
**Standard First Aid & Personal Safety**
Chapter 5, pages 92-94
and
**Advanced First Aid & Emergency Care**
Chapter 6, pages 84-94

# 5 Drowning Emergencies

Drowning is the third leading cause of accidental deaths in the United States each year. Among adults, alcohol intoxication is a factor in about one-third of all drownings. In addition, approximately 9,000 near-drowning incidents occur every year in the United States. Five times as many males drown as females. Male drowning mortality peaks at fifteen to nineteen years, with the highest female mortality showing at the preschool

**DROWNING**

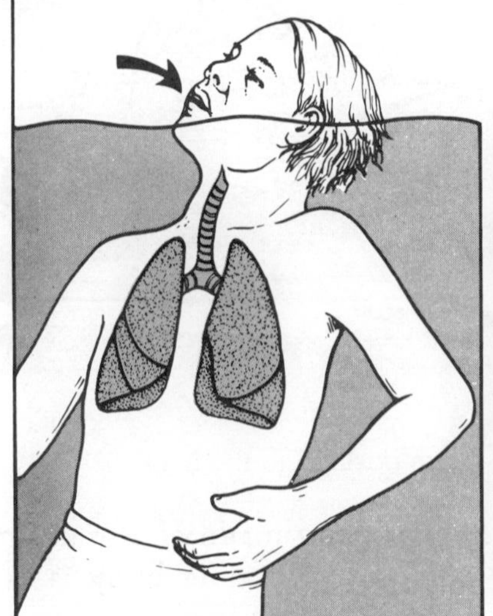

Drowning is a major source of accidental death and can be a result of cold, fatigue, injury, disorientation, intoxication, etc., or of the victim's own limited swimming ability.

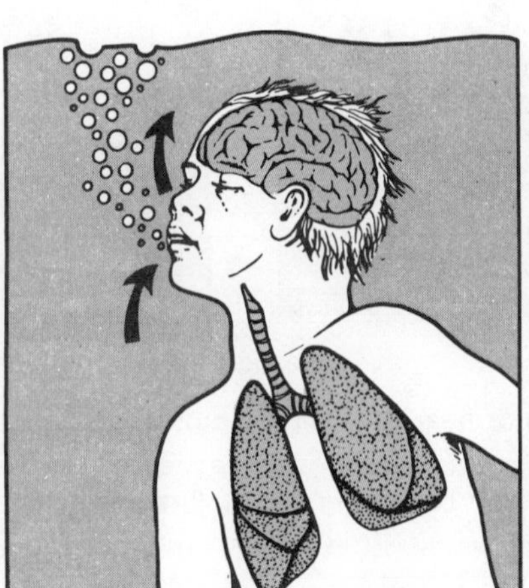

The drowning victim struggles to inhale air as long as possible, but eventually he goes beneath the water where he must exhale air and inhale water.

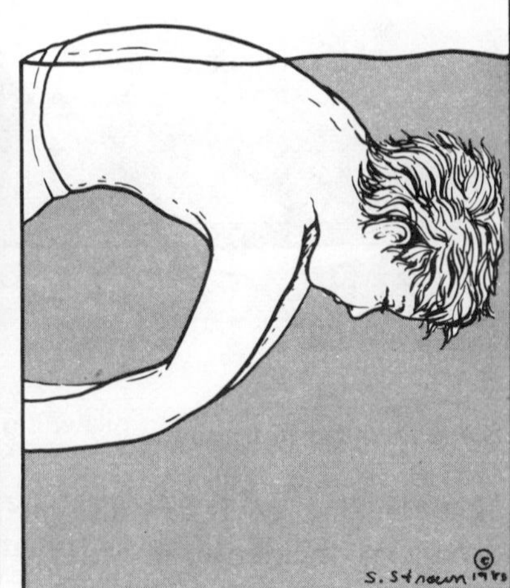

Loss of consciousness, convulsions, cardiac arrest and death follow.

In about 10% of all drownings, a muscle spasm of the larynx closes the victim's airway, causing him to die of asphyxiation without ever inhaling water.

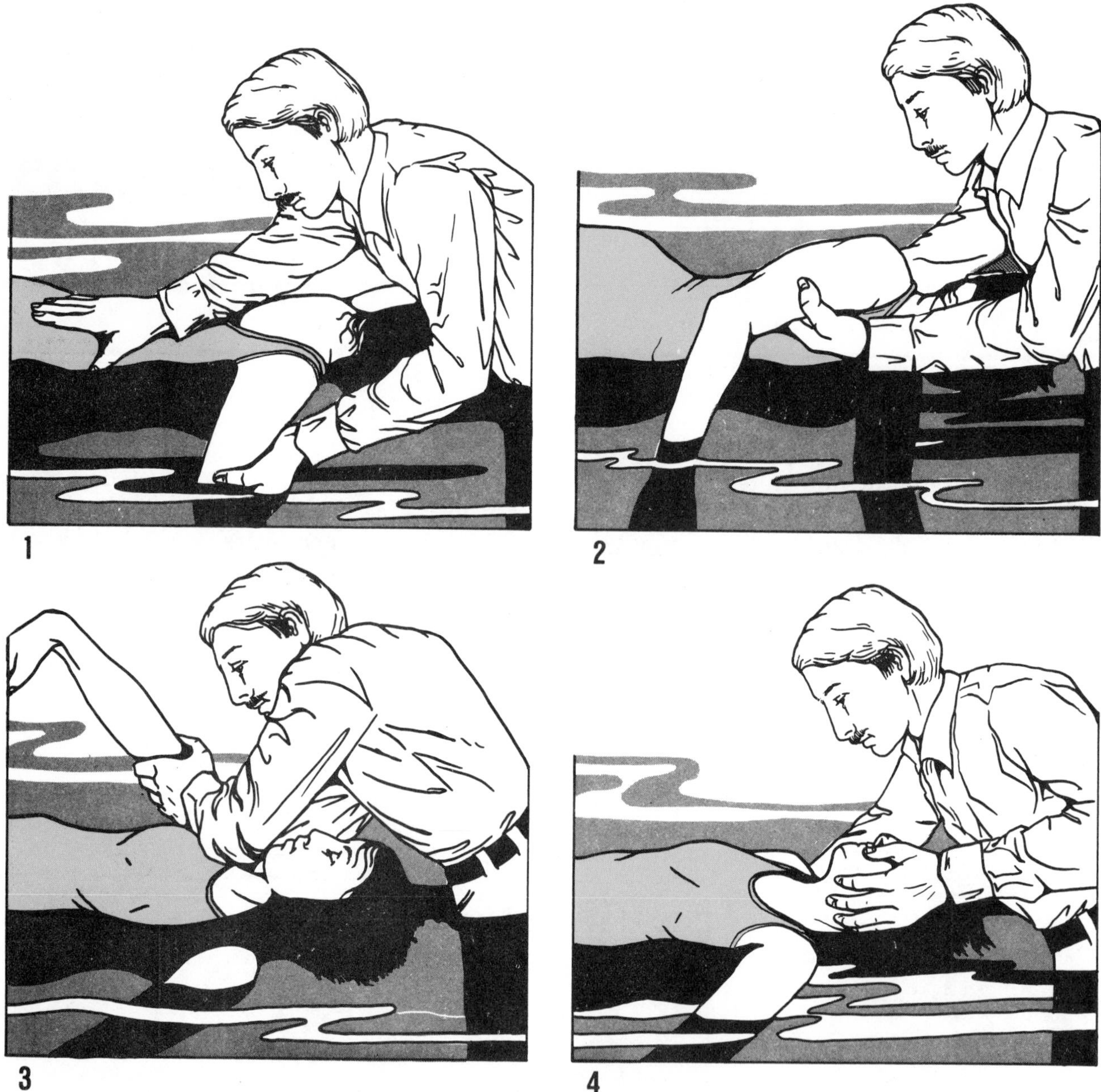

Steps involved in turning a drowning or near-drowning victim from a face-down position to the back.

ages of one to four. The major causes of drowning incidents, in order, are:

1. Becoming exhausted while swimming, skin diving, or attempting a rescue.
2. Losing control and getting swept into water that is too deep.
3. Losing a support (sinking or capsizing).
4. Getting trapped or entangled while in the water.

First Aiders who may need to perform rescues around large water body areas should always have a rescue buoy and swimming fins. The buoy is usually made of aluminum or synthetic polyurethane. The buoy is attached to a six-foot towline with a nylon or canvas strap on the opposite side to slip over the First Aider's shoulder. This, in essence, becomes a "towline" for the First Aider. The proper methods for rescues will not be discussed here but can be obtained from the Council for National Cooperation in Aquatics and the National Surf Life Saving Association of America.

Today, increasingly more head and spinal injuries are occurring due to water accidents, such as diving injuries. Four basic rules should be used when aiding a possible head- or spinal-injured victim in the water.

1. Do not remove the injured from the water.
2. Keep the injured floating on his/her back.
3. Wait for help.
4. Always support the head and neck level with the back.

There are two major aspects to handling an injury in the water — the proper stabilization of the victim in the water, and the proper removal of the victim from the water. The American National Red Cross suggests that the victim not be removed from the water until a backboard or other rigid support be used to splint him/her. Many water accident victims may be floating face down and will need to be turned.

To turn a victim, follow these guidelines:

1. Keeping the victim's head and body aligned, place one of your hands in the middle of his/her back, your arm directly over the victim's head.
2. Place your other hand under the victim's upper arm, near the shoulder.
3. Slowly and carefully, keeping the body and head aligned, rotate the victim over in the water by lifting the shoulder up and rotating it over.

## EMERGENCY CARE OF NEAR-DROWNING VICTIMS

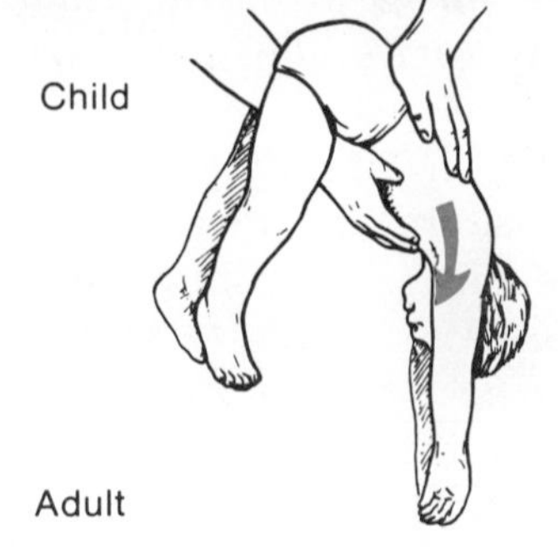


- Use postural drainage to clear water aspiration.
- If in doubt about aspirations, do not waste precious time trying to remove water from the victim's lungs.
- Clear mouth and airway.
- Begin artificial ventilation.
- If airway is obstructed give several abdominal thrusts.
- Be prepared for vomiting.
- Prevent aspiration.
- If carotid pulse absent, begin CPR.

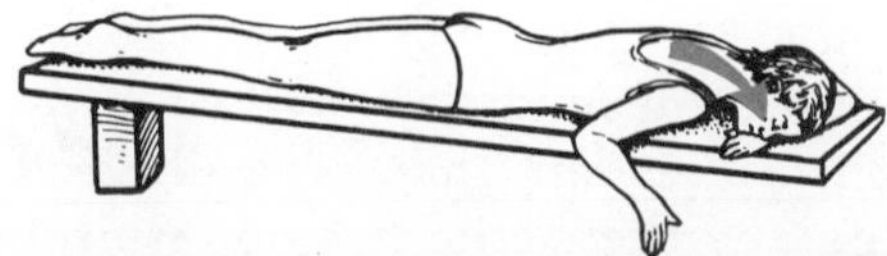

- Anyone submerged long enough to be unconscious and/or require CPR, who has been under water less than one hour, should be resuscitated.
- If under water for more than one hour, no attempt at resuscitation should occur.
- If you do not know how long the person has been under water, consider them under one hour.
- There is no difference between fresh and salt water near-drowning in regard to emergency care.
- These principles apply to any near-drowning, not just those in cold water. The difference between warm and cold water is that in long submersions (greater than 6 minutes), the chance for survival in warm water is much less than in cold water. The colder the water, the better the chance for survival.
- It is very important to clear a blocked airway with the Heimlich Maneuver/abdominal thrusts. (Turn patient's head sideways.)
- CPR must be started immediately.
- Assess carefully for associated injuries.

4. If you suspect a spinal injury, do not attempt to move the victim from the water until a spineboard can be used to immobilize the spine. Other emergency procedures — such as mouth-to-mouth resuscitation — can be accomplished while the victim is supported in a neutral position in the water.
5. Use a spineboard or other rigid support — such as a water ski, a surfboard, a picnic bench, an ironing board, or a wooden plank — to immobilize the spine. Slide it underneath the victim, and let it float up until it is snugly against the victim's back. Use several large towels to secure the victim to the spineboard if you do not have anything else. Never try to support the victim's spine with anything that might bend or break, such as an air mattress or a styrofoam float.

After the initial rescue attempt, initiate lifesaving procedures immediately — never draw hasty conclusions about a victim being dead.

The key to saving a near-drowning victim is:

1. Understanding the **cause** and **pathophysiology** of drowning and near-drowning.
2. Applying the proper resuscitation techniques.

The physiological changes that take place in a near-drowning victim are dependent upon the quantity, type (salt or freshwater), and amount of fluid aspirated. A near-drowning victim has also been subjected to suffocation. It is estimated that 10 percent of drowning victims do not aspirate water, but die from acute asphyxia due to the larynx closing off. Those who do aspirate water have a different physiological experience, depending on whether the water is fresh or salty.

In freshwater drowning, water passes through the lungs into the circulation and may cause dilution of the blood. The degree of blood dilution, however, is directly dependent on the volume of water taken in.

In saltwater drowning, salt from the aspirated water causes the loss of large amounts of fluid from the circulation into the lungs. The result is water accumulation in the lungs, and death.

The basic differences between saltwater and freshwater drowning are related to the salt content of the body fluid compared to that of the water. In saltwater drowning, the water is saltier than body fluids, so water "leaves" the blood and enters the lungs to dilute the salt concentration. The air in the lungs mixes with the fluids and forms a frothy foam, which is a barrier to oxygen diffusion.

In freshwater drowning, there is less salt in the water than in the body fluids, so the water "leaves" the lungs and enters the blood. This causes serious chemical imbalances in the blood, may rupture red blood cells, and will interfere with oxygen exchange and delivery. Do not assume that danger is over once the victim has resumed breathing.

The changes in near-drowning victims will depend on how fast and far the physiologic events that normally lead to death occur. If the victim has not aspirated water, complete recovery usually results if proper resuscitative methods are begun.

## Work Exercises

Drowning is the third leading cause of accidental deaths in the United States each year. The major causes of drowning are becoming exhausted while swimming, skin diving, or attempting a rescue; losing control and getting swept into water that is too deep; losing a support; getting dropped or entangled while in the water.

There are two major aspects to handling an injury in the water: proper ______________ of the victim in the water and the proper ______________________ of the victim from the water. The American National Red Cross suggests that a victim not be removed from the water until ____________________________________________.

What is the difference between freshwater and saltwater drowning?

What are five guidelines for emergency care of drowning victims?

1.

2.

3.

4.

5.

## SELF-TEST

### Part I: True and False

If you believe the statement is true, circle the T. If you believe the statement is false, circle F.

T F 1. Death from drowning always results from a victim inhaling water, and a drowning victim's lungs always contain water.

T F 2. Reflex spasm of the larynx can occur immediately if a swimmer plunges into cold water.

T F 3. The physiological processes that occur during drowning in fresh water and salt water are completely different.

T F 4. Abdominal thrusts are an effective way of forcing water from a drowning victim's air passages.

T F 5. If you suspect that a drowning victim has sustained a neck or back injury, you should move him/her carefully from the water before strapping him to a backboard.

T F 6. A drowning victim may still die up to two days following successful resuscitation, so close monitoring (preferably in a hospital) is essential.

T F 7. If a victim is in trouble near a deck or the pool's edge, you should be able to easily rescue him/her by getting into the water yourself.

T F 8. The First Aider should use postural drainage to clear water aspiration.

T F 9. There is a distinct difference in emergency care given for fresh vs. saltwater near-drowning.

T F 10. A spinal injury victim who is in the water should be removed from the water immediately, then splinted on the shore.

### Part II: Multiple Choice

Circle the answer that best reflects an accurate statement.

1. When rescuing a drowning victim, you should ordinarily begin mouth-to-mouth resuscitation:
   a. as soon as you remove the victim from the water
   b. in the water as soon as you have checked for other injuries
   c. in the water as soon as you reach the victim
   d. as soon as you remove the victim from the water and have had a chance to check for other injuries

2. To remove swallowed water from the victim's stomach: (no spinal injury involved)
   a. use abdominal thrusts
   b. lie the victim on his/her side and exert firm pressure on the stomach
   c. turn the victim quickly onto the stomach and use your hands to "lift" the stomach

3. A swimmer who hyperventilates (takes excessively deep breaths) before going underwater is in danger of drowning because:
   a. he/she may damage lung tissue
   b. he/she may become mentally confused and, eventually, unconscious
   c. he/she may overestimate his/her ability
   d. none of the above

4. Drowning is the __________ leading cause of accidental death in the U.S.
   a. 3rd
   b. 5th
   c. 10th
   d. 12th

5. The American Red Cross suggests that the victim *not* be removed from the water:
   a. until you know what caused the drowning
   b. until you have put a life jacket on the victim
   c. until there are two First Aiders who can get the victim out of the water
   d. until a backboard or other rigid support is used to splint the victim

Corresponds with:
**American Red Cross**
**Standard First Aid & Personal Safety**
Chapter 2, pages 22-29
and
**Advanced First Aid & Emergency Care**
Chapter 2, pages 28-38

# 6 Control of Bleeding

## CIRCULATORY SYSTEM

The life processes depend on an adequate and uninterrupted blood supply. An understanding of what blood is and how it is circulated will help explain why and how blood loss must be stopped quickly and effectively.

In order to function, a person's body must receive a constant supply of nourishment (oxygen, heat, etc.), which is distributed to the blood. If the supply of blood is cut off for any period of time, the tissues in the body will die for want of nourishment.

The **circulatory system,** by which blood is carried to and from all parts of the body, consists of the heart and blood vessels. Through the blood vessels, blood is circulated to and from all parts of the body under pressure supplied by the pumping action of the heart.

## BLOOD

Blood is composed of **serum** or **plasma, red cells, white cells,** and **platelets.** Plasma is a fluid that carries the blood cells and transports nutrients to all tissues. It also transports waste products resulting from tissue activity to the organs of excretion. Red cells give color to the blood and carry oxygen. White cells aid in defending the body against infection. Platelets are essential to the formation of blood clots, which are necessary to stop bleeding. Clotting normally takes six to seven minutes.

The process whereby body cells receive oxygen and other nutrients and wastes are removed is called **perfusion.** An organ is perfused if blood is entering through the arteries and leaving through the veins.

One-twelfth to one-fifteenth of the body weight is blood. A person weighing 150 pounds will have approximately ten to twelve pints of blood. If the blood supply is cut off from tissues, they will die from lack of oxygen. The loss of two pints, 8 to 10 percent of the body's blood, by an adult, usually is serious, and the loss of three pints may be fatal if it occurs over a short time, such as one to two hours. At certain points in the body, fatal **hemorrhages** may occur in a very short time. The cutting of the principal blood vessels in the neck, in the arm, or in the thigh may cause hemorrhage that will prove fatal in one

**DISTRIBUTION OF BLOOD IN THE BODY**

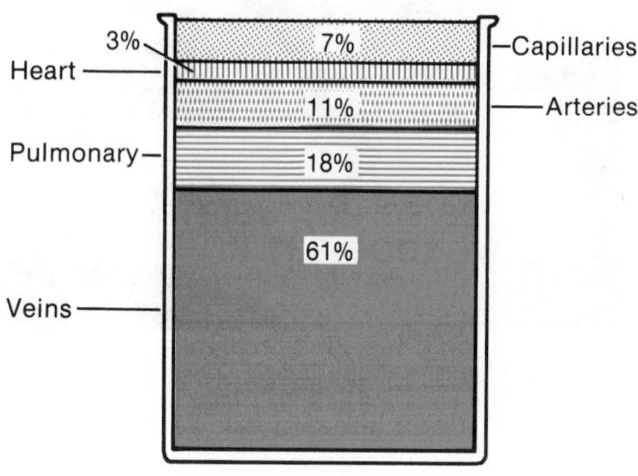

to three minutes or even less. Rupture of the main trunk blood vessels of the chest and abdomen may cause fatal hemorrhage in less than thirty seconds.

The loss of blood causes a state of physical **shock.** This occurs because there is insufficient blood flowing through the tissues of the body to provide food and oxygen. All processes of the body are affected. When a person is in shock, vital body functions slow down. If the conditions causing shock are not reversed, death may result.

## BLOOD VESSELS

Oxygenated blood is carried from the heart by a large artery called the **aorta.** Smaller arteries branch off from this large artery, and those arteries in turn branch off into still smaller arteries. These arteries divide and subdivide until they become very small, ending in threadlike vessels known as **capillaries,** which extend into all the organs and tissues. Through the very thin capillary walls, oxygen, carbon dioxide, and other substances are exchanged between body cells and the circulatory system.

After the blood has furnished the necessary nourishment and oxygen to the tissues and organs of the body, it takes on waste products, particularly carbon dioxide. The blood returns to the heart by means of a different system of blood vessels known as **veins.** The veins are connected with the arteries through the capillaries. Veins collect deoxygenated blood from the capillaries and carry it back to the heart.

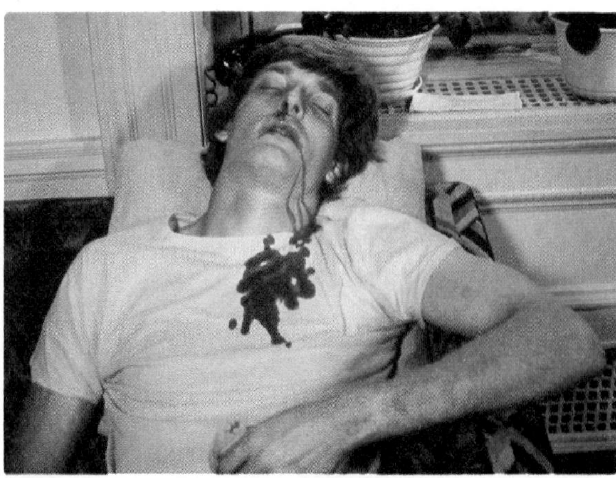

Bleeding from the mouth and/or nose in an unconscious victim can be a serious threat to respiration if proper precautions are not taken for drainage and suctioning.

Very small veins join, forming larger veins, which, in turn, join until the very largest veins return the blood to the heart. While the blood is returning to the heart, it passes through the **kidneys,** where waste products are removed. When the blood from the body reaches the heart, carbon dioxide and other volatile waste products contained in the blood but not removed by the kidneys must be eliminated, and the oxygen used by the body replaced. The heart pumps the blood delivered to it by the veins into the lungs, where it flows through another network of capillaries. There, the carbon dioxide and other waste products are exchanged for oxygen through the delicate walls of air cells. Thus, the blood is oxygenated and ready to return to the heart, which recirculates it throughout the body. The time taken for the blood to make one complete circulation of the body through miles and miles of blood vessels is approximately seventy-five seconds in an adult at rest.

## HEMORRHAGE OR BLEEDING

### Procedures

Hemorrhage or bleeding is a flow of blood from an artery, vein, or capillary. In severe bleeding:

- Place the victim in such a position that he/she will be least affected by the loss of blood.
- Lie the victim down, and elevate the legs in a semi-flexed position. This prevents aggravation of spinal injury or breathing impairment.
- Control the bleeding.
- Maintain an open airway, and give the victim plenty of fresh air.
- Prevent the loss of body heat by putting blankets under and over the victim.
- The victim should be kept at rest, as movement will increase heart action, which causes the blood to flow faster and perhaps interfere with clot formation or dislodge a clot already formed.

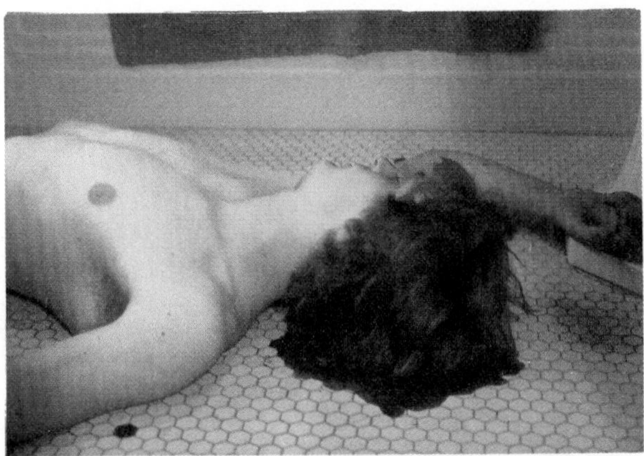

Detecting and controlling profuse bleeding are part of the primary survey.

## Effect of Hemorrhage

- The loss of red blood cells causes a lack of oxygen to the body systems.
- A decrease in **blood volume** causes a decrease in **blood pressure.**
- The heart's pumping rate increases to compensate for reduced blood pressure.
- The force of the heartbeat is reduced, since there is less blood to pump.

## Effect of Unchecked Hemorrhage

If the bleeding is unchecked, the above symptoms quicken, and shock deepens.

- The loss of two pints in the average male (15 percent of blood volume) produces moderate shock.
- Loss of 30 percent or more of blood volume produces severe or fatal shock.

## Bleeding from an Artery

When bright red blood spurts from a wound, an artery has been cut. The blood in the arteries comes directly from the heart and spurts at each contraction. Having received a fresh supply of oxygen, the blood is bright red.

## Bleeding from a Vein

When dark red blood flows from a wound in a steady stream, a vein has been cut. The blood, having given up its oxygen and received carbon dioxide and waste products in return, is dark red.

## Bleeding from Capillaries

When blood oozes from a wound, capillaries have been cut. There is usually no cause for alarm; relatively little blood can be lost. Usually, direct pressure with a compress applied over the wound will cause the formation of a clot. Where a large skin surface is involved, the threat of infection may be more serious than the loss of blood.

## "Bleeders"

Some persons' blood will not clot. Such people are **hemophiliacs,** commonly called "bleeders." They may bleed to death even from the slightest wounds where blood vessels are cut. In addition to applying a compress bandage or gauze, such persons should be rushed to the nearest hospital, where medical treatments may be quickly administered.

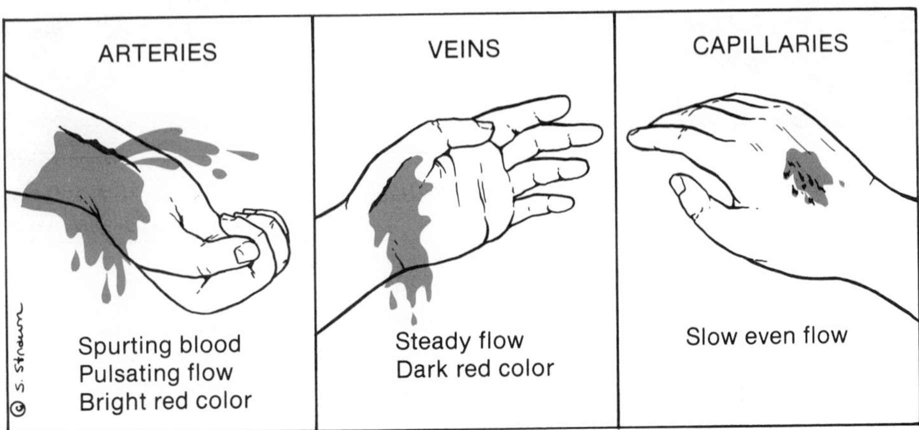


Bleeding characteristics.

## CONTROL OF BLEEDING FROM LACERATED WOUND

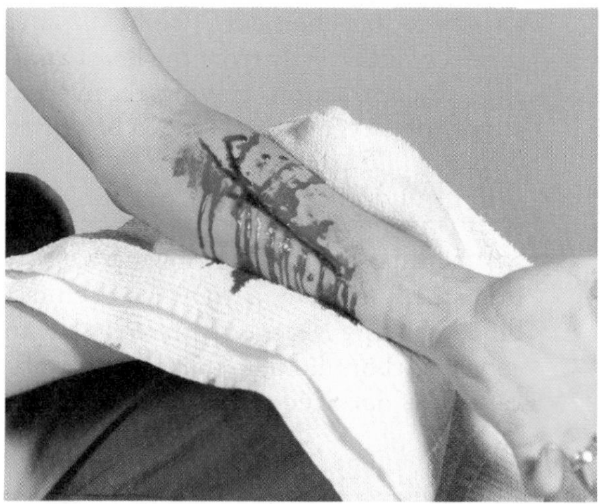

1
Bleeding from a lacerated wound on the forearm.

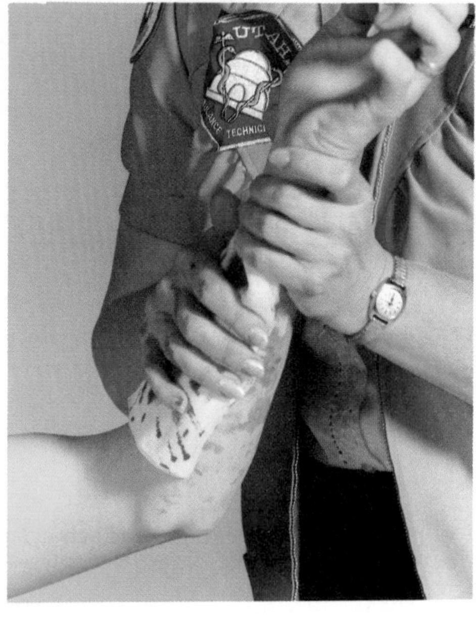

2
Control bleeding with direct pressure and elevation. If necessary, use your bare hand.

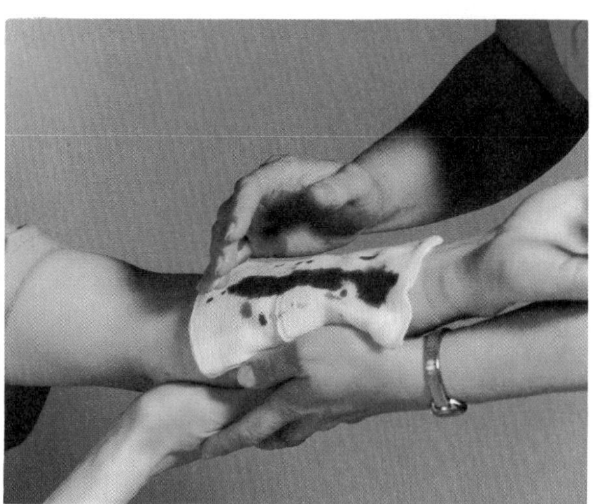

3
If bleeding soaks through the dressing, do not remove the original dressing.

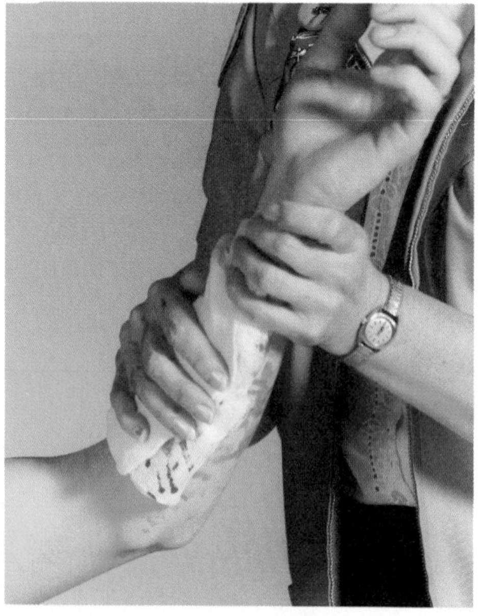

4
Add a new dressing on top of the original and continue with direct pressure and elevation. After bleeding is under control, bandage the dressing in place.

## METHODS OF CONTROLLING BLEEDING

Bleeding control is often very simple. Most external bleeding can be controlled by applying direct pressure to the open wound. Direct pressure permits normal blood clotting to occur.

In cases of severe bleeding, the First Aider may be upset by the appearance of the wound and the emotional state of the victim. It is important to keep calm. Control of bleeding is secondary only to maintenance of air passages and restoration of breathing.

A person's survival can be threatened by loss of a quart or more of blood. Bleeding from a combination of internal and external injuries or from a main artery can be so rapid and extensive that death can result almost immediately.

When a large blood vessel is completely severed, the natural elasticity of the vessel walls tends to retract cut ends. The blood flow may slow down and begin to clot because of the smaller escape opening. A partially severed vessel, however, will not retract, and bleeding continues unless clotting occurs or blood pressure diminishes.

In injuries where severe bleeding is expected but little or no loss of blood is evident, the victim may already be in a state of advanced shock. Such injuries should be watched closely, because when measures are taken to combat the shock and restore normal blood circulation, rapid bleeding may begin.

### Direct Pressure

The best all-around method of controlling bleeding is applying pressure directly to the wound. This is best done by placing gauze or the cleanest material available against the bleeding point and applying firm pressure with the hand until a bandage can be applied. If the dressing and/or bandage soaks through with blood, do not remove the dressing; simply put on another layer and apply pressure. The bandage knot should be tied over the wound unless otherwise indicated. The bandage supplies direct pressure and should not be removed until the victim is examined by a physician. When air splints or pressure bandages are available, they may be used over the heavy layer of gauze to supply direct pressure.

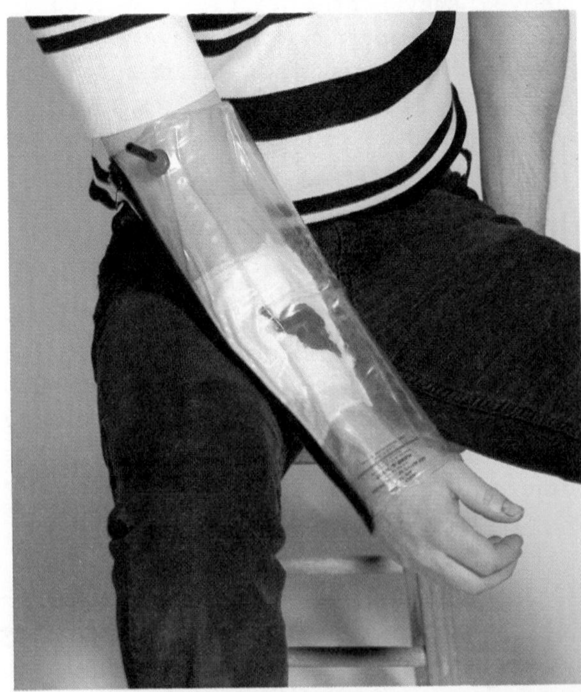

Air splints can be used to apply pressure and control bleeding from an extremity.

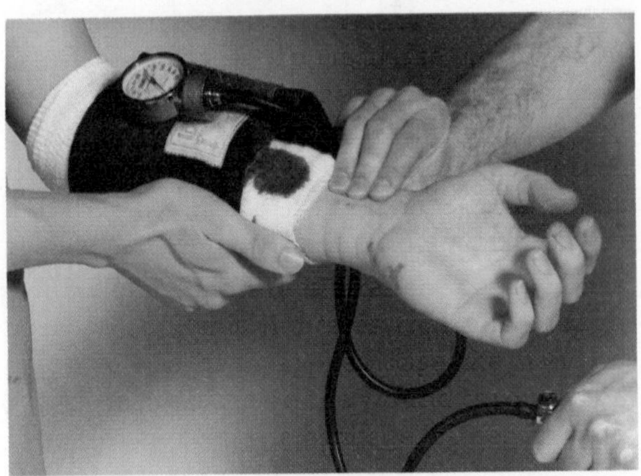

A blood pressure cuff can be used to apply pressure and control bleeding in an extremity.

If bleeding continues after the bandage has been put on, this indicates that not enough pressure has been applied. Use the hand to put more pressure on the wound through the gauze, or tighten the bandage. Either method should control the bleeding. In severe bleeding, if gauze or other suitable material is not available, the bare hand should be used to apply direct pressure immediately.

## Elevation

Elevating the bleeding part of the body above the level of the heart will slow the flow of blood and speed clotting. Elevation should be used together with direct pressure when there are no unsplintable fractures, and when it will cause no pain or aggravation to the injury.

## Indirect Pressure

Arterial bleeding can be controlled by digital thumb or finger pressure applied at **pressure points.** Pressure points are places over a bone where arteries are close to the skin. Pressing the artery against the underlying bone can control the flow of blood to the injury.

In cases of severe bleeding where direct pressure is not controlling the bleeding, digital pressure must be used. Pressure points should be used with caution, as indirect pressure may cause damage to the limb as a result of an inadequate flow of blood. When the use of indirect pressure at a pressure point is necessary, indirect pressure should not be substituted for direct pressure; both kinds of pressure should be used. The pressure point should be held only as long as necessary to stop the bleeding. Indirect pressure should be reapplied if bleeding recurs.

Pressure points on the arms (**brachial** pressure point) and in the groin (**femoral** pressure point) are the ones most often used. **These pressure points should be thoroughly understood.**

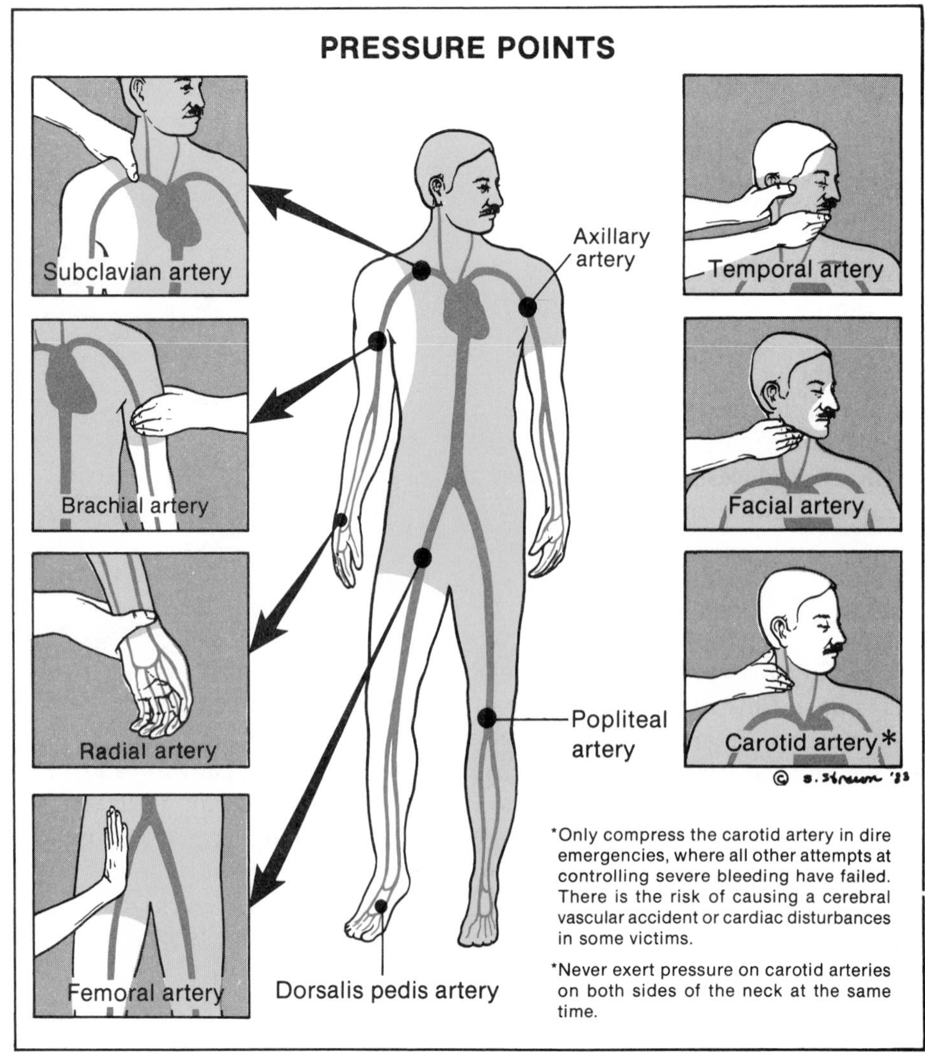

Pressure on the brachial artery is used to control severe bleeding from an open wound on the upper extremities. This pressure point is located in a groove on the inside of the arm between the armpit and the elbow. To apply pressure:

- Grasp the middle of the victim's arm with the thumb on the outside of the arm and the fingers on the inside.
- Press the fingers toward the thumb.
- Use the flat, inside surface of the fingers, not the fingertips. This inward pressure closes the artery by pressing it against the humerus.

The use of the carotid pressure point is of questionable value. If it is to be used, caution must be exercised. Pressure should not be applied to both carotids at the same time, since such **occlusion** may restrict blood flow to the brain.

The femoral artery is used to control severe bleeding from a wound on the lower extremity. The pressure point is located on the front center part of the crease in the groin area. This is where the artery crosses the pelvic basin on the way into the lower extremity. To apply pressure:

- Position the victim flat on his/her back, if possible.
- Kneeling on the opposite side from the wounded limb, place the heel of one hand directly on the pressure point, and lean forward to apply the small amount of pressure needed to close the artery.
- If bleeding is not controlled, it may be necessary to press directly over the artery with the flat surface of the fingertips and apply additional pressure on the fingertips with the heel of the other hand.

## Tourniquet

A **tourniquet** is a device used to control severe bleeding. It is used as a *last resort* after all other methods have failed. First Aiders should thoroughly understand the dangers and limitations of its use.

A tourniquet should normally be used only for severe, life-threatening hemorrhage that cannot be controlled by other means. A tourniquet may be dangerous. Its improper use by inexperienced, untrained persons may cause tissue injury or loss of a limb. It may completely shut off the blood supply to a limb, and the pressure device itself often cuts into or injures the skin and underlying tissues and nerves. It is rarely required and should be used only when large arteries are severed, or when bleeding is uncontrollable.

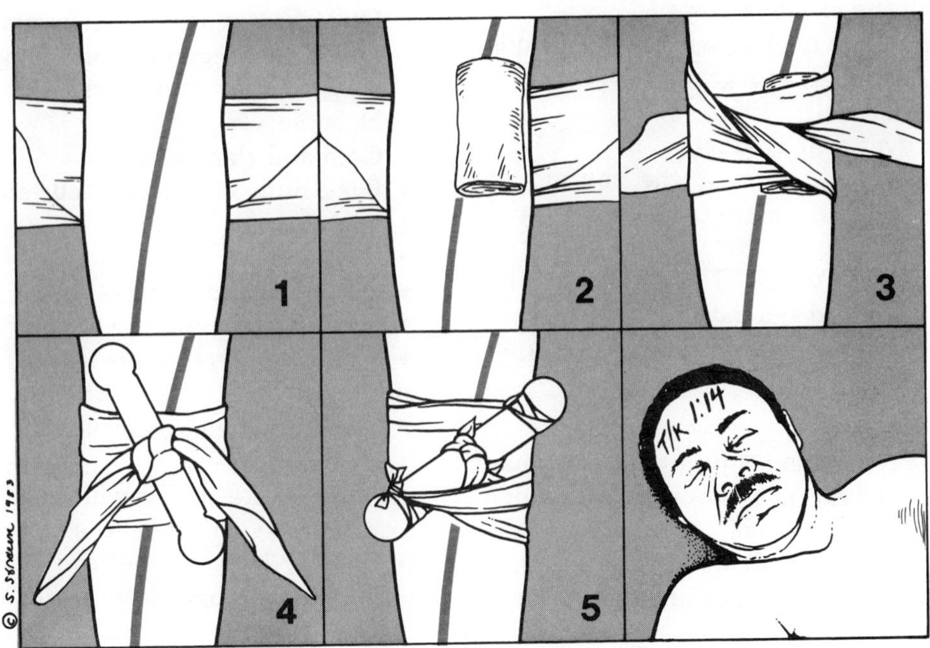


Application of a tourniquet.

The standard tourniquet usually is a piece of web belting about thirty-six inches long, with a buckle or snap device to hold it tightly in place when applied. A tourniquet can be improvised from a strap, belt, suspender, handkerchief, towel, necktie, cloth, or other suitable material. A tourniquet should be at least three to four inches wide to distribute pressure over tissues. A blood pressure cuff can often be used as a tourniquet. However, secure it well so that the *Velcro* does not pop open with additional pressure. Never use wire, cord, or anything that will cut into the flesh. A cravat bandage may also be used as a tourniquet.

The procedure for applying a tourniquet is as follows:

- While the proper pressure point is being held to temporarily control the bleeding, place the tourniquet between the heart and wound, with sufficient uninjured flesh between the wound and tourniquet.
- Apply a pad over the artery to be compressed.
- In using an improvised tourniquet, wrap the material tightly around the limb twice and tie in a half-knot on the upper surface of the limb.
- Place a short stick or similar stout object at the half-knot, and tie a full knot.
- Twist the stick to tighten the tourniquet only until the bleeding stops.
- Secure the stick in place with the base ends of the tourniquet, another strip of cloth, or suitable material.
- Do not cover a tourniquet.
- Make a written note of the tourniquet location and the time it was applied, and attach the note to the victim's clothing. Alternatively, make a "T" or "TK" on the victim's forehead and indicate time applied.
- Get the victim to a medical facility as soon as possible.

Once the tourniquet is tightened, it should not be loosened except by or on the advice of a doctor. The loosening of a tourniquet may dislodge clots and result in sufficient loss of blood to cause severe shock and death.

A deep wound high up on the arm or an amputation at the upper part of the arm may require a tourniquet at the armpit to control bleeding. If needed, apply as follows:

- Place the center of a narrow cravat bandage in the armpit over a firm pad or padded object.
- Cross the ends on the shoulder over a pad.
- Carry the ends around the back and chest to the opposite side, and tie them over the pad.
- To tighten, insert a small stick or similar object under the cross of the bandage on the shoulder and twist. Twist only until the bleeding is controlled. Then secure or anchor the stick to prevent untwisting.
- Loosen the tourniquet only on a doctor's advice.

## INTERNAL BLEEDING

**Internal bleeding** in the chest or abdominal cavities generally results from hard blows or certain fractures. Internal bleeding is usually not visible, but it can be very serious, even fatal. Internal bleeding may be determined by the following signs and symptoms:

- Pain, tenderness, or discoloration where injury is suspected.
- Bleeding from mouth, rectum, or other natural body openings.
- Dizziness, without other symptoms. Dizziness when going from lying to standing may be the only early sign of internal bleeding.
- Cold and clammy skin.
- Eyes dull, vision clouded, and pupils enlarged.
- Restlessness and anxiety.
- Weak and rapid pulse.
- Nausea and vomiting.
- Shallow and rapid breathing.
- Thirst.
- Weak and helpless feeling.

Serious internal bleeding can result from fractures. As an example, a fractured shaft of the femur (thigh bone) can result in an internal loss of one liter of blood. The most serious blood loss from a fracture occurs in fractures of the pelvis.

The most common cause of internal bleeding due to trauma is a fracture, and the most severe blood loss occurs in fracture of the pelvis.

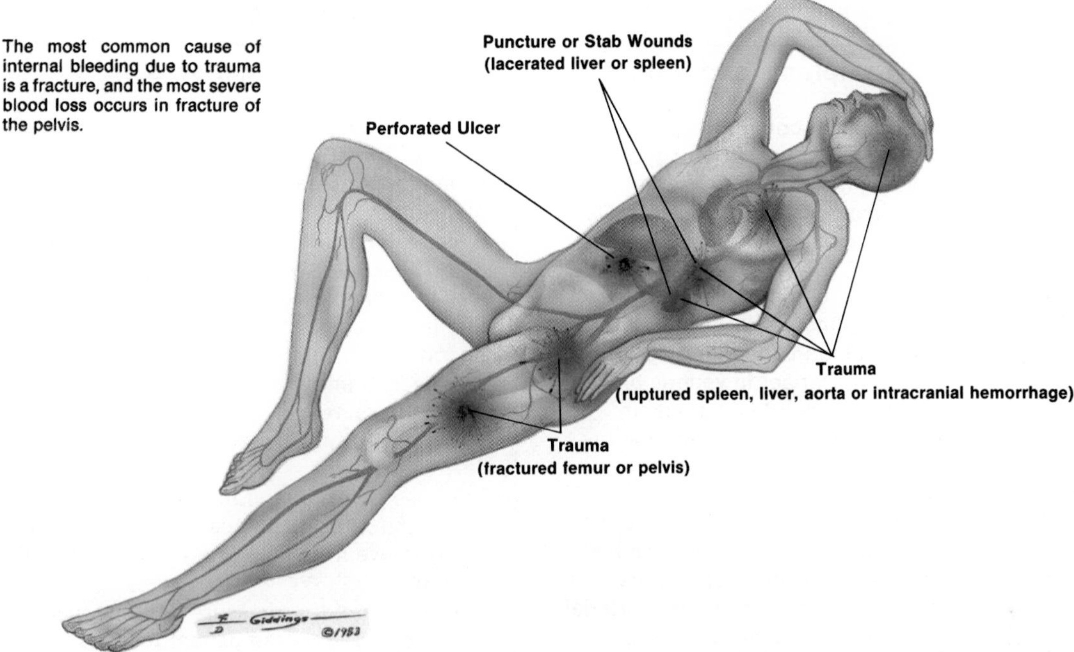


COMMON SITES OF INTERNAL BLEEDING

Emergency care for internal bleeding is to secure and maintain an open airway and treat for shock. Never give the victim anything by mouth.

Anyone suspected of having any internal bleeding should be transported to a medical facility as quickly and safely as possible. When blood or vomit is coming from the mouth, the injured person should be kept on his/her side. For chest injuries, place the victim on the injured side. Be gentle with the victim and call for emergency help as soon as possible.

If the internal bleeding is into an extremity, apply pressure to the injured place with a snug bandage or an air splint over a heavy pad. Elevate the part after it has been immobilized. Pressure will tend to close off the ends of the bleeding vessels. If it is possible that a closed fracture has caused the bleeding, care must be taken in applying any pressure dressing. Application directly over the fracture site might further injure tissue or complicate the fracture.

## NOSEBLEEDS

Nosebleeds are a relatively common source of emergencies. They can result from an injury, disease, activity, the environment, and other causes. Generally, they are more annoying than serious, but enough blood may be lost to cause a slight degree of shock. Bleeding from the nose can be caused by the following:

- Facial injuries, including those caused by a direct blow to the nose.
- A cold, sinusitus, infections, or other abnormalities of the inside of the nose.
- High blood pressure.
- Strenuous activity.
- Exposure to high altitudes.
- Fractured skull.

If a fractured skull is suspected as the cause of a nosebleed, do not attempt to stop the bleeding. To do so might increase the pressure on the brain. The victim should be treated for a fractured skull.

Nosebleed from other causes may be treated as follows:

1. Keep the victim quiet and in a sitting position, leaning forward. If the sitting position is not possible because of other injuries, place the victim in a reclining position with head and shoulders raised.
2. Apply pressure by pinching the nostrils.
3. Apply cold compresses to the nose and face.

<table>
<tr><th colspan="3">SUMMARY — CONTROL OF EXTERNAL BLEEDING</th></tr>
<tr><th>Type</th><th>Symptoms and Nature</th><th>Emergency Care</th></tr>
<tr><td>Capillary</td><td>Oozing, most common type of external hemorrhage. This type of bleeding is expected in all minor cuts, scratches, and abrasions. Dark bluish-red color.</td><td rowspan="3">External bleeding is bleeding that can be seen coming from a wound. Excessive external bleeding can create a crisis situation: the platelets, which usually help the blood clot, aren't effective in cases of severe bleeding or when the blood vessels have been damaged. Serious blood loss is defined as one liter in an adult and half a liter in a child. If the bleeding remains uncontrolled, shock and death may result.<br>Elevate Extremity<br>Direct Pressure<br>1. Apply direct pressure against the bleeding site.<br>2. Use a dressing; if necessary, even your bare hand. If dressing soaks through do not remove it; put another on top and continue applying pressure.<br>3. Maintain firm pressure until the bleeding stops or until the patient reaches the hospital.<br>4. If the wound is on an extremity, elevate it while you apply direct pressure.<br><br>Pressure Points<br>The most important arteries used in pressure point control include:<br>The brachial artery, along the inside of the upper arm midway between the elbow and the shoulder; compression will stop or control bleeding below the pressure point.<br>The femoral artery, in the groin, slows bleeding in the leg on the appropriate side.</td></tr>
<tr><td>Venous</td><td>Slow, even blood flow. Occurs when a vein is punctured or severed. Venous blood is dark in color (maroon). Danger in venous bleeding from neck wound is that an air bubble may be sucked into the wound.</td></tr>
<tr><td>Arterial</td><td>Occurs when an artery is punctured or severed. Not common because arteries are located deep in the body and are protected by bones. Arterial bleeding is characterized by spurting of bright red blood. Common arteries injured in accidents: carotid, brachial, radial, femoral.</td></tr>
<tr><td colspan="3">Splints<br>In cases of open fractures, splintered bone ends can damage tissue and cause external bleeding. Properly applied splints can immobilize the fracture and lessen the chance of further injury.<br><br>Tourniquet<br>Use of a tourniquet is rarely warranted, because control of external bleeding can almost always be achieved by using some other means. Tourniquets should be used as a last resort only, and only after trying all other methods of control.</td></tr>
</table>

4. If this does not control the bleeding, insert a small clean pad of gauze into one or both nostrils and again apply pressure with the thumb and finger pinching the nostrils. A free end of the gauze must extend outside the nostril so that the pad can be removed later.
5. If the person is conscious, it may be helpful to apply pressure beneath the nostril above the upper lip.
6. Instruct the victim to avoid blowing, the nose for several hours, as this could dislodge the clot.
7. If bleeding continues, obtain medical assistance.

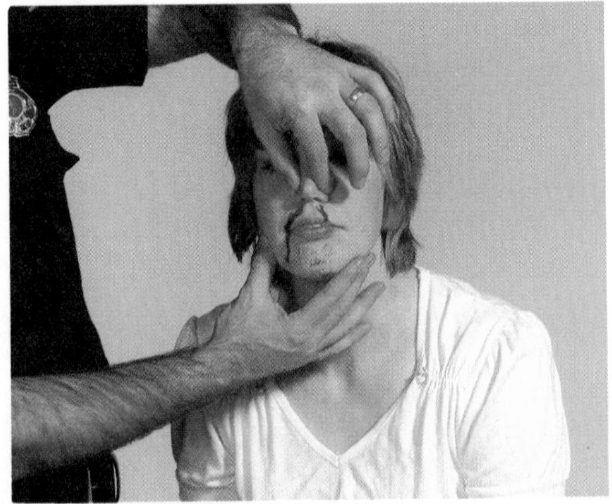

Apply pressure by pinching the nostrils and, if necessary, apply cold compresses to the nose and face.

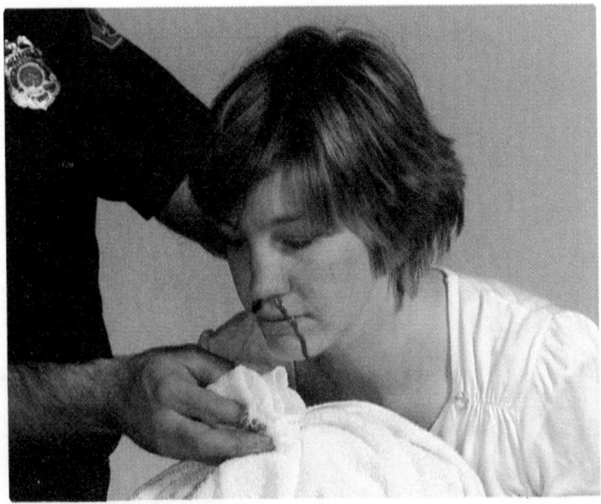

For a nosebleed victim, keep the victim quiet and leaning forward in a sitting position.

## SUMMARY — EMERGENCY CARE FOR INTERNAL BLEEDING

Internal bleeding is an extremely serious condition. It is just as dangerous as external bleeding and, when uncontrolled, can lead to death due to shock. It may be caused by a tearing or bruising force that actually ruptures or tears apart one of the internal organs or tissues. Pressure on nerves from internal bleeding can cause great pain or paralysis. The most common cause of internal bleeding due to trauma is a fracture. The most severe blood loss occurs in fracture of the pelvis. Extensive swelling can cut off blood circulation to a limb. Internal bleeding is often hard to assess and can prove rapidly fatal. The signs of internal bleeding are similar to those of shock — look for restlessness, anxiety, cold, clammy skin, weak, rapid pulse, rapid breathing, and, ultimately, a drop in blood pressure. In addition, the patient may cough up or vomit bright red blood, vomit dark blood (the color of coffee grounds), pass dark stools, pass bright red blood, or have a tender, rigid abdomen that enlarges.

| Common Causes | Signs and Symptoms | Emergency Care |
|---|---|---|
| Hard blow to any part of the body will cause contusions and/or rupturing of internal organs. | A fractured bone, hard blow, or other force may cause internal bleeding and swelling. A closed fracture may cause loss of blood internally. | Internal bleeding usually requires surgical correction.<br>1. Activate the EMS system immediately.<br>2. If bleeding originates in an extremity, elevate it.<br>3. Application of a splint or pressure dressing may also help. |
| Fractured ribs causing puncture of lungs. Fractured sternum from too vigorous CPR. | Bright red frothy blood coughed up usually means bleeding from the lungs. Pale, moist skin; weak, rapid pulse; shallow, rapid respiration. | |
| Bleeding ulcer. Ingestion of a sharp object. i.e. glass. | Vomiting bright red blood may indicate stomach bleeding. Blood which has been in stomach a longer time will resemble coffee grounds. | |
| Disease corroding intestines, tapeworms, blow to abdominal area, appendicitis. | Slow bleeding in the intestinal tract above the sigmoid colon will cause the stools to be jet black (tar color). Hardness or spasm of abdominal muscles accompanies. | |
| Blockage of urethra may result in rupture of bladder, causing internal bleeding; multiple trauma may cause fractured pelvis, which may puncture kidneys. | Blood in urine may indicate bladder rupture or injury to the urinary tract. Urine may be a smoky color. | |

## Work Exercises

There are two types of hemorrhage, external and internal. External hemorrhage is bleeding that can be seen coming from a wound.

Place the following list of things to do in case of severe hemorrhage in the correct order: (1-7)

_________ Control the bleeding by direct pressure

_________ Open airway

_________ Keep the patient at rest

_________ Maintain an open airway

_________ Place the patient in such a position that he will be least affected by the loss of blood

_________ Elevate the injured limb to help control bleeding

_________ Prevent loss of body heat by putting blankets over and under the patient

### Pressure Points

Order the following procedures for application of a tourniquet. (1, 2, 3, etc.)

_________ Secure the stick in place.

_________ Wrap the tourniquet around the limb twice and tie in a half knot on the limb's upper surface.

_________ Do not cover a tourniquet.

_________ Twist the stick to tighten the tourniquet only until bleeding stops.

_________ Place the tourniquet between the heart and the wound.

_________ Get the patient to a medical facility as soon as possible.

_________ Place a short stick at the half knot and tie a full knot.

_________ Make a written note of the location and the time the tourniquet was applied.

## Pressure Points

Label each of the pressure points illustrated.

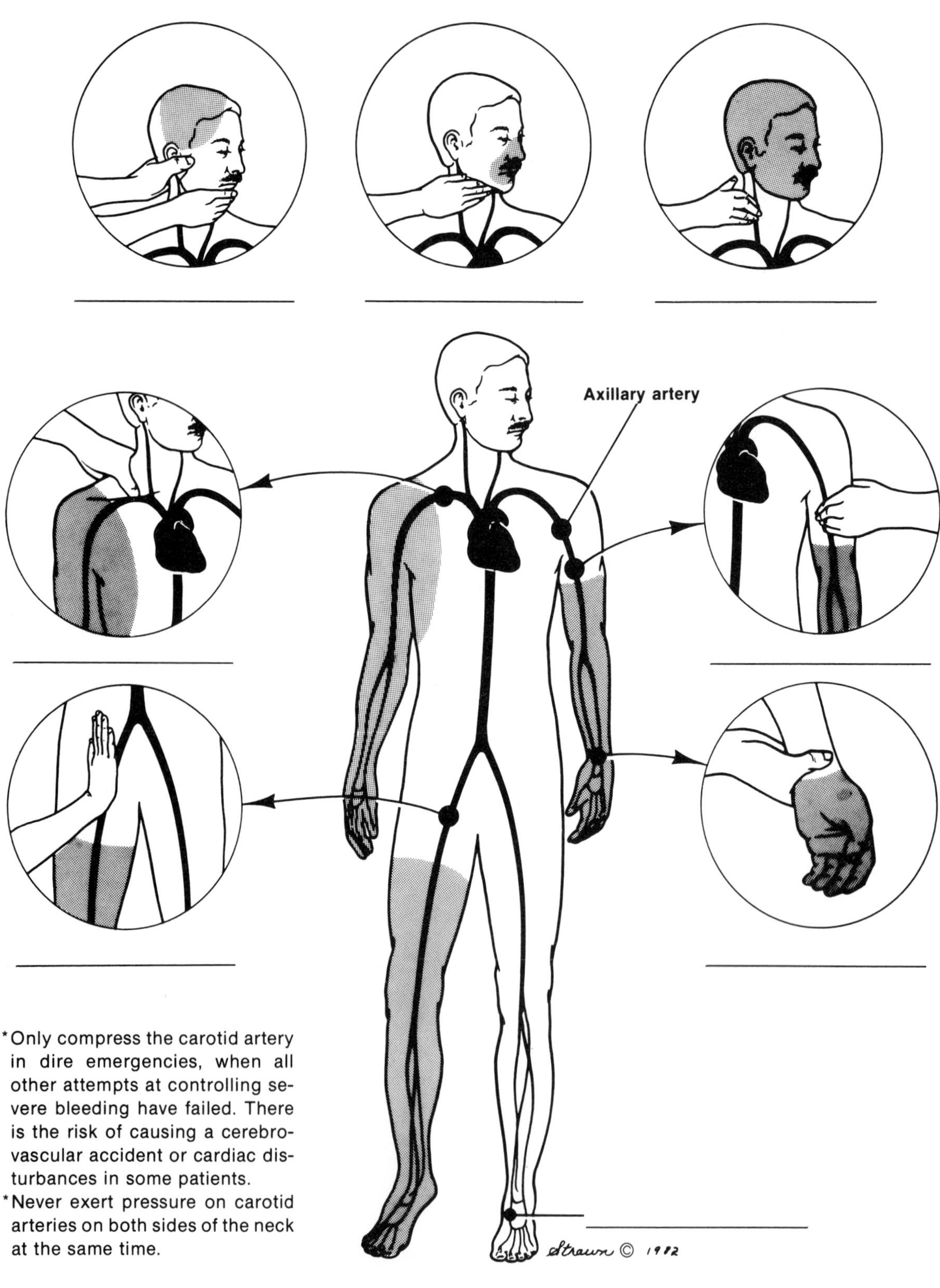


*Only compress the carotid artery in dire emergencies, when all other attempts at controlling severe bleeding have failed. There is the risk of causing a cerebrovascular accident or cardiac disturbances in some patients.

*Never exert pressure on carotid arteries on both sides of the neck at the same time.

## SELF-TEST

### Part I: True and False

If you believe the statement is true, circle the T. If you believe the statement is false, circle F.

T F 1. Loss of a quart of blood is a serious threat to a person's survival.

T F 2. When a large blood vessel is completely severed, the flow of blood may slow down enough to permit clotting.

T F 3. If a large blood vessel is only partially cut, bleeding will usually continue and clotting will be difficult.

T F 4. Severe bleeding from an open wound usually can't be controlled by direct pressure only.

T F 5. You should never attempt to control bleeding with just your bare hand.

T F 6. If blood soaks through a compress, the compress should be removed and a new, heavier one should be used.

T F 7. For a severely bleeding open arm wound, pressure over the radial artery will help control bleeding.

T F 8. The major and most easily located artery of the leg is the fibial.

T F 9. A person with internal bleeding will usually have a rapid, weak pulse and pale, moist skin.

T F 10. Once a bad (deep) wound has stopped bleeding, remove the dressing and clean the wound thoroughly to prevent infection.

T F 11. The signs of internal bleeding are similar to those of shock.

T F 12. The application of cold to a wound causes the blood vessels to constrict.

T F 13. First aid for internal bleeding usually means keeping the victim in a supine position.

T F 14. You should elevate a bleeding limb even if it is fractured — control of bleeding is the top priority.

T F 15. Never raise a severely bleeding limb higher than the rest of the body.

### Part II: Multiple Choice

Circle the one answer that best reflects a true statement.

1. Which of the following is *not* a component of blood?
   a. platelets
   b. capillaries
   c. white cells
   d. plasma

2. What component of blood is essential for the formation of blood clots?
   a. platelets
   b. white blood cells
   c. red blood cells
   d. plasma

3. How long does clotting take in most instances?
   a. 1-2 minutes
   b. 6-7 minutes
   c. 10-12 minutes
   d. 18-20 minutes

4. Perfusion means:
   a. the process of blood clotting
   b. manufacture of red blood cells
   c. another word for transfusion
   d. circulation of blood within an organ

5. The loss of __________ of the body's blood may be fatal if it occurs in a very short time.
   a. 3 pints
   b. 2 pints
   c. 1 pint
   d. ½ pint

6. Which of the following may be a sign of internal bleeding?
   a. vomiting of bright red blood
   b. pale, moist skin
   c. black stools
   d. blood in the urine
   e. all of the above

7. A person who has lost a large amount of blood should always be treated for:
   a. respiratory failure
   b. cardiac arrest
   c. anemia
   d. shock

8. Keeping a hemorrhaging victim quiet will encourage:
   a. rational behavior from the First Aider
   b. other victims to remain calm
   c. formation of a clot in the wound
   d. natural cleansing of the wound

9. Which of the following characterizes arterial bleeding?
   a. dark red color and spurting flow
   b. bright red color and spurting flow
   c. dark red color and steady flow
   d. bright red color and steady flow

10. Once you have applied a tourniquet to control bleeding, you should:
    a. cover it to prevent it from being jarred loose
    b. loosen it briefly once every two to three minutes
    c. immediately seek help from a physician
    d. all of the above

11. To control arterial bleeding in the neck, first:
    a. pack the area with ice
    b. apply a firm pressure dressing
    c. elevate the head and shoulders
    d. apply digital pressure to the carotid artery

12. When a dressing becomes saturated with blood, you should:
    a. remove it and apply a new dressing
    b. apply a tourniquet
    c. leave the dressing in place and apply an additional dressing on top of it
    d. tie the knot on the bandage tighter

13. How is direct pressure applied to control bleeding?
    a. by a compress and pressure on the wound
    b. by a compress and tourniquet on the wound
    c. by manual pressure at the appropriate pressure point
    d. by a tourniquet at the appropriate pressure point

14. If direct pressure does not succeed in stopping bleeding, what should be tried next?
    a. apply a tourniquet below the wound
    b. elevate the bleeding part
    c. apply pressure at the appropriate pressure point
    d. apply a tourniquet above the wound

15. What is a pressure point?
    a. a point where the blood pressure drops low enough to stop bleeding
    b. a place where the artery is protected on all sides by bone and muscle
    c. a place where an artery is close to the skin surface and over a bone
    d. a point where an artery is near the wound

16. Which of the following is *not* a guideline in using the carotid arteries as pressure points?
    a. improper use of carotid pressure points can cause a cerebrovascular accident or cardiac disturbances in some patients
    b. use only one carotid pressure point at a time
    c. use carotid pressure points only in cases of dire emergency
    d. if bleeding is extremely severe, compress the carotid arteries on both sides

17. Which pressure points are most often used?
    a. brachial, femoral
    b. ulnar, carotid
    c. subclavian, axillary
    d. temporal, dorsalis pedis

18. Severe bleeding from the upper arm may be controlled by finger pressure on the:
    a. femoral artery
    b. temporal artery
    c. radial artery
    d. brachial artery

19. One of the greatest dangers in bleeding from a neck wound is:
    a. an air bubble that may be sucked into the wound
    b. shock
    c. you cannot apply a tourniquet or use pressure points
    d. later infection

20. Use a tourniquet only if:
    a. there is severe hemorrhage
    b. bleeding cannot be controlled by direct pressure
    c. bleeding cannot be controlled by pressure at the appropriate pressure point
    d. bleeding cannot be controlled by any other means

21. When it becomes necessary to apply a tourniquet, you should place it between the wound and the heart. You should also make sure that it is:
    a. well away from the wound, and as tight as possible without causing severe pain
    b. well away from the wound, and only tight enough to stop bleeding
    c. as close to the wound as is practical and as tight as possible without causing severe pain
    d. as close to the wound as is practical and only tight enough to stop bleeding

22. Which of the following could be used as the band in an improvised tourniquet?
    a. rope
    b. string
    c. wire
    d. stockings

23. Once the tourniquet is tightened, it should:
    a. be loosened every 20 minutes so there will be adequate circulation to prevent limb loss
    b. not be loosened except by, or on the advice of, a physician
    c. be loosened if the bleeding appears to stop
    d. be loosened every two hours

24. Which of the following may *not* be a sign of internal bleeding:
    a. vomiting of bright, red blood
    b. pale, moist skin
    c. strong, bounding pulse
    d. dizziness

Corresponds with:
**American Red Cross**
**Standard First Aid & Personal Safety**
Chapter 4, pages 60-65
and
**Advanced First Aid & Emergency Care**
Chapter 4, pages 59-64

# 7 Shock

## DEFINITION OF SHOCK

**Shock** is a serious condition that can cause death. You should assume it to be present in all victims of injury and serious illness. Only the management of breathing, cardiac arrest, and bleeding emergencies should have priority over the emergency care of shock. It is important for you as a First Aider to realize that the classical signs and symptoms of shock may not appear until the condition is severe. You should anticipate shock before it develops and assume that every victim is in shock until proven otherwise.

Shock, a state of circulatory deficiency associated with depression of vital bodily processes, occurs when the cardiovascular system fails to provide sufficient blood circulation to all parts of the body. When blood is circulating normally throughout an organ, the cells of the organ are kept healthy — they receive oxygen and other nutrients from the incoming blood, and the blood that leaves the organ through the veins carries off waste products. This process of blood circulation within an organ is called **perfusion** and may become disrupted due to shock. Many lives have been lost due to reaction of the body to physical and/or emotional trauma. Although only one area of the body may be injured, the body as a whole reacts to the injury and attempts to recover as a whole.

Shock, then, is a **syndrome** (a collection of symptoms) that results from a decrease in effective circulating blood volume through blood loss and/or peripheral **vascular collapse** and from the body's efforts to compensate for this decrease. Some degree of shock occurs with every illness and trauma situation.

Shock is, in effect, an alarm reaction and a defensive mechanism. It may appear suddenly after trauma, or it may develop very gradually. Its leading characteristic is a reduction in the volume of the circulating blood accompanied by **constriction** of the blood vessels. This is followed by **dilation** of the vessels, low blood pressure, rapid heartbeat, and mental and physical collapse. The initial circulatory deficiency is rapidly complicated by widespread oxygen deprivation and by a lessening of function of all tissues, especially of the brain, liver, heart, and kidneys.

Three chief dangers are associated with shock:

1. Early loss of consciousness that mainly involves the nervous system and that may be fatal.
2. Progressive loss of blood from the active circulation, which may lead to failing heart output and insufficient oxygen to cells that are vital for survival.
3. Sustained lowered blood pressure, which may lead to liver and kidney failure.

## PROCESS OF SHOCK

Whatever the cause of shock, a deteriorating cycle develops unless correction is immediate. Diminished tissue perfusion (circulation of blood within the organ) is soon followed by decreased return of blood to the heart through the veins. This, in turn, results in lessened

## CAUSES OF SHOCK

Some of the major causes of shock are as follows:

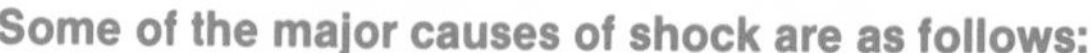

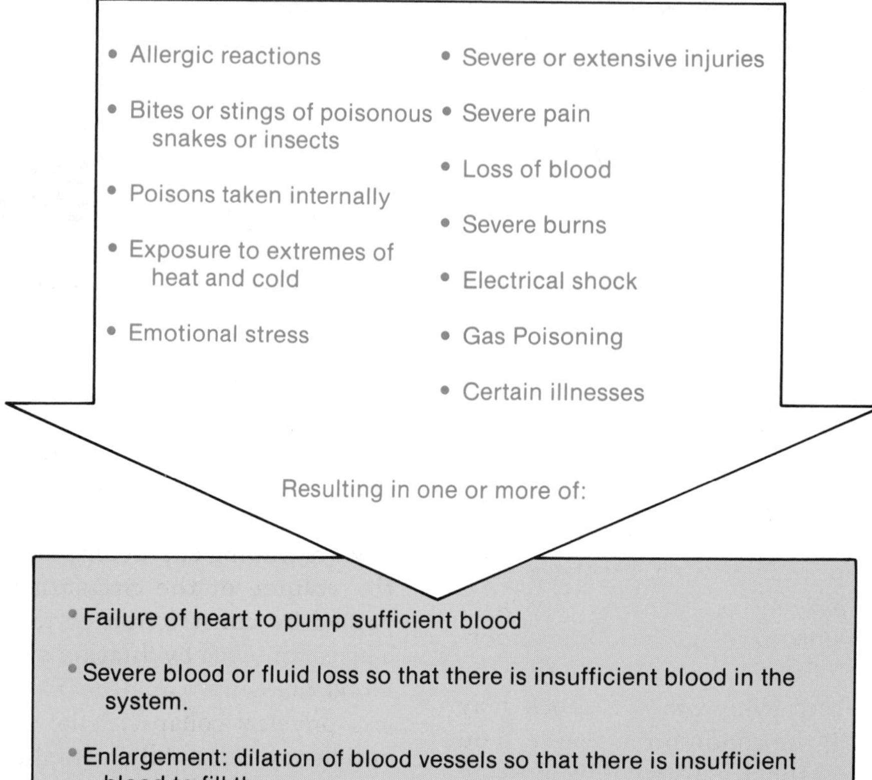


**RESULT:** No matter what the reason, the result is the same: all normal bodily processes are affected. There is insufficient blood flow (perfusion) to provide nourishment and oxygen to all parts of the body.

cardiac output and further impairment of blood circulation in the tissues.

Shock does not happen all at once, but rather develops in distinct stages as the body reacts to and assesses the injury. Although shock is a series of stages, it can progress rapidly (especially in the event of major injury). Shock progresses in the following way:

1. Blood flow in the entire body is disrupted.
2. With less blood flow to the heart, the heart beats faster, blood vessels near the skin and in the arms and legs constrict, sending most of the available blood supply to the vital organs of the body and to the nerve centers of the brain that control all vital functions.
3. While blood rushes to the brain and other vital organs, the other body cells do not receive enough blood and therefore do not get enough oxygen or nutrients.
4. The blood vessels, like the rest of the body, suffer from this lack of oxygen, and eventually they lose their ability to constrict.
5. When blood vessels lose their ability to constrict, the vital organs and the brain do not receive enough blood, and shock worsens.
6. As the blood supply is shut off to the internal organs and to the brain, the cells — because of an oxygen deprivation — begin to die. As the shock gets worse, this condition progresses.

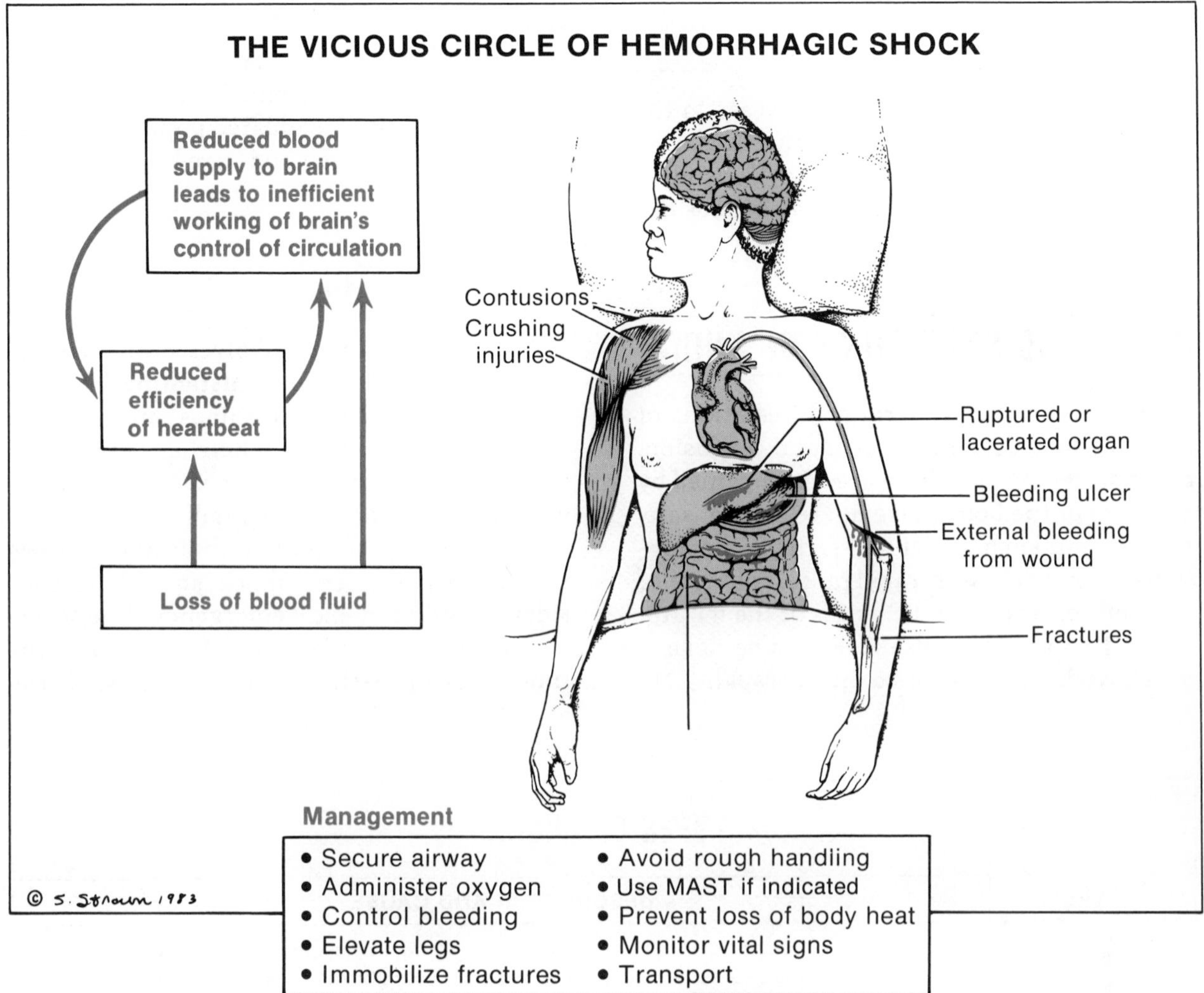


7. The brain suffers from a lack of oxygen-rich blood and loses its ability to function. The victim's powers of reasoning and expression are decreased.
8. If shock is not reversed, the internal organs and brain eventually die.

## FACTORS INFLUENCING THE DEGREE OF SHOCK

Some degree of shock occurs from all injuries; its severity depends on the stability of the victim's nervous system. What might cause a mild case of shock in one person could cause a severe case in another.

The following factors may have a significant effect on the degree of shock induced by trauma and disease:

1. **Pain.** Pain can produce or increase the severity of shock.
2. **Physical condition.** People who have been starved, deprived of water, or exposed to extremes of cold or heat go into shock very easily.
3. **Fatigue.** Excessive fatigue can increase the severity of shock.
4. **Disease.** As a general rule, people who have any kind of **chronic** illness go into shock more easily than healthy people.
5. **Individual reaction.** Some unexplained differences exist between individuals regarding their resistance to shock. An injury that might cause serious, perhaps even fatal, shock in one person may cause only mild shock in another.
6. **Improper evaluation/care/movements.** Shock may be increased by rough handling and by delay in treatment.

## TYPES OF SHOCK

Any injury that results in a decrease in the amount of blood that is effectively circulating will produce symptoms of shock. Depending on the type of injury, eight types of shock can be identified.

## SIGNS AND SYMPTOMS OF SHOCK

The most common early manifestations of shock include restlessness, mental confusion, and disorientation. These are accompanied by evidence of the body's attempt to compensate, resulting in such associated signs and symptoms as skin paleness, rapid pulse, coldness of extremities, thirst, and dryness of the mouth. In early shock, the pulse rate may be normal or slowed, or it may be quite rapid. Late symptoms of shock include low or unobtainable blood pressure; rapid, "thready," or unobtainable pulse; a bluish or purplish discoloration of the skin; dilated pupils; faintness or unconsciousness; and irregular, gasping respirations.

## ANAPHYLACTIC SHOCK

Anaphylactic shock involves a massive release by the body of toxic **histamine**-like substances when a victim comes into contact with something to which he/she is extremely allergic. These act as tissue poisons in causing widespread dilation of the capillaries and pooling of blood. Anaphylactic shock follows rapidly. Anaphylactic shock should be considered a grave medical emergency. The severity of the reaction is inversely related to the time elapsing between the contact with the

| | TYPES OF SHOCK |
|---|---|
| **TYPE** | **DESCRIPTION AND CAUSE** |
| **Hemorrhagic (Hypovolemic** or **Traumatic)** | Loss of blood resulting in not enough blood going to tissues, i.e., wounds, internal bleeding. Possible causes — multiple trauma and severe burns. There is insufficient blood in the system to provide adequate circulation to all body organs. |
| **Respiratory** | There is an insufficient amount of oxygen in the blood because of inadequate breathing or respiratory arrest due to:<br>a) spinal injury resulting in damage to respiratory controlled nerves<br>b) obstruction of airways — mucous plug, foreign body<br>c) chest trauma, flail chest, punctured chest, etc. |
| **Neurogenic** | Spinal or head injury resulting in loss of nerve control and thus **integrity** of blood vessels. The nervous system loses control over the vascular system — the blood vessels dilate and there is insufficient blood to fill them. |
| **Psychogenic** | Something psychological affects the patient, i.e., the sight of blood, loved one injured, etc.; blood drains from the head and pools in the abdomen, person faints due to lack of blood in the brain because of a temporary dilation of blood vessels. |
| **Cardiac** | Cardiac muscle not pumping effectively due to injury or previous heart attack. The heart muscle no longer imparts sufficient pressure to circulate the blood through the system. |
| **Metabolic** | Loss of body fluids with a change in biochemical equilibrium.<br>Example: insulin shock or diabetic coma, vomiting, diarrhea. |
| **Septic** | Severe infection. Toxins cause pooling of blood in capillaries with dilation of blood vessels; not enough blood to tissues. Bacteria attack small blood vessel walls so that they lose blood and plasma and can no longer constrict. |
| **Anaphylactic** | Severe allergic reaction of the body to sensitization by a foreign protein, such as insect sting, foods, medicine, ingested, inhaled or injected substances. It can occur in minutes or even seconds following contact with the substance the patient is allergic to. |

## SIGNS AND SYMPTOMS OF SHOCK

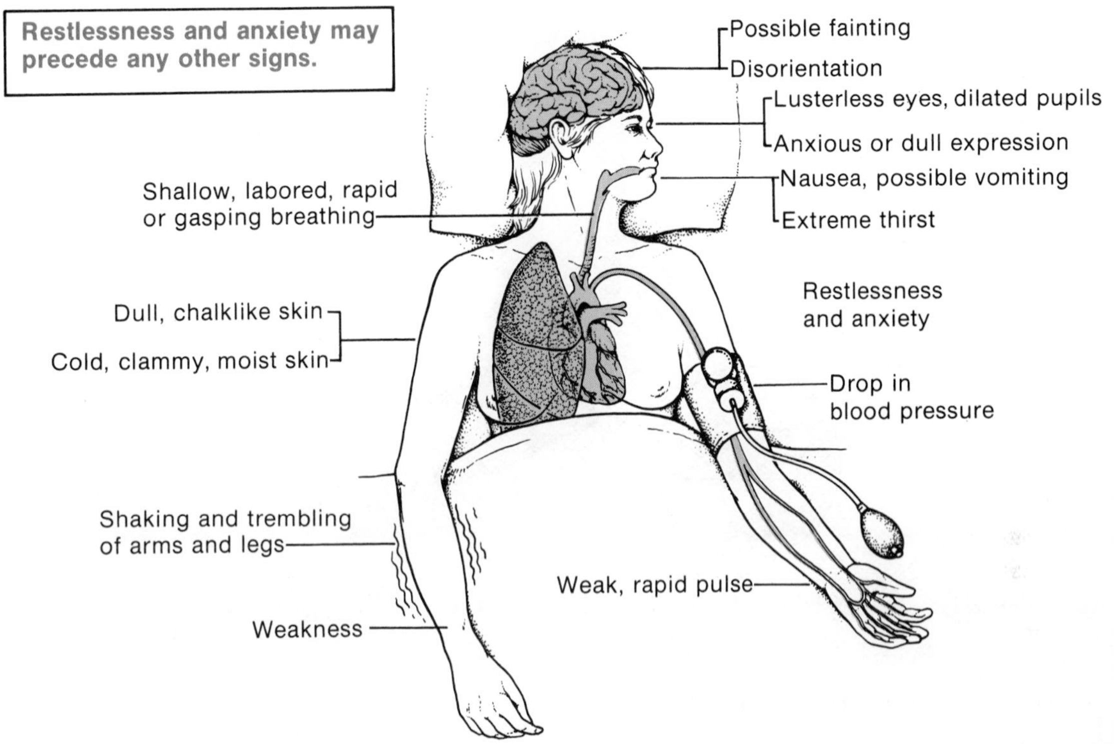

Restlessness and anxiety may precede any other signs.
Possible fainting
Disorientation
Lusterless eyes, dilated pupils
Anxious or dull expression
Nausea, possible vomiting
Extreme thirst
Shallow, labored, rapid or gasping breathing
Restlessness and anxiety
Dull, chalklike skin
Cold, clammy, moist skin
Drop in blood pressure
Shaking and trembling of arms and legs
Weak, rapid pulse
Weakness
© S. Sönnen '83

## DETERMINING SHOCK IN A DARK-SKINNED PERSON

Skin around mouth and nose is gray
Lips are blue
Tongue is blue
Mucous membranes of mouth are blue
Nailbeds are blue
© S. Sönnen '83

A healthy person with dark skin will usually have a red undertone and show a healthy pink color in the nailbeds, lips, mucous membranes of the mouth, and tongue. However, a Black victim in shock from a lack of oxygen does not exhibit the marked skin color changes. Rather, the skin around the nose and mouth will have a grayish cast, the mucous membranes of the mouth and tongue will be blue (cyanotic), and the lips and nailbeds will have a blue tinge. If shock is due to bleeding, the mucous membranes in the mouth and tongue will not look blue but will have a pale, graying, waxy pallor. Other landmarks include the tips of the ears, which may be red during fever.

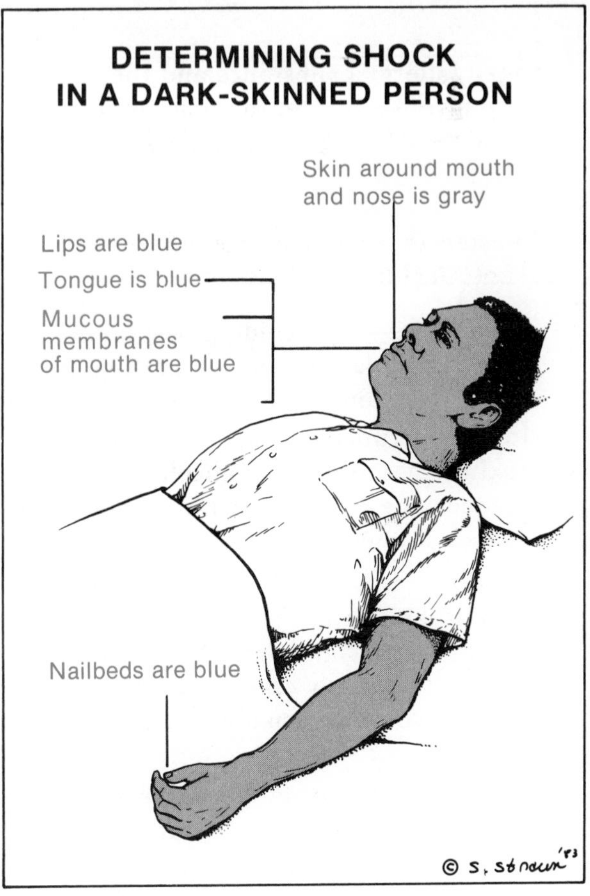

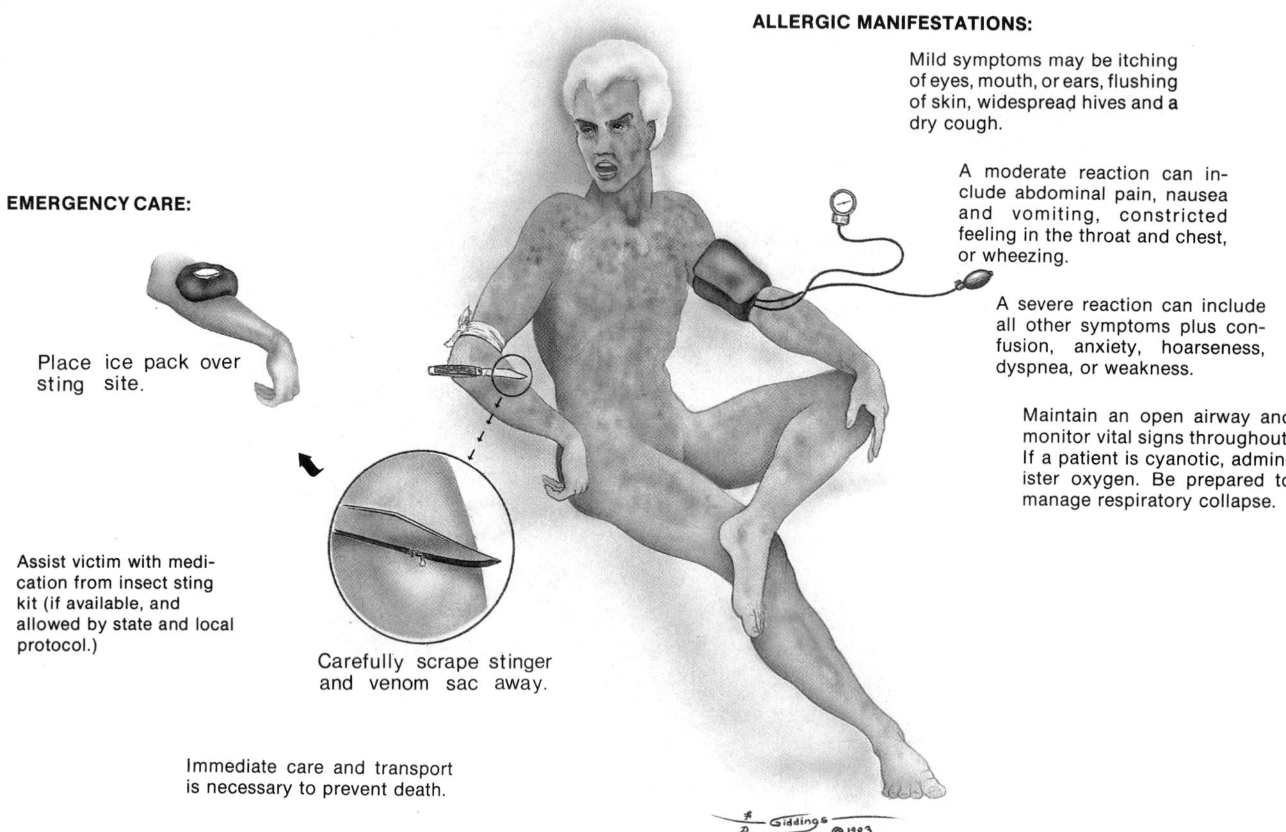


**ALLERGIC REACTION TO INSECT VENOM**

**antigen** (allergic) substance and the onset of symptoms. The shorter the time before symptoms appear, the greater the risk of a fatal reaction.

Substances commonly producing anaphylactic shock include the following:

1. Insect stings — including bee, wasp, hornet, yellow jacket, and other stinging insects. Reaction is usually severe and rapid.
2. Injected **serums** or drugs. The **tetanus antitoxin** sometimes causes anaphylactic shock, as does the drug **penicillin** (whether ingested or injected, although the reaction is more rapid from injection.
3. Foods. Common foods that may cause anaphylactic shock include shellfish, fish, berries (especially strawberries), and milk. The reaction is usually gradual but can become very severe.
4. Drugs. Depending on the sensitivity of the person, a simple drug like aspirin can cause fatal anaphylactic shock.
5. Inhaled substances. If a person is allergic to them, inhaled substances such as ragweed, pollens, animal hair, and dust can produce anaphylactic shock.

People are sensitized when they become allergic to a material that they have previously contacted. Unlike a simple allergy, however, where **hives** and itching, sneezing, and nasal drainage are the usual symptoms, an anaphylactic reaction produces a sudden, dramatic drop in blood pressure and can rapidly result in death.

1. **Signs and symptoms involving the skin:**
   - Itching and burning of the skin with flushing, especially around the face and chest.
   - Blueness (cyanosis) around the lips.
   - Raised, hivelike patches with severe itching.
   - Swelling of the face and tongue.
   - Paleness.
   - Swelling of the blood vessels just underneath the skin.

2. **Signs and symptoms involving the heart and circulation:**
   - Weak, rapid pulse.
   - Low blood pressure.
   - Dizziness.
   - Restlessness.
   - Diminished stroke volume and cardiac output.
3. **Signs and symptoms involving the respiratory tract:**
   - Spasm of the bronchioles.
   - A painful, squeezing sensation in the chest.
   - Difficulty in breathing.
   - Coughing, bronchial obstruction.
   - Swelling of the larynx.
   - Swelling of the epiglottis.
   - Respiratory wheezes.
4. **Signs and symptoms involving the gastro-intestinal tract:**
   - Nausea.
   - Vomiting.
   - Abdominal cramps.
   - Diarrhea.

Consult the section on Management of Shock in this chapter for special emergency procedures involved in anaphylactic shock.

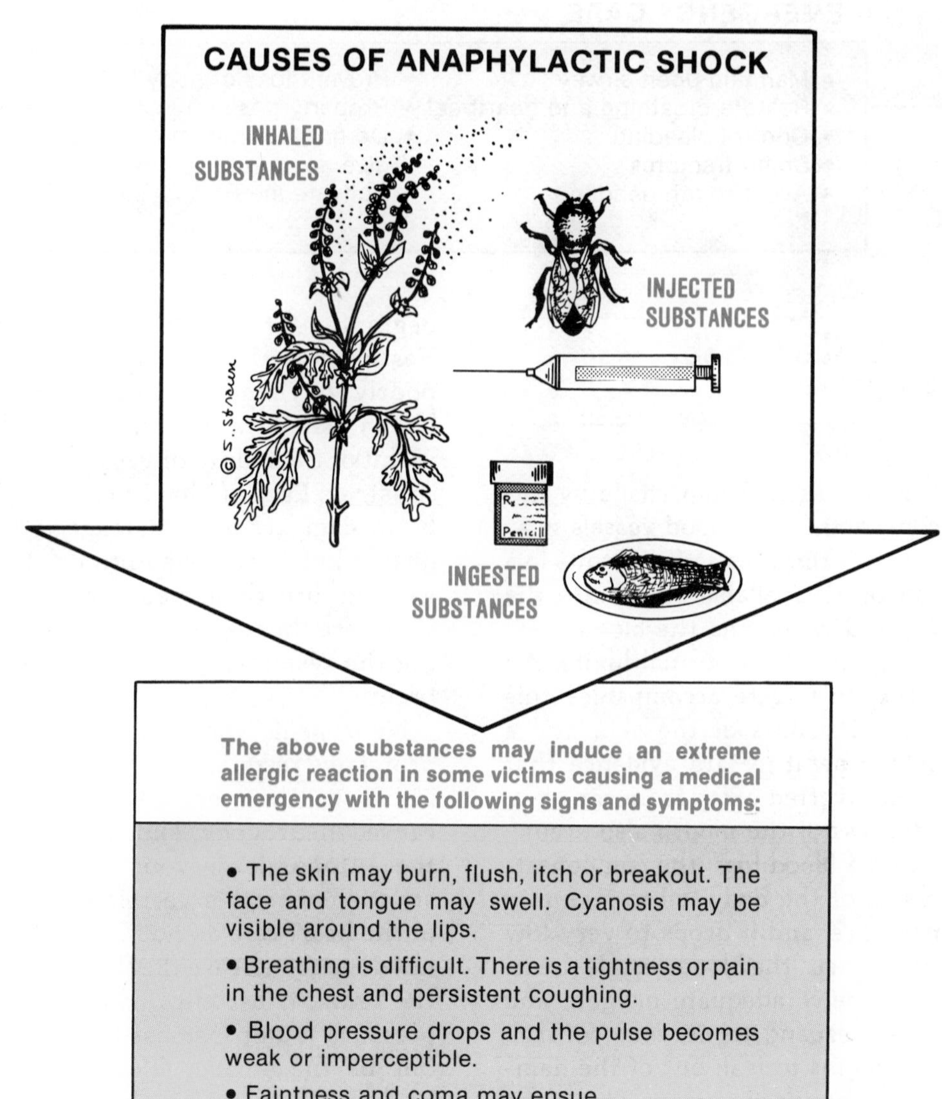


**The above substances may induce an extreme allergic reaction in some victims causing a medical emergency with the following signs and symptoms:**

- The skin may burn, flush, itch or breakout. The face and tongue may swell. Cyanosis may be visible around the lips.
- Breathing is difficult. There is a tightness or pain in the chest and persistent coughing.
- Blood pressure drops and the pulse becomes weak or imperceptible.
- Faintness and coma may ensue.

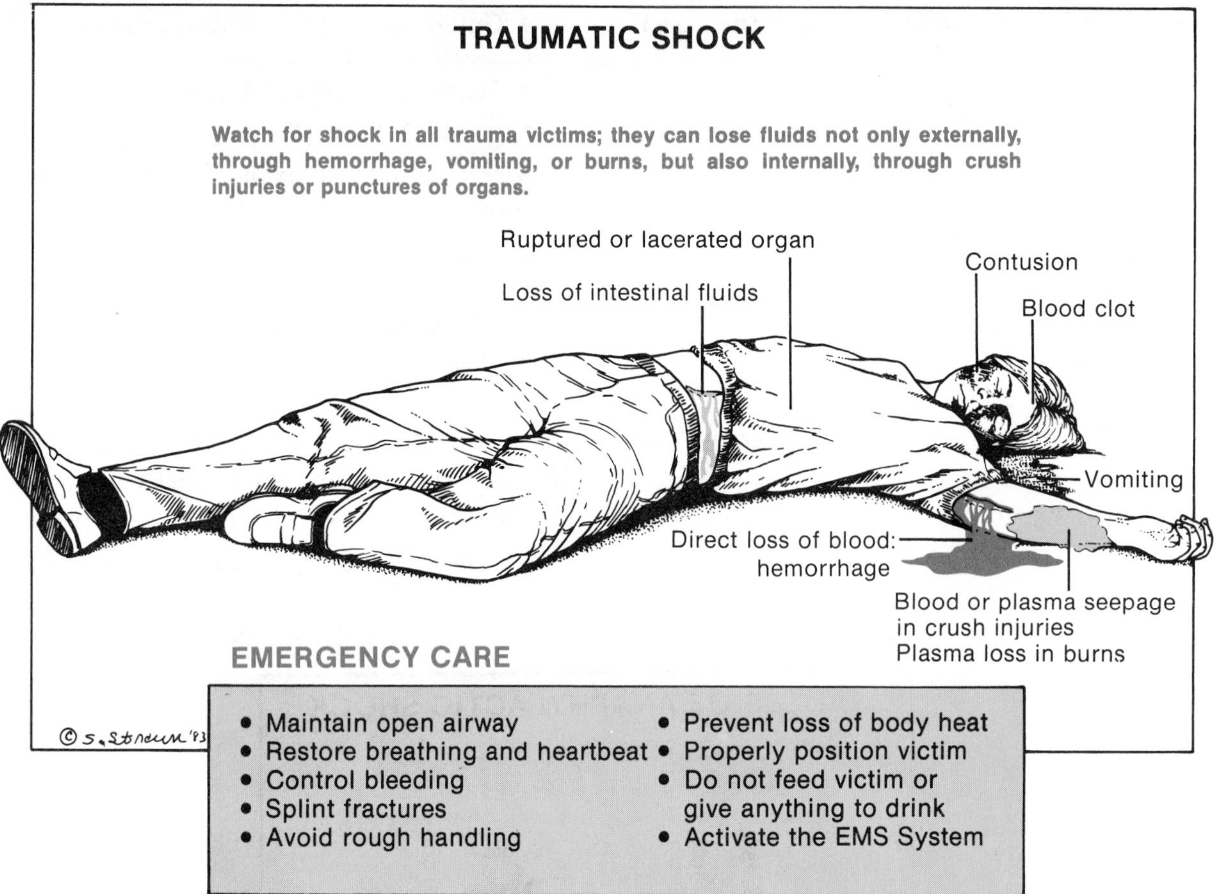


## PROTECTIVE RESPONSE OF THE BODY

The body responds to hemorrhage by immediately constricting the blood vessels near the surface of the skin. This action results in a concentration of all available blood into the main arteries and veins, and the blood pressure is maintained within normal limits. An increase in the pulse rate accompanies this initial reaction. Paleness of the skin and a drop in skin temperature are evidence that blood has been diverted away from the skin. Thirst and dryness of the mouth also occur.

With continued blood loss, the compensating mechanisms of the body fail to maintain the blood pressure, and it drops to very low levels. At these levels, the blood vessels themselves do not receive adequate oxygen, and they no longer respond to nervous control. Blood plasma begins to leak out of the damaged vessels and into tissue spaces. This is the beginning of so-called **irreversible shock.** Vessels near the skin now dilate and fill with poorly oxygenated blood. The slate-gray, bluish skin of a patient in late shock is the result of the failure of vessels near the skin to constrict. Lack of blood to the brain results in brain damage; brain damage is indicated by dilated pupils and convulsions. The irregular, gasping breathing seen in victims of late shock are the result of a lack of oxygen affecting the respiratory center at the base of the brain.

Neurogenic shock is serious because the protective response of the body is absent. The stress to the nervous system, which has caused neurogenic shock, has also affected the autonomic nervous system: reflex constriction of smaller vessels and reflex increase in the heart rate do not occur. If something is not done to increase the flow of blood through the brain, it becomes damaged. If the blood pressure is not increased, plasma soon leaks out of the smaller blood vessels, and the pattern of irreversible shock begins to appear.

## MANAGEMENT OF SHOCK

Much of the emergency care for shock involves nothing more complicated than caring for the injury causing the shock and applying the following general principles:

1. Establish an airway. This takes precedence over everything else. Breathing should be constantly monitored; check for obstructions in the throat.
2. Assist breathing as necessary.
3. Stop bleeding if it is present. Use gentle, firm, **direct pressure** with sterile gauze compresses and then bandages over the site of bleeding from arteries or oozing from veins.
4. Elevate the lower extremities and maintain a head-low position except when other wounds or discomfort do not make it possible.
5. Immobilize fractures; this lessens damage to soft tissues from splintered bone ends, preventing further hemorrhage. Immobilizing fractures also makes the victim more comfortable and increases the safety of transport.
6. Avoid any rough or excessive handling.
7. Activate the EMS System.
8. Keep the victim's temperature normal. Sponge him if he/she is feverish, but do not overdo it. Avoid intense cooling, which causes shivering. Put blankets underneath and over the patient if he/she is cool. Prevent loss of heat, but do not add more heat. It is better for the victim to be slightly cool than to be too warm.
9. Monitor the victim's state of consciousness and pulse, and record at five-minute intervals. Keep checking vital signs every five minutes until the emergency team arrives.
10. Do not feed the victim or give him/her a beverage. Give nothing.

The most important single requirement in the management of shock is to arrest and reverse progressive deterioration by prompt and adequate restoration of the circulatory system.

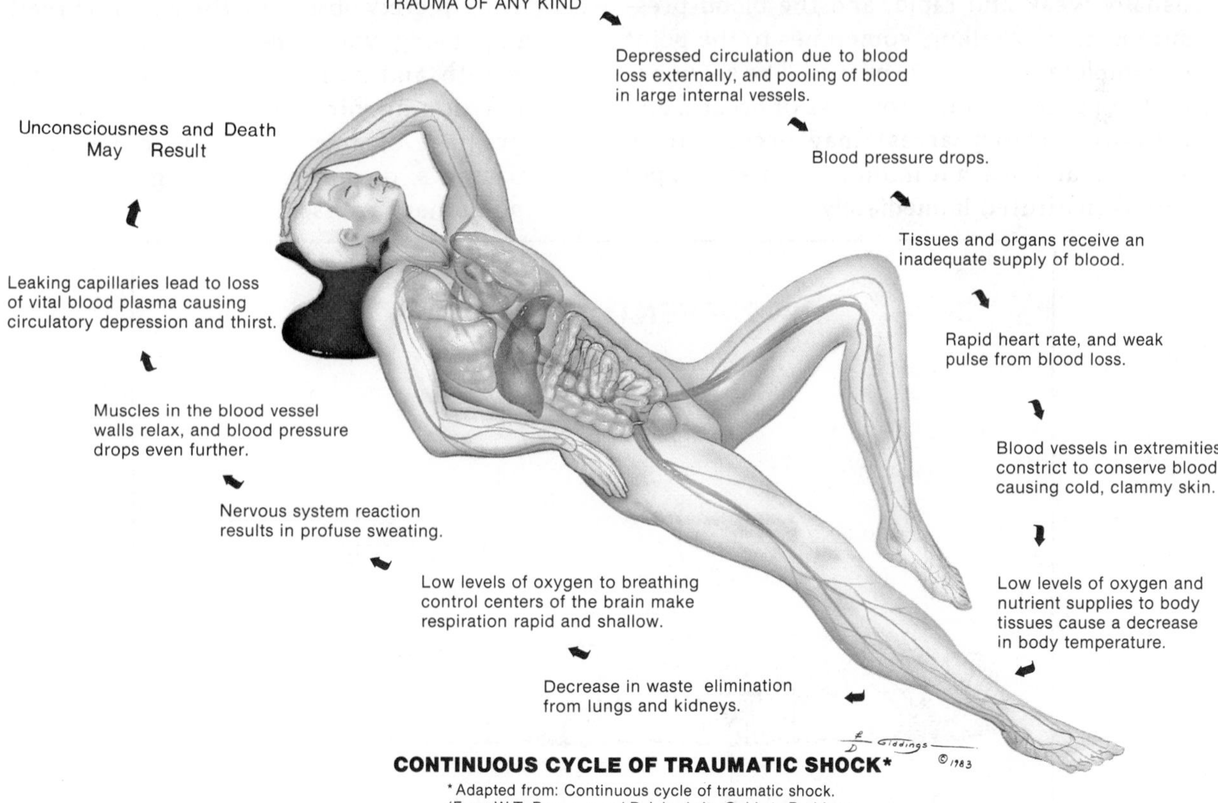


**CONTINUOUS CYCLE OF TRAUMATIC SHOCK***

*Adapted from: Continuous cycle of traumatic shock. (From W.T. Brennan and D.J. Ludwig, Guide to Problems and Practices in First Aid and Emergency Care. Dubuque, Iowa: William C. Brown Company, Publisher, 1976, Pg. 48) 3rd. Edition.

Deleterious effects of injury and the system's reactions to them are continuing processes. Observations of the victim should also be a continuing process, not a single act. The victim may pass through more than one pattern of shock and may change abruptly from one condition to another, even though general measures for the prevention of shock were successful at the time that they were applied.

## Management of Anaphylactic Shock

The victim in anaphylactic shock will experience shortness of breath and often sneezing, wheezing, or coughing up of blood-tinged sputum. He/she will frequently complain of tightness in the chest or a sensation that his/her throat is closing. The face may be flushed or ashen, with marked facial swelling, especially noticeable around the eyes. Sometimes he/she will complain of severe itching, either generalized or localized to the throat area. Hives are often present, or the skin may simply take on a red, inflamed appearance. Abdominal cramps followed by nausea, vomiting, and diarrhea are common. The pulse is usually weak and rapid, and the blood pressure is usually falling, sometimes to the point of complete circulatory collapse. The sequence of itching, coughing, shortness of breath, and cardiorespiratory arrest may occur within seconds, and death is imminent unless proper care is instituted immediately.

1. Establish an airway and administer CPR if necessary.
2. Activate the EMS System.
3. If the reaction is due to an insect sting or injection, place a constricting band above the site of the injection, if at all possible. (Obviously, this will not be feasible if the injection site is not on an extremity.)
4. Assist the victim in administering his/her medication.
5. The victim should be transported **immediately** to a medical facility for further lifesaving treatment.

# PREVENTING SHOCK

**The following preventive measures should be carried out in all cases of impending shock** except those in which the specific measure would be against the best interests of the victim.

1. Control hemorrhage. Use direct pressure and a pressure dressing, elevate the part, or apply a **tourniquet** as appropriate.
2. Assure adequate breathing. This may involve merely observing the victim's breathing, using your finger to sweep his/her mouth and clear it of foreign matter, or positioning him/her to assure adequate drainage of any fluid obstructing the air passages; or it may involve giving cardiopulmonary resuscitation.

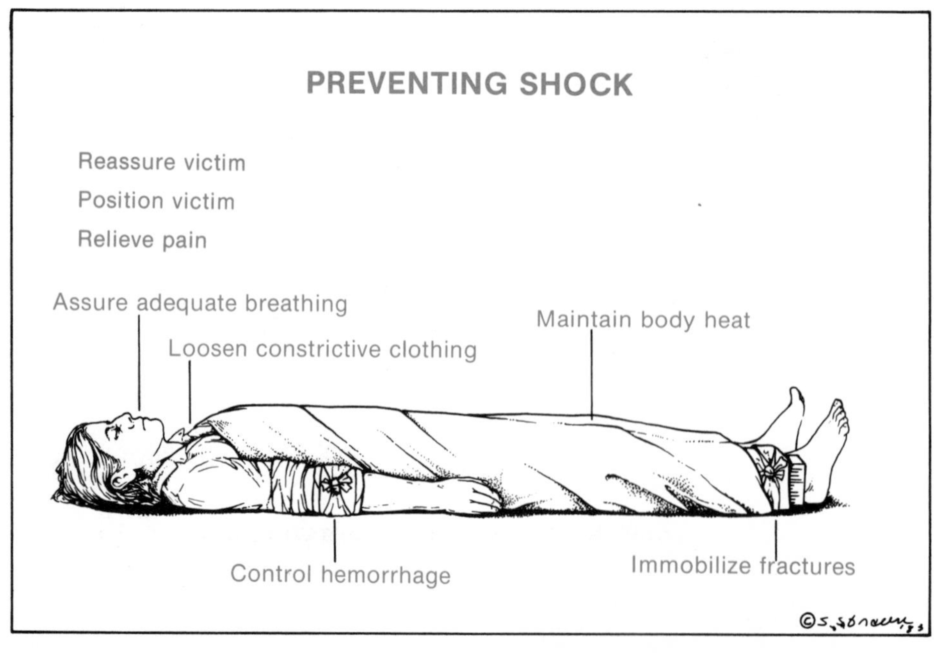

3. Loosen constrictive clothing, especially at the neck, the waist, and other areas in which it tends to bind the victim. Loosen, but do not remove, shoes.
4. Reassure the victim. You can do this by reassuring yourself. Remember — if personnel better qualified to give emergency medical care were available, you would not be attending the victim. Self-confidence and an attitude of expectancy of success, along with gentle, yet firm, actions in giving that care do much to reassure the patient. Jokes, ridiculous promises, and unneeded questions are as much out of place as rough handling, indecision, and predictions of impending doom. Acknowledge the victim's return to mental clarity with a nod of your head and brief look into his/her eyes, then continue with emergency care. Be receptive and accessible, but initiate conversation only to give instructions or warnings or to take necessary information. Answer the victim's questions in as brief and straightforward a way as possible in keeping with the situation.
5. Splint and immobilize fractures.
6. Relieve pain. Proper dressing, bandaging, splinting, and positioning of the victim are the best measures for relieving pain.
7. Position the victim. When his/her condition indicates that a lying down position will best serve his/her interest, either the semi-prone or the head-low position should generally be used. Other positions are discussed in connection with the special injuries with which they are used. In all instances, small amounts of soft material should be placed beneath the victim so that the bony prominences, such as those of the cheek, elbow, shoulder, hips, or knees, do not press against the ground, or other unyielding support.

**BODY POSITIONING FOR SHOCK**

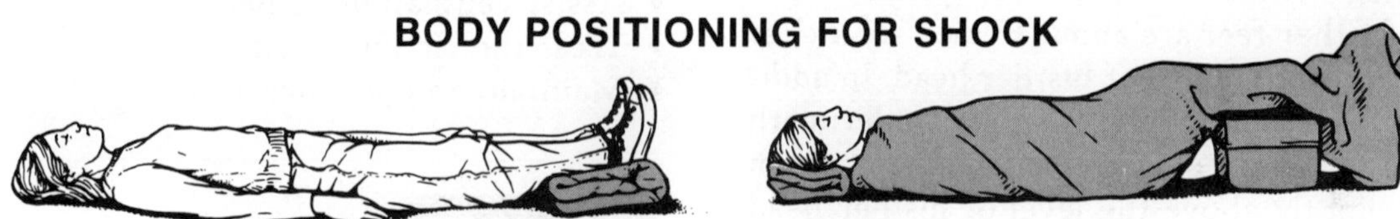

Normally, the lower extremities should be elevated. By gravity this will reduce the blood in the extremities and may improve the blood supply to the heart. If the victim has leg fractures, the legs should not be elevated unless they are well splinted.

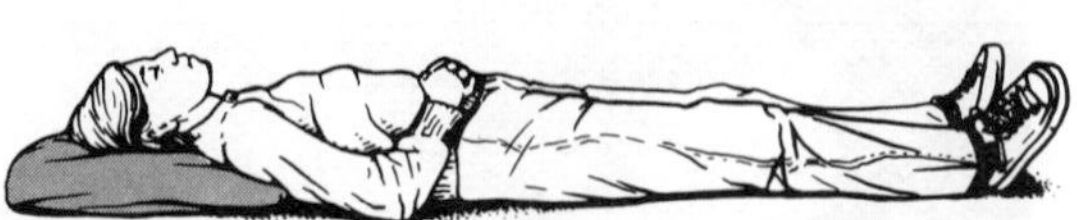

If there are indications of head injuries, the head could be raised slightly to reduce pressure on the brain. The feet may also be elevated. The head should not be elevated if there is mucus in the throat.

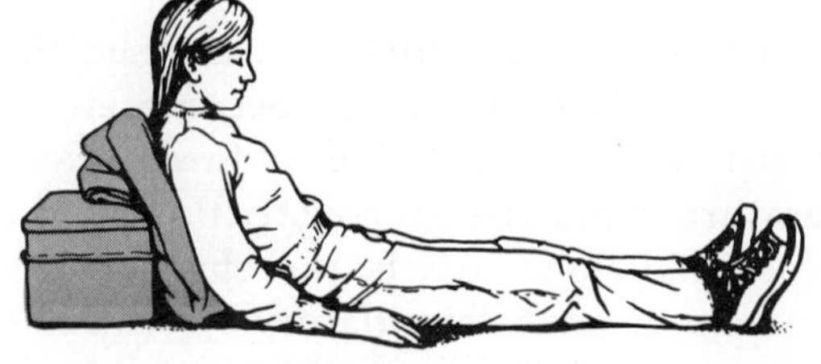

If there are breathing difficulties, the victim may be more comfortable with the head and shoulders raised, that is, in a semi-sitting position.

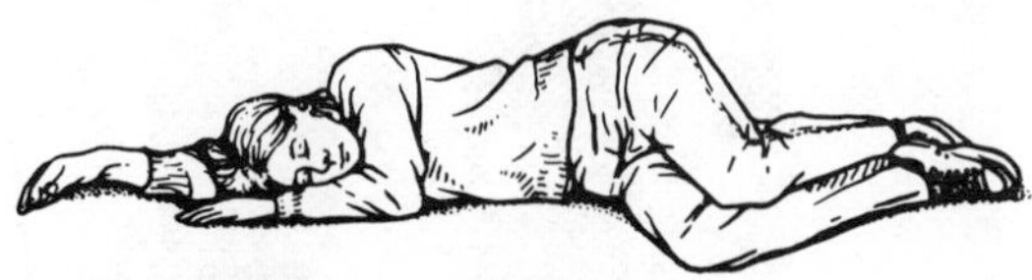

If the victim is unconscious, she should be placed on her side in coma position.

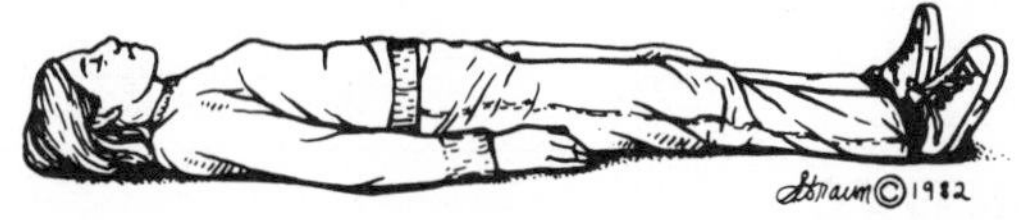

If circumstances indicate, the individual should be left in the position found.

- The semiprone **(coma)** may be used when the victim is unconscious; when the victim is wounded in the head, face, neck (except fracture), or chest; or when vomiting is likely. When the victim is in this position, drainage from the respiratory tract is possible.
- The head-low position may be used when the conscious victim has no external injury or has a wound of the limbs. The head-low position is not used with victims under the conditions discussed for the coma position nor with victims who have fractures of the neck or spine. In the head-low position, the victim is on his/her back with feet elevated approximately six inches above the level of the head. This position aids the flow of blood back to the heart and the brain. If no bed is available, the head-low position or its physiologic equivalent may be accomplished by elevating and then supporting the victim's legs with soft or padded material so that his/her feet are about five or six inches above the level of his/her head. In addition, padding may be placed underneath the victim's buttocks to raise them slightly above the level of his/her head and shoulders. Alternately, the victim may be placed in a head-low position on a slightly inclined slope.

8. Keep the victim comfortably warm; he/she should not be allowed to become either cooled or overheated. A drop in skin temperature gives rise to constriction of the superficial blood vessels, thereby reducing the volume of the **circulatory system.** In a cool or cold atmosphere, the victim's body and limbs should be covered with blankets. Wet clothing should be removed and blanket coverings tucked close to the victim's skin. Sweating should be watched for and differentiated from signs of chilling by assessing the victim's skin temperature.

## FAINTING

Fainting is a temporary loss of consciousness due to an inadequate supply of oxygen to the brain and is a mild form of shock. Fainting may be caused by the sight of blood, exhaustion, weakness, heat, lack of air, or strong emotions such as fright or joy. Some people faint more easily than others.

The signs and symptoms of fainting are as follows:

- The victim may feel weak and dizzy and may see black spots before his/her eyes.
- The face becomes pale and the lips blue.
- The forehead is covered with cold perspiration.
- The pulse is rapid and weak.
- The breathing is shallow.

The care for fainting is as follows:

- The victim should lie down with the head lower than the feet, or sit with the head between the knees.
- If the victim is unconscious for more than a short time, something may be seriously wrong. The victim should be taken to a medical facility as quickly as possible.
- Assist ventilations if necessary.
- Treat the victim for shock.
- Maintain an open airway.

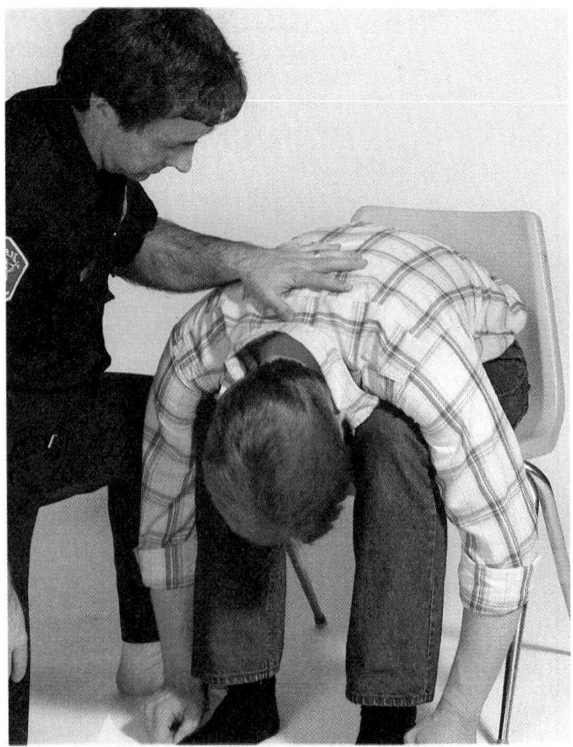

A conscious victim who feels faint may sit with the head between the knees.

## Work Exercises

Shock is a life-threatening condition. You should assume it to be present in all victims of injury and serious illness. Only the management of breathing, cardiac arrest, and bleeding emergencies should have priority over the emergency care of shock.

Shock means a state of ______________________________ associated with

______________________________________________. It occurs when the

______________ system fails to provide sufficient ______________

to ______________ of the body.

Shock does not happen all at once. It occurs in stages and can progress rapidly. Arrange the following progression of shock in the correct order: (1, 2, 3, etc.)

_________ Vital organs and brain do not receive enough blood.

_________ If shock is not reversed, internal organs and brain will eventually die.

_________ Brain suffers from lack of oxygen-rich blood and loses ability to function.

_________ Heart beats faster, blood vessels near skin and in arms and legs contract, sending blood to vital organs and brain.

_________ Blood vessels lose their ability to contract.

_________ Blood flow in the entire body is disrupted.

_________ Some degree of shock occurs from all injuries.

_________ Cells in internal organs and brain begin to die because of oxygen deprivation.

_________ Other body cells do not receive enough blood, oxygen, and nutrients.

The collapse of the cardiovascular system that occurs in shock may be a result of four conditions that typically follow major causes of shock. These conditions are:

1.

2.

3.

4.

Complete the following table by describing the condition that may occur in each of the areas if shock is present.

**SIGNS/SYMPTOMS OF SHOCK**

| Area | Descriptive Condition That May Occur if Shock is Present |
|---|---|
| Skin | |
| Temperature | |
| Blood Pressure | |
| Consciousness | |
| Breathing | |
| Pulse | |
| Gastrointestinal | |
| Thirst | |
| Orientation | |
| Blood Flow to Brain | |
| Blood Flow to Lungs | |
| Blood Vessels | |
| Blood Flow to Heart | |

Shock is a condition that can be reversed if recognized early and treated effectively. Indicate which of the following emergency care procedures are true or false:

## Emergency Care For Shock

| True/False | Emergency Procedure |
|---|---|
| 1. ______ | Normally the lower extremities should be elevated. |
| 2. ______ | If there are possible head injuries, always raise the feet. |
| 3. ______ | Give the victim fluids if he is conscious. |
| 4. ______ | Monitor the victim's vital signs and state of consciousness every 20 minutes until emergency team arrives. |
| 5. ______ | If victim is unconscious, put in semi-reclining position. |
| 6. ______ | Avoid rough handling. |
| 7. ______ | Never attempt to remove dentures; it changes contour of mouth. |
| 8. ______ | Waiting a short time before controlling bleeding can help the blood vessels regain their ability to contract. |
| 9. ______ | Keep victim dry and attempt to raise body temperature above normal to compensate for lack of blood flow to extremities. |
| 10. ______ | Openly discuss injuries with the victim. |
| 11. ______ | Immobilize fractures. |
| 12. ______ | Loosen clothing around neck and chest but not waist. |
| 13. ______ | Calm and reassure victim. |

## Anaphylactic Shock

Anaphylactic shock involves a massive release of histamine-like substances by the body when a victim comes into contact with something to which he/she is extremely allergic. Indicate which of the following are true signs and symptoms of anaphylactic shock.

| True/False | Signs-Symptoms |
|---|---|
| 1. ______ | Easy breathing. |
| 2. ______ | Nausea and vomiting. |
| 3. ______ | Swelling of skin on arms and legs. |
| 4. ______ | Itching or burning skin. |
| 5. ______ | Convulsions. |
| 6. ______ | Bounding, strong pulse. |
| 7. ______ | Tightening or pain in chest. |
| 8. ______ | Pale face. |
| 8. ______ | Hives. |

## Positioning the Shock Victim

Match the correct body position for shock with the correct injury.

| | |
|---|---|
| 1. ______ Nauseated. | a. Semi-sitting position. |
| 2. ______ Wound of limbs. | b. Elevate lower extremities. |
| 3. ______ When circumstances indicate. | c. Victim on side — coma position. |
| 4. ______ Breathing difficulties. | d. Slightly elevated head. |
| 5. ______ Victim has no external injury. | e. Victim left in position found. |
| 6. ______ Head injuries. | |
| 7. ______ Unconscious. | |

The signs and symptoms of shock change as shock progresses. Review the signs and symptoms listed below, and label each **E** (occurs during early stages of shock), **L** (occurs during late stages of shock), or both.

| | |
|---|---|
| ______ bluish skin | ______ pale skin |
| ______ rapid breathing | ______ dilated pupils |
| ______ unresponsiveness | ______ rapid pulse, indiscernible at wrist |
| ______ skin cold to the touch | ______ sunken eyes, vacant expression |
| ______ apathy | ______ nausea and/or vomiting |
| ______ shallow, irregular breathing | ______ moist, clammy skin |
| ______ mottled appearance of skin | ______ lowered temperature |
| ______ anxiety and restlessness | ______ thrashing around |
| ______ loss of consciousness | ______ severe drop in blood pressure |
| ______ severe thirst | |
| ______ weakness | |

Generally, the most satisfactory position for a shock victim is lying flat on the back (supine); however, you may need to position an injured shock victim differently, depending on the injury. For each type of injury listed below, describe the preferred position.

a. unconscious victim ______________________________

b. victim of neck or spine injuries ______________________________

c. victim of head injury ______________________________

d. victim with severe jaw and lower face injuries ______________________________

e. victim of breathing difficulties ______________________________

## SELF-TEST

### Part I: True and False

If you believe the statement is true, circle the T. If you believe the statement is false, circle F.

T F 1. Shock may appear immediately following an injury or may not show up until hours later.

T F 2. The degree of shock may be increased by abnormal changes in body temperature.

T F 3. The degree of shock may be increased by rough handling or delay in treatment.

T F 4. A slow, strong pulse is a good indication of shock.

T F 5. A victim of hemorrhagic shock may complain of thirst and nausea.

T F 6. Warm, dry skin is one of the most common symptoms of shock.

T F 7. Shock can be fatal even when the victim's injuries themselves are not life-threatening.

T F 8. Pain can produce or increase the severity of shock.

T F 9. Respiratory shock is caused by insufficient oxygen in the blood.

T F 10. Cardiogenic shock is caused by severe infection.

T F 11. When caring for shock, the First Aider should keep the victim cool — covering the victim with blankets will increase shock.

T F 12. A shock victim should be kept lying flat with his/her feet raised for all types of injuries, including head injuries.

T F 13. Fainting is a temporary loss of consciousness due to an inadequate supply of oxygen to the brain.

T F 14. Itching, burning, and flushed skin are symptoms of anaphylactic shock.

T F 15. Difficulty in breathing and chest pains are symptoms of anaphylactic shock.

T F 16. Anaphylactic shock is a very serious, acute, allergic reaction.

T F 17. Death can result within minutes from anaphylactic shock.

T F 18. Anaphylactic shock can be caused by a food or drug allergy or an insect bite.

T F 19. The prime objective in first aid for anaphylactic shock is to maintain body heat.

T F 20. Shock is rarely a serious problem in first aid situations.

T F 21. You should always wait for symptoms to appear before you begin treating a victim for shock.

T F 22. Shock can result in death.

T F 23. It is important to help a shock victim maintain body heat, but you can greatly endanger him/her by adding extra heat.

### Part II: Multiple Choice

Circle the one answer that best reflects a true statement.

1. Shock is defined as a condition in which:
   a. there is too much carbon dioxide in the blood
   b. there is too little oxygen in the blood
   c. there is a complete stoppage of blood flow
   d. there is a disturbance of the blood flow

2. Which of the following signs and symptoms is *not* an indication of shock?
   a. dull and lackluster eyes
   b. constricted pupils
   c. shallow respiration, possibly irregular or labored
   d. cold and clammy skin

3. Which of the following symptoms is an indication of anaphylactic shock?
   a. itching or burning skin
   b. swelling of the face and tongue
   c. tightening or pain in the chest
   d. all of the above

4. The primary goal in shock treatment is to:
   a. keep the victim conscious
   b. avoid dehydration by administering fluids
   c. keep the victim warm
   d. improve and maintain circulation

5. Which of the following is *not* an objective in shock treatment?
   a. improve circulation of the blood
   b. replace or maintain body fluids
   c. ensure adequate oxygen supply
   d. maintain normal body temperature

6. Management of *all but one* of the following emergencies should precede shock:
   a. bleeding
   b. burns
   c. cardiac arrest
   d. breathing stoppage

7. Which of the following shock processes occurs first?
   a. brain loses its ability to function
   b. vital organs and brain do not receive enough blood
   c. blood rushes to the brain and vital organs thus depriving other body cells of oxygen and nutrients
   d. internal organs and brain cells begin to die

8. Which of the following is *not* a type of shock?
   a. hypothermic
   b. metabolic
   c. septic
   d. respiratory

9. When does anaphylactic shock occur?
   a. when a person contacts something to which he is extremely allergic
   b. it follows every major injury to some degree
   c. it is a psychological reaction to the injury
   d. it follows excessive blood loss

10. Anaphylactic shock should be considered:
    a. a true medical emergency
    b. an emergency only in a sensitized person
    c. an emergency only if the person has been stung on the face or hand
    d. a non-emergency situation

11. In anaphylactic shock, the shorter the time before symptoms appear:
    a. the greater the chance of a recovery in a short time
    b. the greater the chance of swelling of the larynx
    c. the greater the risk of a fatal reaction
    d. the greater the chance of an antigen-antibody reaction

12. A person may be in anaphylactic shock from which preceding event?
    a. sight of a bloody accident
    b. eating berries
    c. head injury
    d. severe illness

13. What are the signs of anaphylactic shock?
    a. strong, bounding pulse; heavy breathing; dizziness
    b. weak pulse, itching or burning skin, swelling of the tongue and face
    c. fever, sweating, chest pains, pale coloring
    d. increased blood pressure; rapid, strong pulse; convulsions

14. The body's response to shock can be observed by summarizing the general signs and symptoms of shock. *All but one* of the following are signs and symptoms of shock:
    a. restlessness and anxiety
    b. weakness
    c. feeling of impending doom
    d. bounding pulse

15. How does the body compensate when it loses large amounts of blood:
    a. circulating blood to the entire body in smaller volumes
    b. supplying blood only to the brain, heart, lungs, and kidneys
    c. constriction of vessels near the skin surface so available blood is concentrated in the main arteries and veins
    d. pumping the remaining blood harder and faster throughout the body

16. Which of the following procedures for management of shock comes first?
    a. prevent loss of body heat
    b. establish an airway
    c. monitor the victim's state of consciousness
    d. elevate lower extremities except when contraindicated

17. The most important single requirement in management of shock is to:
    a. reassure the victim so neurogenic shock does not complicate the victim's condition
    b. establish an airway, stop bleeding, and prevent loss of body heat
    c. arrest and reverse progressive deterioration and restoration of the circulatory system
    d. treat the injuries quickly and efficiently

18. Which of the following is *not* a means of preventing shock?
    a. keep the victim's body temperature above normal
    b. reassure the victim
    c. loosen constrictive clothing
    d. control hemorrhage by direct pressure, elevation, or pressure points

19. Coma position should *not* be used with a victim who:
    a. has a neck fracture
    b. is very nauseated
    c. is unconscious
    d. has a head injury

Corresponds with:

**American Red Cross**

**Standard First Aid & Personal Safety**

Chapter 2, pages 18-36 and, Chapter 3, pages 45-47, 53, 58-59, Chapter 13, pages 177-194

and

**Advanced First Aid & Emergency Care**

Chapter 2, pages 24-45, Chapter 3, pages 46-48, 52, 53, 57-58, and Chapter 14, pages 202-224

# 8 Wounds and Bandaging

In the injured victim, the skin not only reflects blood circulation but may itself (as well as underlying structures) be the site of damage. The entire surface of the body must therefore be inspected for **soft tissue** injuries. Although this type of injury may be the most obvious and dramatic, it is seldom the most serious unless it compromises the airway or is associated with massive hemorrhage.

Soft tissue injuries are those that involve the skin and underlying **musculature.** An injury to these tissues is commonly referred to as a **wound**. More specifically, a wound is a physically caused injury to the body that disrupts the normal **continuity** of the tissue, organ, or bone affected.

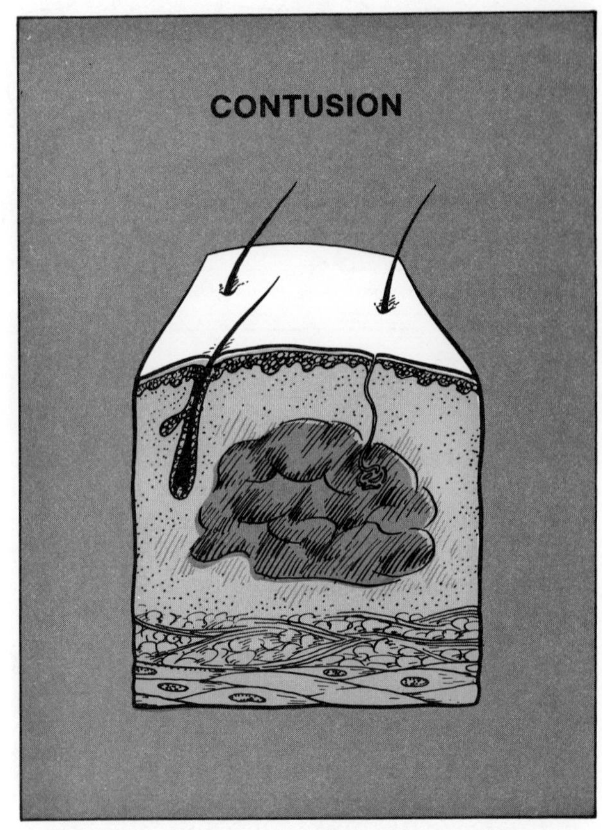


## CLOSED WOUNDS

In a closed injury, such as a **bruise,** or **contusion,** soft tissues beneath the skin are damaged, but the skin is not broken. Contusions are marked by local pain and swelling. If small blood vessels beneath the skin have been broken, the victim will also exhibit **ecchymosis** (black and blue coloring). If large vessels have been torn beneath the bruised area, a **hematoma,** or collection of blood beneath the skin, will be evident as a lump with bluish discoloration. Closed wounds should be given cold applications to minimize swelling but otherwise require no specific care. For severe injuries, bleeding may be controlled by **counterpressure.** If internal bleeding is suspected, treat for shock.

## OPEN WOUNDS

In an open wound, the skin is broken, and the victim is susceptible to external hemorrhage and **contamination.** An open wound may be the only surface evidence of a more serious injury such as a fracture. Open wounds include **abrasions, incised wounds, lacerations, puncture wounds,** and **avulsions.**

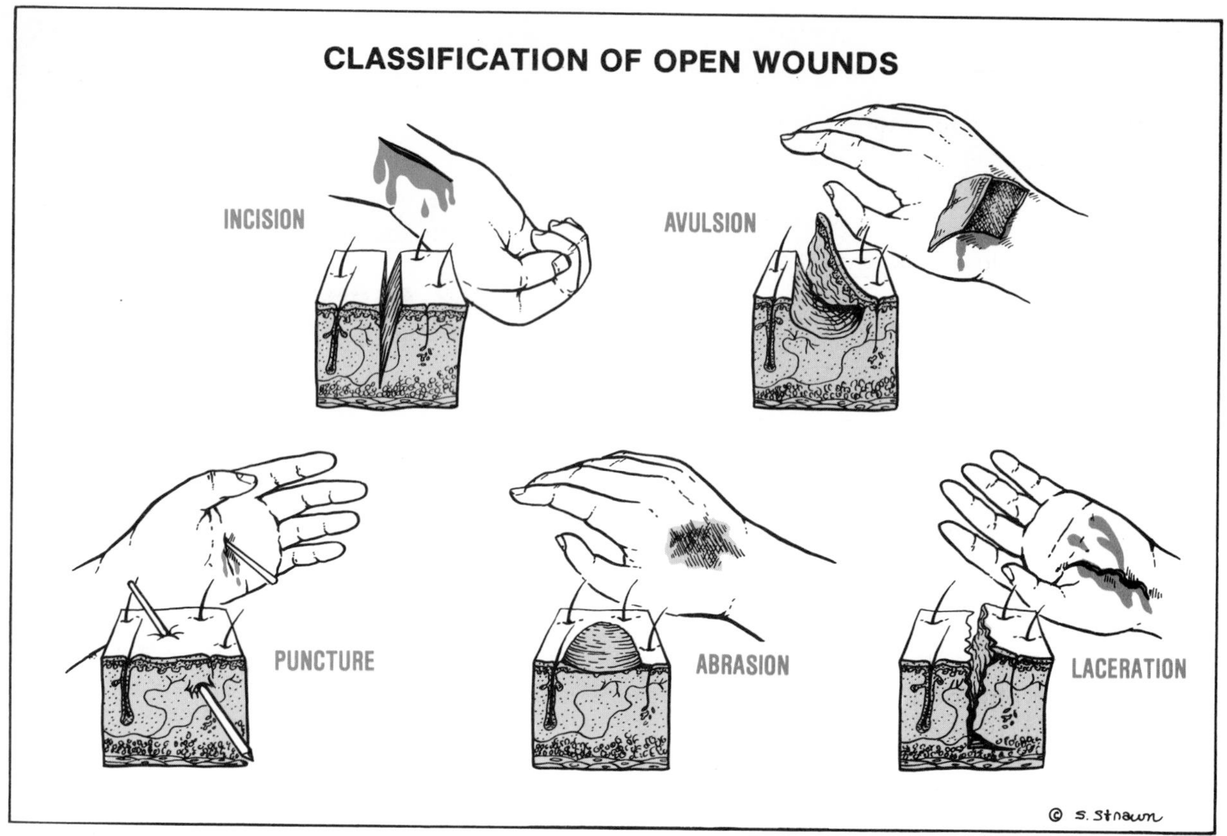


## Abrasions

An abrasion is a **superficial wound** caused by rubbing or scraping in which part of the skin surface has been lost. Cover the abrasion with a sterile dressing.

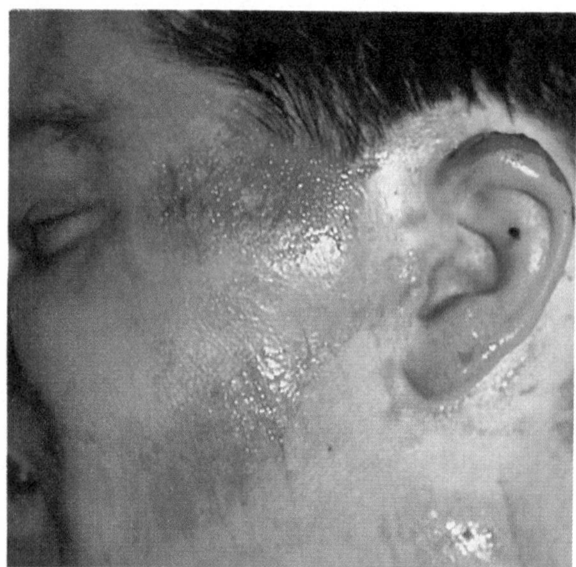

Abrasions.

## Incised Wounds

Incised wounds are sharp, even cuts that tend to bleed freely because the blood vessels and tissue have been severed. They are caused by any sharp, cutting object, such as a knife, razor blade, or broken glass. The greatest dangers with an incised wound are severe bleeding and cut **tendons** and **nerves.**

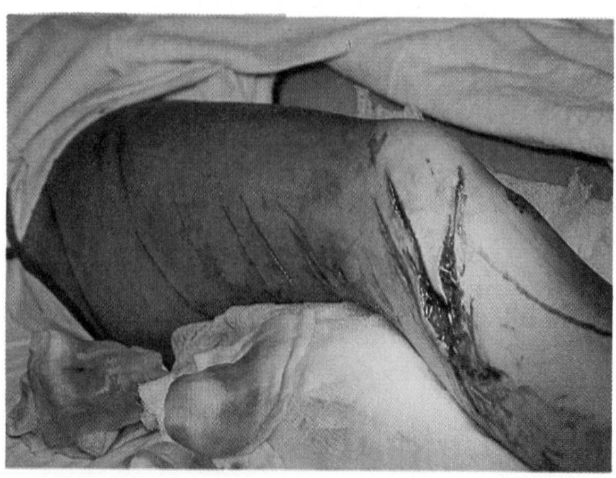

Incision and lacerations.

The first priority in caring for an incised wound is to control bleeding by **direct pressure.** Then draw the wound edges together and secure them with **butterfly strips** where appropriate. Apply a **sterile pressure dressing,** and give emergency care for shock.

## Lacerations

A laceration is a cut inflicted by a sharp, uneven instrument (such as a broken glass bottle) that produces either a clean or jagged incision through the skin surface and underlying structures. Tissue tearing through force also produces a laceration.

Lacerations may cause significant bleeding if the sharp instrument also cuts the wall of a blood vessel, particularly an artery. This is especially true in regions where major arteries lie close to the surface, such as in the wrist. Skin and tissue may be partly or completely torn away.

A laceration may contain **foreign matter** that can lead to infection. Apply the same care as for an incised wound.

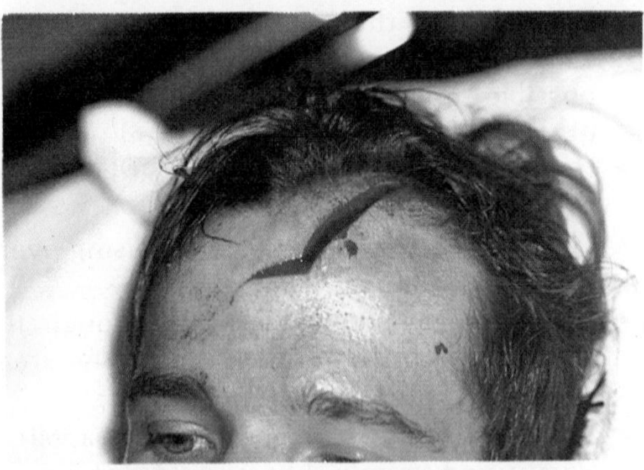

Laceration of the forehead and scalp.

## Puncture Wounds

A puncture wound is caused by a stab from a pointed object, such as a nail. A special type of puncture wound occurs when a foreign object that causes the injury remains imbedded in the wound. The opening in the skin may appear small, but the wound can be very deep and pose a serious infection problem. Internal organs can also be injured by this type of wound.

A puncture wound usually does not cause a bleeding problem, but it needs to be **irrigated** with water for cleaning. Any foreign object that causes a large, penetrating puncture wound should be stabilized and left intact. Cover the wound with a sterile dressing and give the victim emergency care for shock. Immobilize the injured area in a comfortable position. If there is an **impaled object, do not remove it.** Efforts to do so may cause severe hemorrhage and additional injury to underlying structures. Always check for an **exit wound.**

Control hemorrhage by direct pressure, but do not apply pressure on the impaled object itself or on immediately adjacent tissues. Stabilize the impaled object with a bulky dressing. Unless the object is extremely unwieldy, do not attempt to shorten it, for motion may further damage nerves, blood vessels, and surrounding tissues. Simply surround the protruding end of the object with bulky dressings and bandage them in place.

## Penetrating Objects

Splinters, nails, or thorns protruding from the skin and not penetrating more than one centimeter could be removed. Remove the object carefully, and conduct a prompt assessment to determine whether any of the object might have remained in the wound. Always send the penetrating object with the victim for the benefit of the physician. (Since bodily tissues tend to clamp around penetrating objects and make removal extremely difficult, it is sometimes better to simply send the victim to a physician.

## Avulsions

An avulsion involves the tearing loose of a flap of skin, which may either remain hanging or be torn off altogether. Avulsions concern any part of the body that is completely severed or torn away.

The most commonly **amputated** parts of the body include fingers and toes, hands, forearms, legs (above, through, or below the knee), feet, ears, nose, and penis. Most often, the victim with an avulsion works with machinery — home accidents involving lawnmowers and power tools are especially increasing in number. Amputations also commonly occur in automobile or motorcycle accidents.

To care for an avulsion, clear the wound surface, fold the skin flap back into normal position, and control bleeding by direct pressure. Apply a bulky, sterile dressing once the bleeding has been controlled. Give the victim emergency care for shock, and get medical assistance.

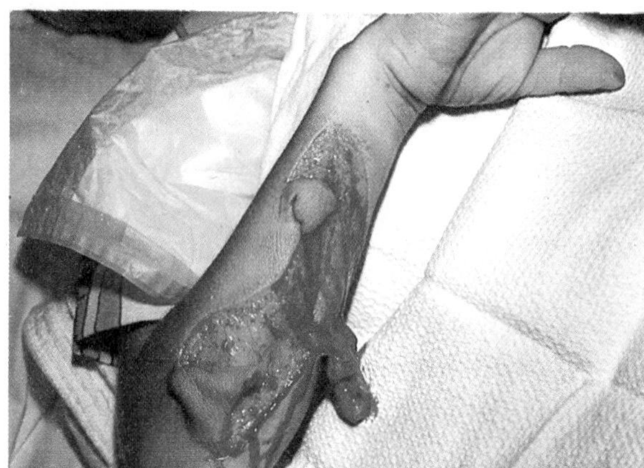

Forearm avulsion.

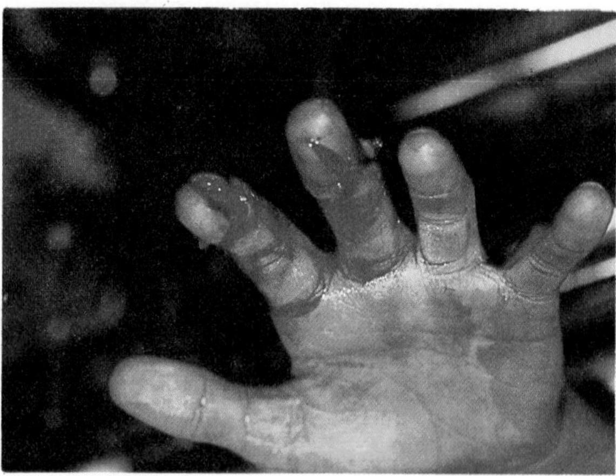

Finger avulsion.

## GENERAL EMERGENCY CARE FOR OPEN WOUNDS

The chief duties of a First Aider in caring for an open wound are to stop bleeding and to prevent **germs** from entering the wound. If germs do not enter, there will be much less chance of infection, and the wound will heal quickly.

- Where there is severe bleeding from an artery, always control it by direct pressure and elevation, and then, only if necessary, at a **pressure point,** and only as a last resort use a tourniquet.
- If a limb is involved, elevation will help to control bleeding.
- Shock usually follows wounds, especially if much blood is lost.
- Carefully cut or tear the clothing so that the injury may be seen.
- If loose foreign particles are around the wound, wipe them away with clean material. Always wipe away from the wound, not toward it.
- Do not attempt to remove a foreign object embedded in the wound, since it may aid the doctor in determining the extent of the injury. Serious bleeding and other damage may occur if the object is removed. Stabilize the object with a bulky dressing.
- Leave the work of cleansing the wound to the doctor.
- Do not touch the wound with your hands, clothing, or anything that is not clean, if possible, and do not pour water or any other liquid into or on the wound.
- Immobilize the injured part, and keep the victim quiet.
- Place a bandage compress or dressing over the wound, and tie it in place.
- All dressings should be wide enough to completely cover the wound and the area around it.
- The dressing and bandage should be applied firmly and snugly, but should not be so tight as to affect the blood supply to the injured part.
- The bandage should be securely tied or fastened in place so that it will not move.
- There should be no loose ends that could get caught on any other object while the victim is being moved.
- Protect all bandages, compresses, or gauze dressings by an outer bandage made from a **roller** or **triangular bandage,** except dressings for wounds of the eye, nose, chin, finger, and toe, or compound (open) fractures

## EMERGENCY CARE FOR OPEN WOUNDS

**Control Bleeding**

**Prevent further contamination:** all open wounds will already be contaminated but a dressing and bandage will prevent further contamination.

**Do not remove impaled objects:** they may be cut if necessary to move the victim but should remain in place until the victim receives hospital care. The object should be stabilized with bulky dressings.

**Do not try to replace protruding organs:** that is, protruding eyeballs or protruding intestines should be covered as they are and no attempt should be made to replace them in their normal positions within a body cavity. The covering for intestines should be kept moist.

**Immobilize the part and keep the victim quiet.**

**Preserve avulsed parts:** torn off parts should be saved and flaps of skin may be folded back to their normal position before bandaging.

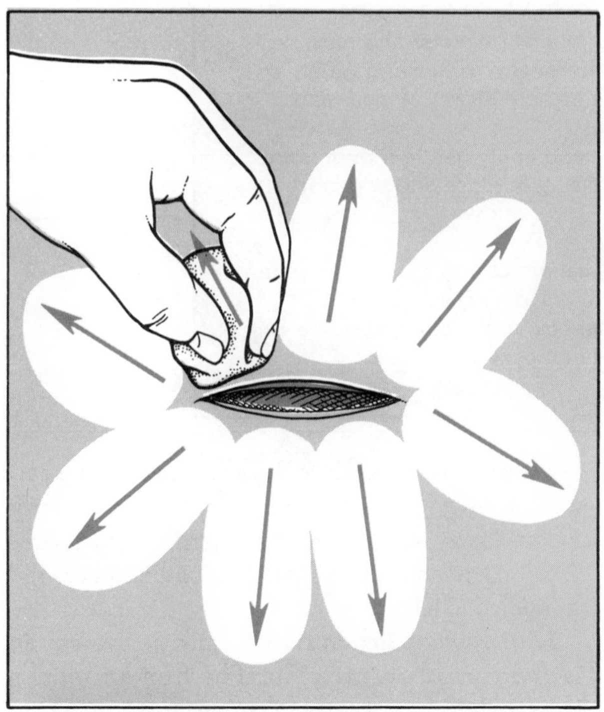

Use separate strokes and wipe away from edges when cleaning area around a wound.

of the hand and foot when splints are applied. If a bandage is used, open it enough to cover the entire dressing.

- Unless otherwise specified, tie the knots of the bandage compress and cover bandage over the wound on top of the compress pad to help in checking the bleeding.
- Preserve all avulsed parts.
- Calm and reassure the victim.

## BITES

Americans experience over one million dog bites and more than two thousand snakebites every year. The number of human bites is not recorded. If the number were known, it would probably be staggering. People are also bitten by cats, rats, bats, and birds. Although a bite is handled similarly to any other wound of the same type, you should have some ground information and a knowledge of care.

Dog bites are the most common. See the accompanying illustration for first aid procedures.

## DOG BITES

Over 1 million people suffer dog bites in the United States annually. The typical victim is male, under 20 years of age, and bitten by his own pet or some "familiar" large dog between 1 and 9 PM during the summer. Facial wounds occur predominantly in young children and teenagers.

Commonly Bitten Areas:

- FACE 11%
- TRUNK 7%
- UPPER EXTREMITIES 28%
- LOWER EXTREMITIES 31%

If possible, ascertain where the dog can be located: If an address is not possible, obtain a description of the dog, where it was encountered, and if the attack was provoked.

- Was its behavior unusual?
- Report immediately to hospital and/or health department.

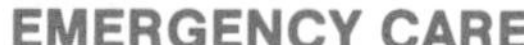

### EMERGENCY CARE

- Wash wound thoroughly with soap and warm water and rinse well.
- If soap is not available, rinse bite thoroughly with warm water.
- In bites of the head, neck and face be sure airway is clear and position for drainage or suctioning.
- Cover wound with a thick dressing and apply gentle firm pressure.
- If wound is deep leave original dressing in place and add more gauze and then bandage in place.
- Immobilize injured part.
- The victim is usually frightened — calm him/her by talking to him while you are giving necessary care.
- If wounds are severe, monitor for shock, and maintain body heat.
- Always have a dog bite victim go to a hospital.

The most difficult bite to handle is the human bite because of the high infection rate associated with it. Human bites usually involve the ears, nose, and fingers. They are inflicted most frequently by children involved in fights or in play, or by people of all ages involved in sexual assault or confined in mental institutions. It is common for police to be bitten while breaking up disturbances or trying to apprehend suspects.

Human bites should be considered as serious wounds. Even though the resulting wound may seem to be only a minor puncture wound, it may also involve badly lacerated tissue.

More serious than tissue damage, however, is the threat of infection. The human mouth is extremely dirty, and massive contamination may result from contact with an open wound. Human bites on fingers have sometimes resulted in loss of the fingers involved and, in some cases, loss of the entire hand.

- Call for emergency medical aid or transport the victim immediately to a hospital, where the wound can be cleaned in a sterile, controlled atmosphere, where unhealthy tissue can be removed, and where a culture can be taken.

- If the victim cannot be transported for some time, wash the wound immediately with an antiseptic soap. If such a soap is not available, rinse the wound continuously with clean, running water. Cover the wound with a sterile dressing; immobilize the injured area.

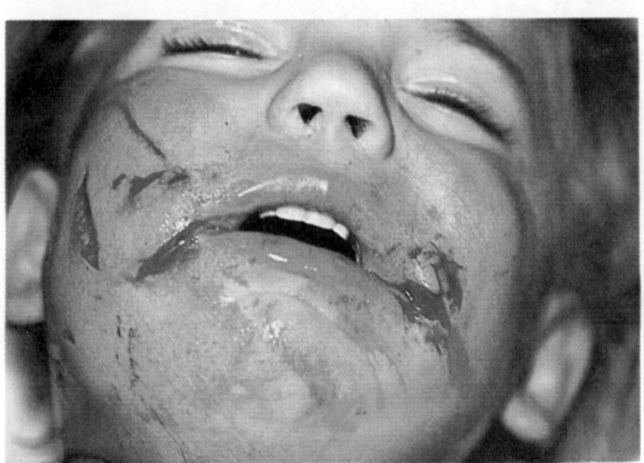

Dog bite.

## TRAUMATIC AMPUTATIONS

The ripping, tearing force of industrial and automobile accidents is great enough to tear away or crush limbs from the body. The victims are usually young males, and the effects can be tragic. Therefore, the initial emergency management of the amputated victim and the dismembered limb is critical. Common types of amputations include:

- digits
- hands
- forearms
- ears
- toes
- below the knee
- through the knee
- above the knee
- penis
- nose

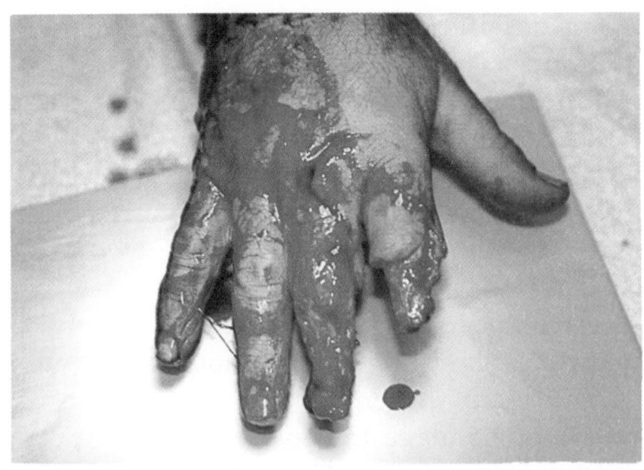

Finger amputation.

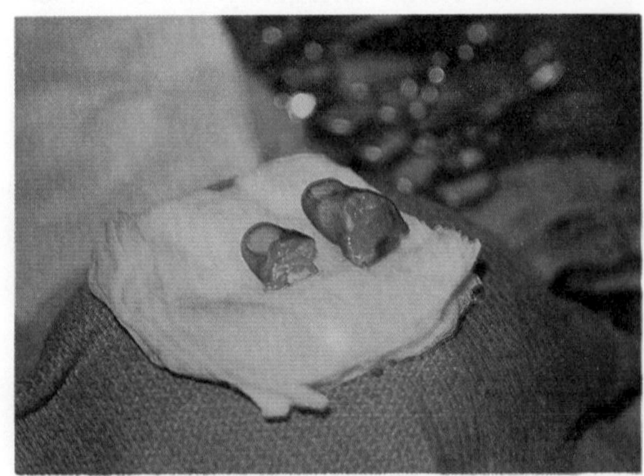

Amputated finger parts.

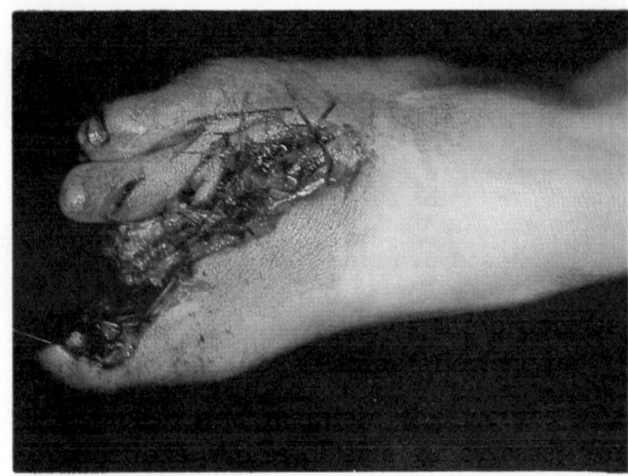

Toe amputation.

The following list reviews the proper sequence of care for the amputation victim.

1. Establish and maintain the victims vital functions (ABCs of emergency care). Remember — trauma great enough to cause

an amputation may also cause other bodily injury.
2. The limb, if crushed, may not bleed a great deal. Any hemorrhage should be controlled. A tourniquet may be necessary, but try direct pressure and pressure points first. Remember — a tourniquet can be dangerous.
3. After bleeding has been controlled, apply a proper dressing to the amputated stump, and wrap the end of the stump with an elastic bandage to replace the hand pressure. Continue to observe the wound for recurring bleeding.
4. Give the victim emergency care for shock.

Try to save the severed part for attachment by:

1. Finding all severed parts.
2. Separating the part from dirt and other foreign matter.
3. Wrapping the part in sterile gauze, a towel, or a clean sheet.
4. Wetting the wrapping with sterile water, if available.
5. Placing the severed part in a plastic bag and sealing the bag shut.
6. Placing the bag in a longer plastic bag containing ice or cold water.
7. Transporting the part with the victim.

Proper handling of a severed part may allow it to be reattached up to twenty-four hours after the trauma.

It is important to **not** do the following with a severed part. **Do not:**

1. Freeze the part.
2. Apply a tourniquet.
3. Make a judgment and throw the part away.
4. Immerse the part in solution bath, soapy water, antiseptic solution, or water of any type.

You may find a victim whose limb has been severely lacerated or mangled but not completely amputated. The limb may be attached by a few strands of soft tissue and a small piece of skin. **Do not complete the amputation.** An important consideration in amputation is to preserve as much as possible of the original length of the limb. Even if a limb has been severely mangled and will eventually require amputation, the flap of skin holding

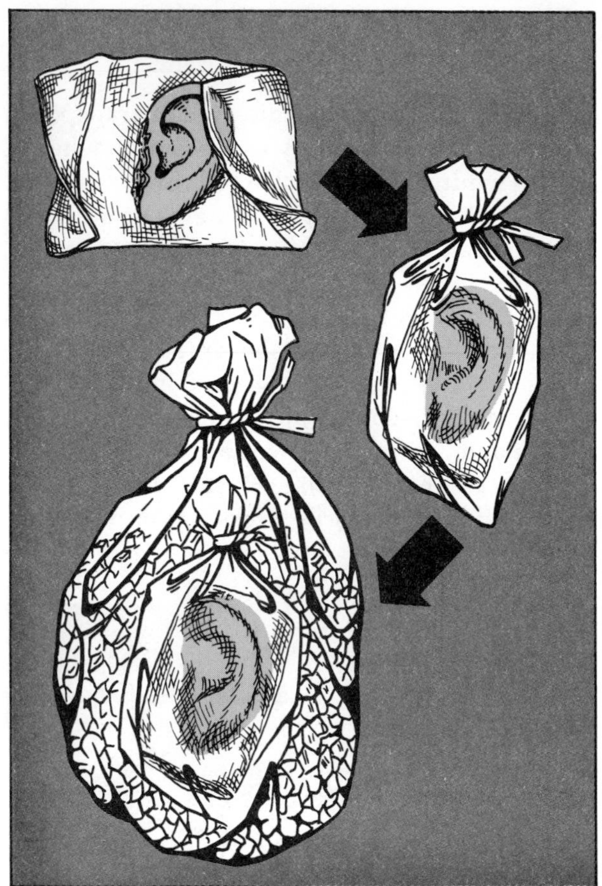

Emergency care for amputated parts consists of the following: (1) Wrap part completely in gauze or towel; wet the wrapping; (2) Place in plastic bag and seal shut; (3) Place bag inside an outer bag filled with ice; seal.

the limb together may be used by the surgeon to cover the end of the stump, thereby a significant amount of limb length to be preserved. In addition, the strands of soft tissue connecting the limb might contain nerves or blood vessels that, with proper surgical management, might help preserve the ability of the limb to survive.

Care for the open wound as previously described. Make sure that the skin bridge is not twisted or constricted by the pressure dressing.

Amputation, especially of the upper extremities, often occurs when a limb is caught in a piece of machinery. The limb will continue to be pulled into the machinery until some major obstruction — like the elbow or shoulder joint — is encountered. At this point, the limb will not progress any further — it will simply be ground up in the machine.

When this happens, immediately shut off the power supply to the machine. If the drive mechanism can be reversed, reverse the gears manually, and slowly remove the limb. If it is impossible to remove the limb, or if the piece of machinery is small, leave the limb in the machinery and disassemble the machinery while sending for emergency medical aid.

## IMPALED OBJECTS

Objects that both penetrate and protrude are impaled. The object may be a stick, glass, arrow, knife, steel rod, etc. that penetrates any part of the body. The skin usually clamps down around an impaled object and the entrance site.

This type of injury requires careful immobilization of the victim and the injured part. Any motion of the impaled object can cause additional damage to the surface wound, and particularly the underlying tissues.

### Emergency Care for Impaled Objects

- Do not remove the impaled object. To do so may cause added bleeding and damage to underlying tissues (muscle, nerves, blood vessels, bones, organs, etc.).
- Remove clothing so that the wound is exposed. Cut it away so that the impaled object is not disturbed.
- Control bleeding with direct pressure, but do not exert any pressure on the impaled object or on the tissue margins around the cutting edge of the object.

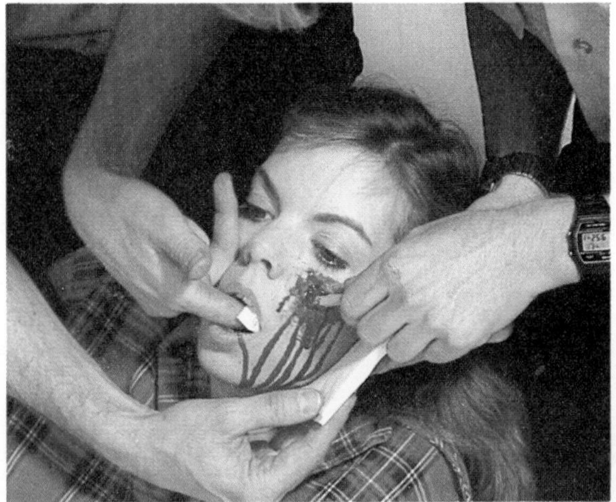

Impaled objects in the cheek may be removed. Dress outside of wound and put dressing on inside wound between cheek and teeth. Hold in place if necessary.

- Stabilize the impaled object with bulky dressings and bandage in place. The objective is to pack dressings around the object and tape securely in place so that motion is reduced to a minimum. The use of a "doughnut" type ring pad may also be useful in stabilization.
- Calm and reassure the victim as you monitor for shock.
- Keep the victim at rest.
- Do not attempt to cut off, break off, or shorten an impaled object unless absolutely necessary. If the object must be cut off, stabilize securely before cutting. Remember — any motion is transmitted to the victim and can cause additional tissue damage and shock.

### IMPALED OBJECT INJURY

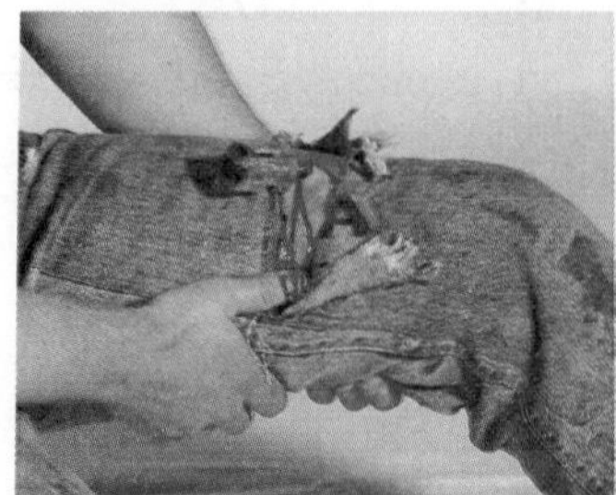

1
Impaled object injury.

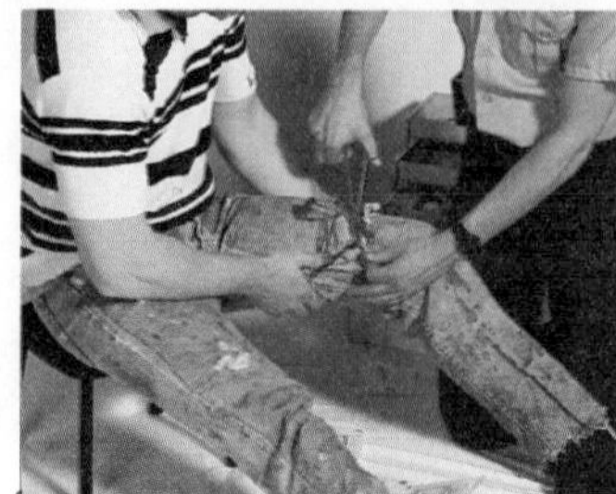

2
Cut or rip away clothing.

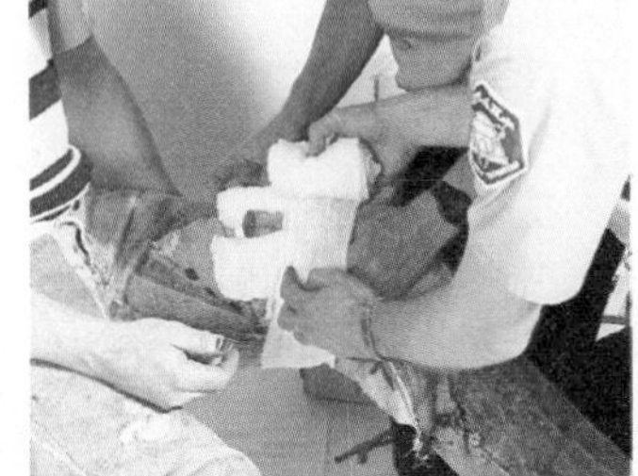

3
Stabilize and bandage impaled object in place.

- Send for emergency medical aid as soon as possible. If help can arrive in a short period, it may be better to wait for the rescue team to immobilize.

# EYE INJURIES

## Foreign Objects in the Eye

Foreign objects, such as particles of dirt, sand, cinders, coal dust, or fine pieces of metal, frequently are blown or driven into the eye and lodge there. They not only cause discomfort, but if not removed can cause inflammation and possibly infection. Fortunately, through an increased flow of tears, nature dislodges many of these substances before any harm is done. In no case should the eye be rubbed, since rubbing may cause scratching of the delicate eye tissues or force a foreign particle with sharp edges into the tissues, making removal difficult. It is always much safer for the First Aider to get help so that the victim can be seen by a physician rather than attempt to remove foreign objects in the eye.

However, if removal of a foreign object is necessary, the procedure is as follows:

1. Flush the eye with clean water, if available, holding the eyelids apart.

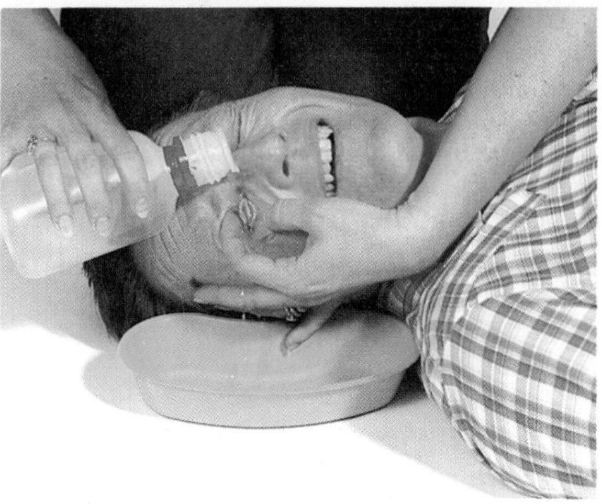

Flushing foreign object out of the eye.

2. Often, a foreign object lodged under the upper eyelid can be removed by drawing the upper lid down over the lower lid; as the upper lid returns to its normal position, the undersurfaces will be drawn over the lashes of the lower lid and the foreign body removed by the wiping action of the eyelashes.
3. A foreign object in the eye may also be removed by grasping the eyelashes of the upper lid and turning the lid over a cotton swab or similar object. The particle may then be carefully removed from the eyelid with the corner of a piece of sterile gauze.

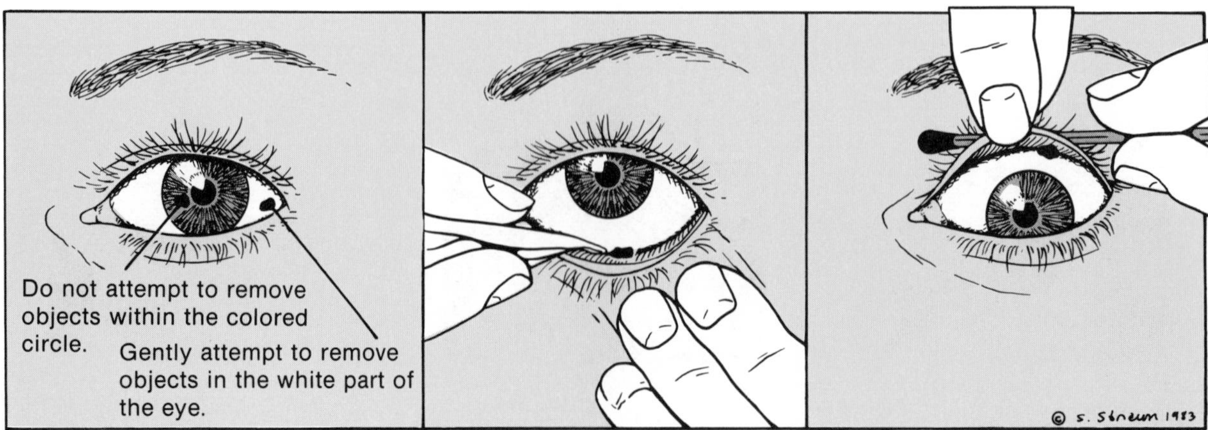


Gently attempt to remove objects in the white part of the eye. Using two fingers, gently pull down the lower eyelid while the victim looks up. Carefully pull up the upper eyelid as the victim looks down. A matchstick can help you to grip the lid as shown.

4. Particles lodged under the lower lid may be removed by pulling down the lower lid, exposing the inner surface. The corner of a piece of sterile gauze can be used to remove the foreign object.

Should a foreign object become lodged in the eyeball, do not attempt to disturb it, as it may be forced deeper into the eye and result in further damage. Place a bandage compress over **both eyes.**

Gentleness is essential in handling eye injuries. Always get medical assistance for an eye injury.

## Lid Injuries

These include ecchymosis (black eyes), burns, and lacerations. In general, little can be done for these injuries in the field beyond gentle patching. First aid care consists of controlling bleeding and protecting the injured tissue and underlying structures.

- Eyelid bleeding can be profuse but can usually be controlled with light pressure. Only a light dressing should be used, and **no** pressure should be used if the eyeball is cut.
- Cover the uninjured eye with a bandage to decrease movement.
- If the eyelids do not cover the eyeball, use a light, moist dressing to prevent drying.

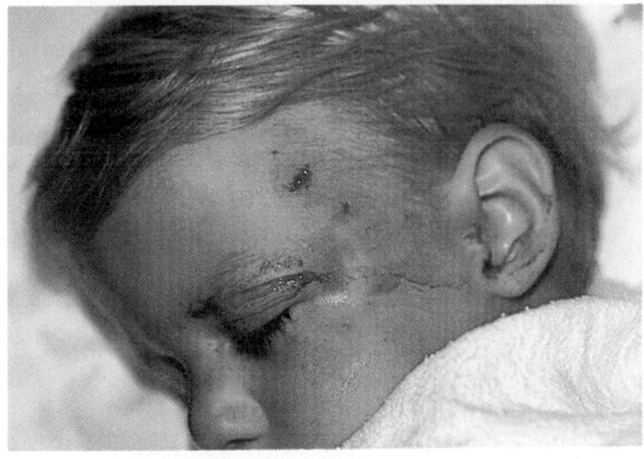

Eyelid injury.

## Impaled Objects in the Eye

Objects impaled or embedded in the eye should be removed only by a doctor. Penetrating objects must be protected from accidental movement or removal until the victim receives medical attention.

- Tell the victim that both eyes must be bandaged to protect the injured eye.
- Encircle the eye with a gauze dressing or other suitable material.
- Position a crushed cup or cone over the embedded object. The object should not touch the top or sides of the cup.
- Hold the cup and dressing in place with a bandage compress or roller bandage that covers both eyes. It is important to bandage both eyes to prevent movement of the injured eye.
- Never leave the victim alone, as he/she may panic with both eyes covered. Keep in hand contact so that the victim will always know someone is there.
- Stabilize the head with sand bags or large pads, and keep victim on his/her back.
- For an unconscious victim, close the eyes before bandaging to prevent drying of tissues.
- Send for emergency medical assistance as soon as possible.

## Eyeball Knocked Out of Socket

During a serious injury, the eyeball may be knocked out of the socket (extruded or avulsed). No attempt should be made to put the eye back into the socket.

- The eye should be covered with a moist covering and a protective cup without applying pressure to the eye.
- A bandage compress or roller bandage that covers both eyes should be applied.
- Keep the victim face up with the head immobilized.
- Send for emergency medical aid immediately.

## IMPALED OBJECT IN THE EYE

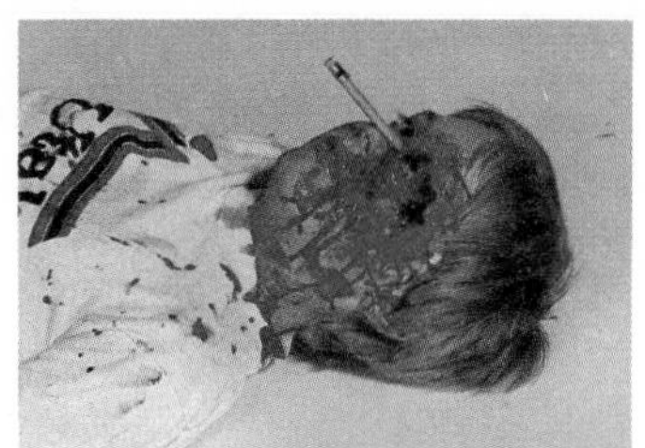

1
Impaled object in eye.

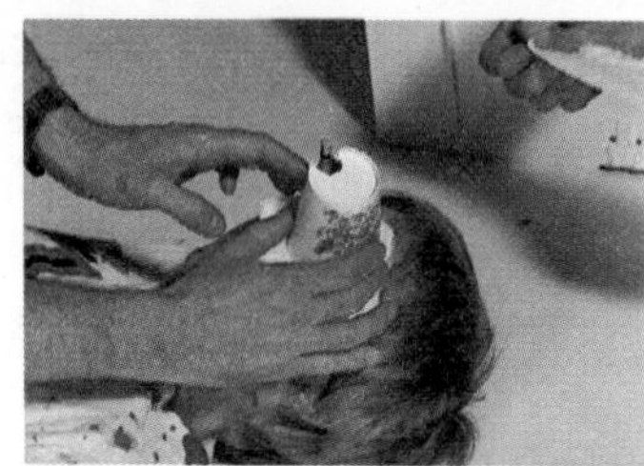

2
Dress and stabilize impaled object.

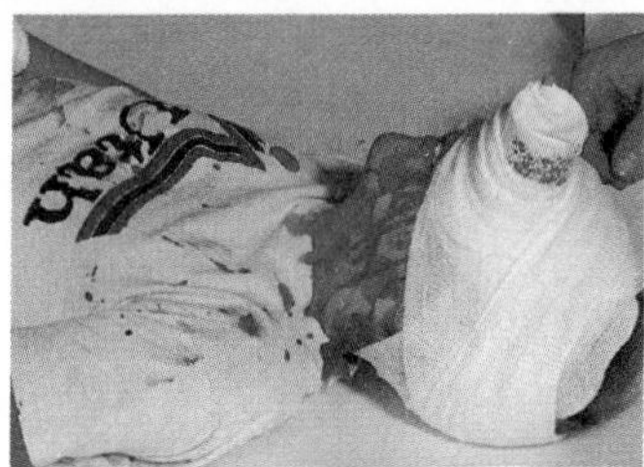

3
Bandage the cup in place.

## Basic Rules for Emergency Eye Care

Remember these basic rules when giving emergency eye care:

1. Do not wash the injured eye. **The obvious exception is a chemical or detergent injury to the eye.** If the injury does not involve chemicals, you will only end up scratching the eye surface. If the eye has been perforated, damage incurred in washing it will be irreversible.
2. Do not put salves or medicine into the injured eye. They will probably do more harm than good.
3. Sponge blood from the face to help keep the victim comfortable. Leave the eye alone.
4. Do not try to force the eyelid open unless you have to wash out chemicals.
5. Make the victim lie down and keep quiet. Never let a victim with an eye injury walk without help, especially up or down stairs.
6. Limit use of the **uninjured** eye. Eyes move together, and if the victim is using one eye, chances are the other one is moving, too.
7. Never panic. It will upset the victim and cause you to lose valuable calmness needed in effective care.
8. An eye emergency should always be seen by a physician.

## When A Tooth Is Knocked Out

- Anyone's teeth can "pop out" under pressure, but it usually happens at an early age when the bone structure is more supple. When an adult's tooth is put under stress, it will often break. If a tooth that is knocked out is properly handled and treated quickly, it may be replanted.
- If the tooth is whole (root not broken off), a dentist may be able to replant it. Some dentists will choose not to replant a young child's "baby" tooth for fear of damaging the permanent teeth, but each case is different — let a dentist make the decision.
- One of the keys to having a knocked-out tooth successfully put back in is *water* to keep the tooth moist until it can be treated. While some dental experts feel the tooth should be put in plain, warm water, and others believe it should be immersed in salt water, all agree the tooth has to be kept moist.
- The second key to a successful replanting is speed in getting to a dentist. The faster the tooth can be treated, the greater the chance the replant will work. Ideally, treatment should take place within 30 minutes of the accident, but replants have worked even after 24 hours.
- The First Aider should take the tooth to the emergency room with the victim, where the emergency room personnel can contact a dentist.
- If the replanted tooth survives the first three to six months, it probably will last for about five to eight years; then the body eventually rejects it. The value of this method, say for a 12-year-old child, is that during that period the youngster's mouth and facial structure have a chance to develop properly and the child is then emotionally old enough to deal with the trauma of receiving a partial denture.

# Face, Scalp, and Neck Wounds

**The face, scalp and neck are richly supplied with arteries and veins, and wounds of these areas bleed heavily.**

## SPECIAL CONSIDERATIONS

- Suspect brain or neck injuries for any wounds of the head, face or neck.
- Check the mouth carefully for any loose objects, such as broken teeth, that might impair the airway. Send any dentures, broken teeth, etc., with the team that transports the victim.
- Check carefully for bleeding into the mouth or throat that might impair the airway.
- Position the victim so blood will drain out of the mouth.
- Cover exposed nerves, tendons, or blood vessels with a moist dressing and bandage.
- Save any avulsed parts.

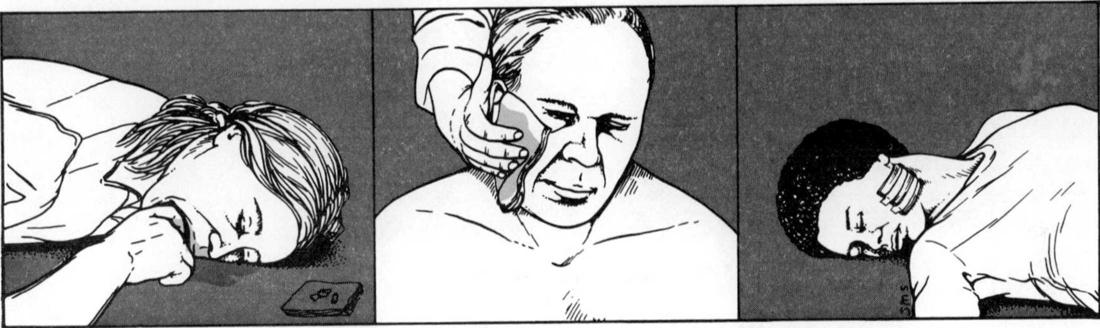

## EMERGENCY CARE

- Control by direct pressure. Be gentle because there may be broken facial bones beneath the wounds.
- For cheek wounds, hold a gauze pad inside the cheek as well as outside if necessary. Do not put dressings in mouth without holding in place.
- Remove any object impaled in the cheek. This is the only exception to the rule of not removing impaled objects. If removal proves difficult, leave object in place and stabilize.
- Control arterial bleeding from the neck by direct pressure without closing airway. If necessary use carotid pressure point. DO NOT apply pressure at the same time to both sides of the neck.
- If a large neck vein is torn, apply pressure above and below the point of bleeding to prevent air from entering the circulatory system - the latter could be rapidly fatal. It is best that these victims remain in a supine (lying) position to reduce the chance of an air embolism.
- For cut lips insert a rolled or folded dressing between the victim's lip and gum.

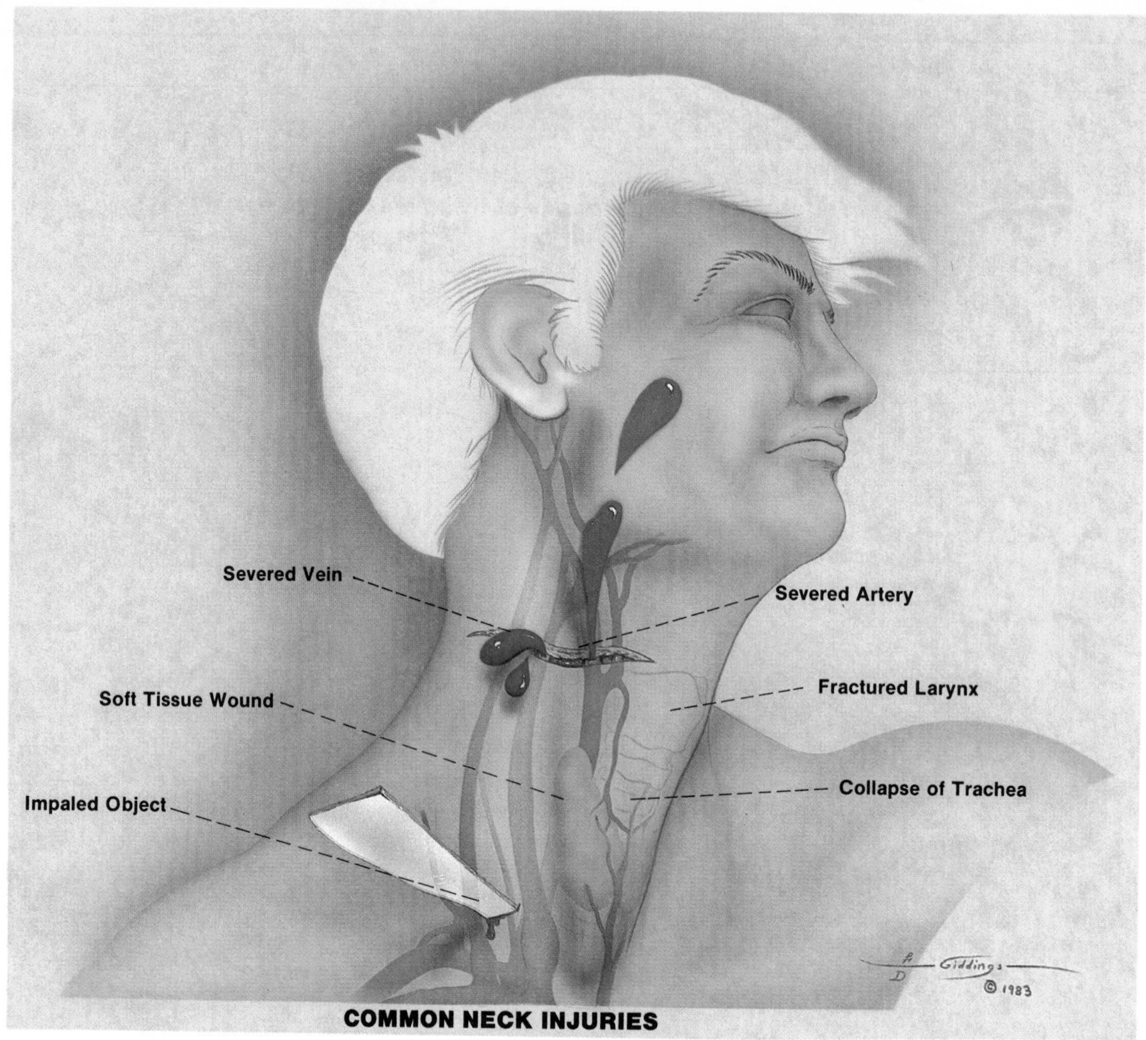


COMMON NECK INJURIES

## BLUNT OR CRUSHING TRAUMA

- Loss of voice.
- Severe airway obstruction even though the mouth and nose are clean and no foreign body.
- Deformity, contusions, or depressions in the neck.
- Swelling in the neck and sometimes face and chest. When the swollen areas are touched there are crackling sensations under the skin due to air leakage in the soft tissues.
- If one of the above signs is present, it is an extreme emergency, and the victim needs to be transported to a medical facility immediately.
- Calm and reassure the victim, encouraging him/her to breathe slowly.
- Maintain airway and assist ventilations if necessary.
- Be alert for possible cervical spine injuries and take necessary immobilization precautions.
- Send for emergency medical aid immediately.

## OPEN INJURIES

**Serious open wounds of the neck can cause profuse bleedings.**

- If an *artery* has been severed and there is bright red spurting blood, apply direct pressure with a sterile (if possible) bulky dressing. If blood soaks through the dressing do not remove it — Just add another dressing on the first one. Maintain firm pressure with your hand until you arrive at the hospital. Caution: Pressure dressing around the neck can compromise the airway.
- Do not apply pressure over the airway or on both sides of the neck at the same time.
- If necessary, apply pressure to the carotid pressure point. Do not apply pressure on both carotid arteries at the same time. If there is an impaled object, stabilize in place with bulky dressings. Do not remove.
- Keep victim supine with legs slightly elevated and transport immediately.
- If a large vein (profuse, steady flow of dark red to maroon-colored blood) is severed, attempt to control bleeding using direct pressure with a bulky dressing. If bleeding is controlled, cover with an occlusive dressing.
- If bleeding is not immediately controlled, apply pressure above and below the point of bleeding. It is imperative that air not be allowed to be sucked into the vein (air embolism) and be carried into the circulatory system. This can be rapidly fatal. This is more likely to occur if the victim is sitting or standing.
- Cover wound with an occlusive dressing or plastic wrap, and tape all edges snugly to form an airtight seal over the severed vein.
- Position the victim on his/her side.
- Monitor airway.
- Send for emergency medical aid immediately.

## COMMON WOUNDS

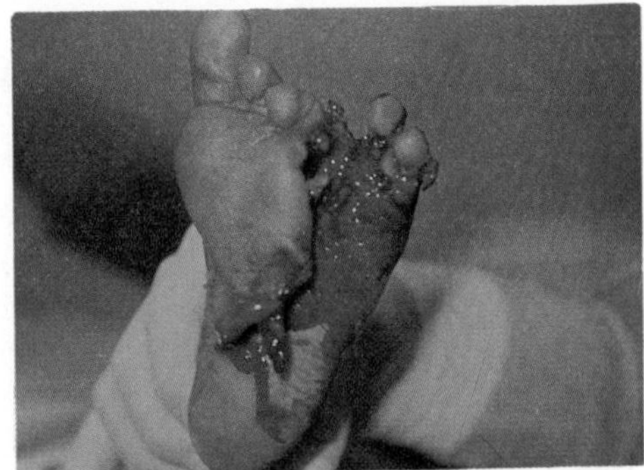
Foot avulsion.

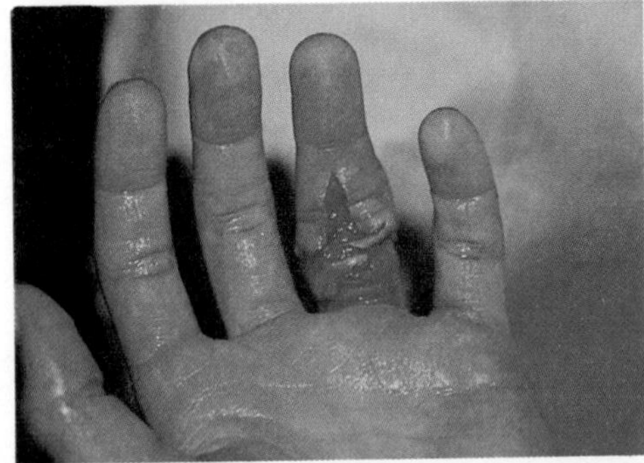
Ring avulsion.

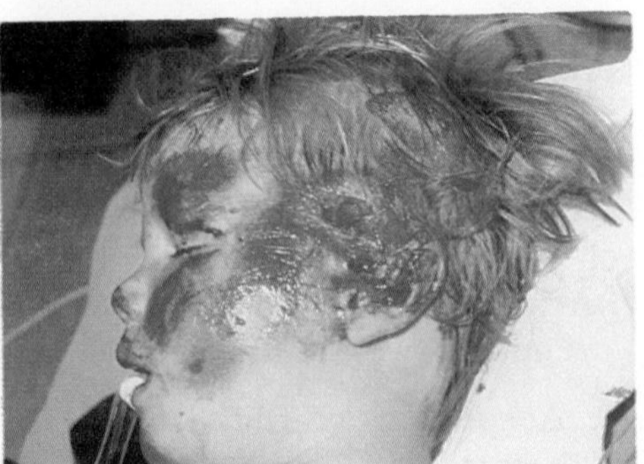
Abrasions and laceration.

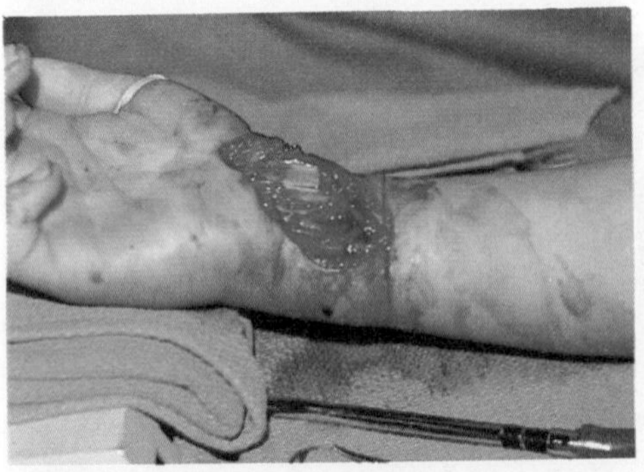
Foreign object (glass) injury.

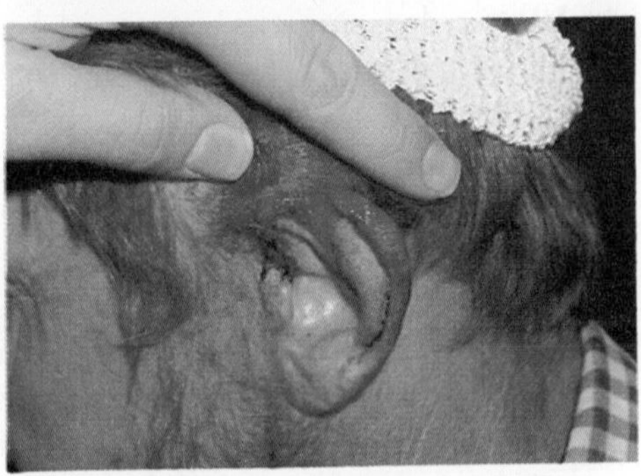
Ear laceration.

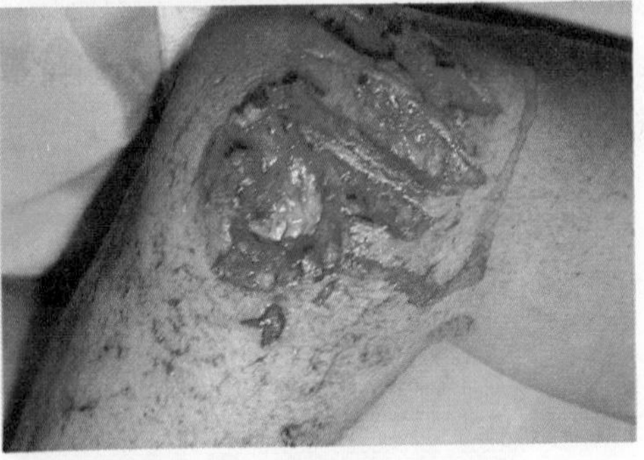
Deep abrasions and lacerations.

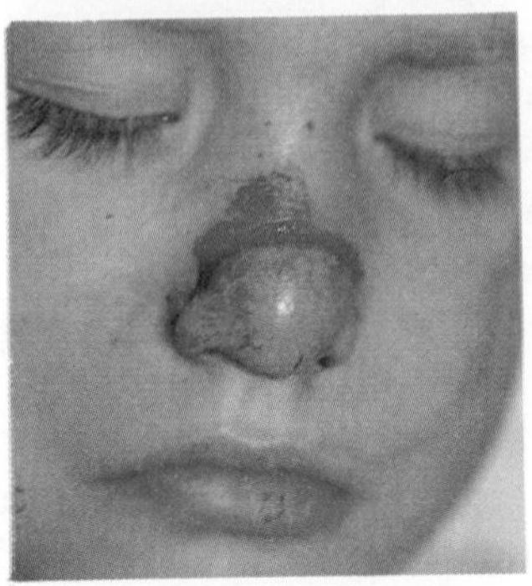
Nose avulsion.

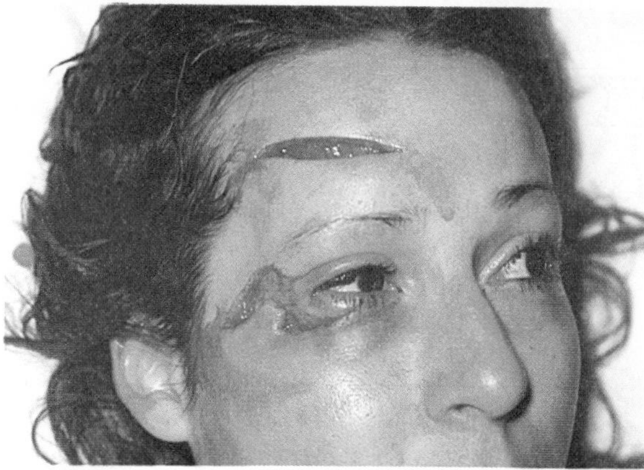
Laceration of head and face.

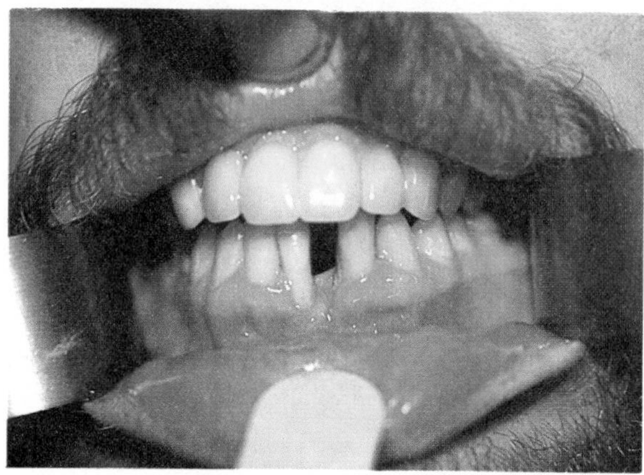
Avulsed tooth.

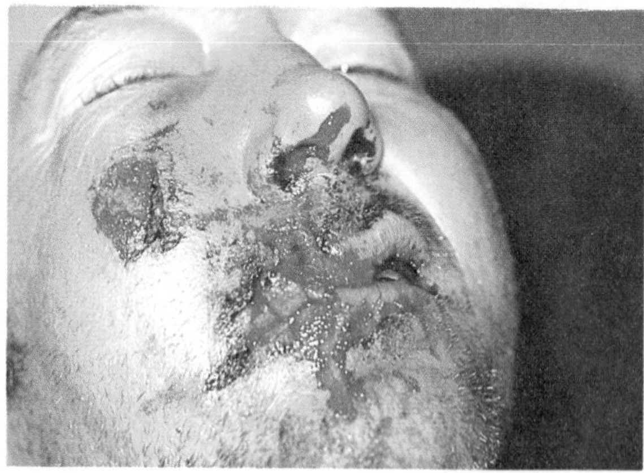
Mouth injury.

## DRESSINGS AND BANDAGES

Once you have controlled hemorrhaging, you are ready to dress and bandage a wound. Proper wound care enhances healing, adds to the comfort of the victim, and promotes rapid recovery. Improper wound care can delay healing, cause severe discomfort to the victim, and, in rare cases, result in the loss of a limb.

### Dressings

A **dressing** is what immediately covers the wound. A **bandage** holds the dressing in place. The dressing should be sterile and held in place snugly enough to control external bleeding but not too tight to stop blood circulation. The ideal dressing should be layered and should consist of coarst-mesh gauze and self-adhesing roller gauze. It should be bulky enough to immobilize the tissues and to give protection to the wound in case of rough handling. This cuts down on renewed bleeding and movement of bacteria into unaffected areas. Dressings, then, prevent introduction of bacteria and provide protection against further injury to the wound.

Types of wound dressings include:

1. **Aseptic:** a sterile dressing (free from bacteria).
2. **Antiseptic:** a sterile dressing containing a substance to kill bacteria.
3. **Wet:** a dressing that may not be sterile.
4. **Dry sterile:** a sterile dressing that is free of moisture.
5. **Petroleum gauze:** sterile gauze saturated with petroleum to prevent the dressing from sticking to an open wound.
6. **Occlusive:** An occlusive dressing is used when an air-tight seal is required, such as for sucking chest wounds and severed neck veins. Occlusive dressings would include plastic wrap, aluminum foil, and petroleum gauze.

When prepared sterile dressings are not available, any piece of cloth is suitable for use as a compress in case of emergency, provided it is as clean as possible.

A **universal dressing** is one that is made from a nine-by-thirty-six-inch piece of thick, absorbent material. It can be folded into a compact size and can be used for wounds and burns, to stabilize impaled objects, and to pad splints. Bedsheets can also be sterilized and kept in plastic wrappers for use on burns.

Dressings are fixed in position either by a bandage or adhesive. Without proper fixation,

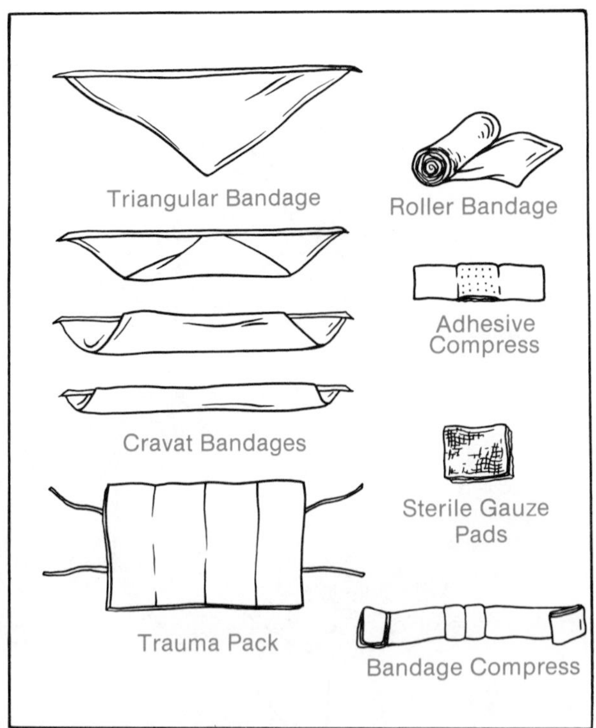


Dressings and bandages.

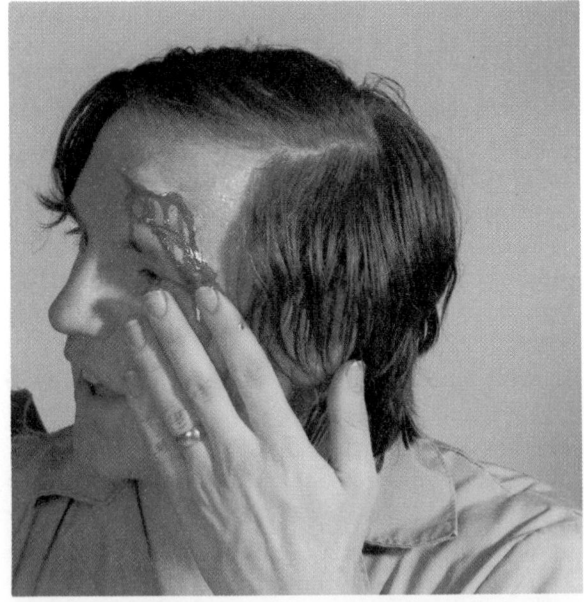

Forehead laceration.

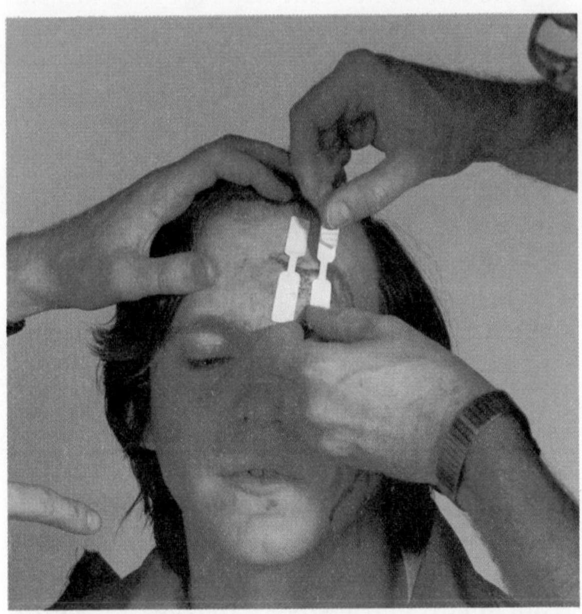

Butterfly strips (commercially prepared or improvised from adhesive tape) may be used to insure wound closure.

the dressing tends to shift out of position, permitting contamination. Once in place, the bandage should not be removed until the victim is in the hands of a physician, and means are available to control hemorrhage.

## Bandages

A bandage is used to hold a dressing in place over a wound, to create pressure over a bleeding wound for control of hemorrhage, to secure a splint to an injured part of the body, and to provide support for an injured part. Properly applied, bandages promote healing, prevent severe complications, and help the victim to remain comfortable during transport.

A bandage should never be applied directly over a wound. It should be used only to hold the dressing in place. A bandage should be applied firmly and fastened securely. It should not be applied so tightly that it stops circulation or so loosely that it allows the dressing to slip. If bandages work themselves loose or become unfastened, wounds may bleed or become infected, and broken bones may become further displaced. It is essential, therefore, that bandages be properly applied and well secured.

**Self-adhesive roller bandages** and **triangular bandages** are the most popular and can be adapted to most of the types of bandages needed. An **air splint** can also be effectively used to hold a dressing in place on an extremity, particularly if a pressure dressing is necessary.

Use care in applying adhesive bandages because of potential skin reaction or allergic sensitivity.

Practice bandaging regularly; practice is the key to developing skill. Avoid the two most common mistakes: bandaging too loosely and bandaging too tightly.

Before you bandage a victim, remove any rings from the fingers, and make sure that you do not apply the bandage over any previous bandage that has been taped. Rings and hidden tape can cause pressure that may stop circulation and lead to **gangrene** that goes unnoticed until the bandage is removed.

If the bandaged part of the body is a **mobile** one, apply the bandage snugly to counter stretching. However, make sure that the bandage is not too tight. Signs that indicate a too-tight bandage are:

1. The skin around the bandage becomes pale or cyanotic (bluish).
2. The victim complains of pain usually only a few minutes after you have applied the bandage.
3. The skin around the bandage is cold.
4. The skin around the bandage is tingling or numb.

## Bandage Compress

A **bandage compress** is a special dressing to cover open wounds. It consists of a pad made of several thicknesses of gauze attached to the middle of a strip of gauze. Pad sizes range from one to four inches. Bandage compresses usually come folded so that the gauze pad can be applied directly to the open wound with virtually no exposure to the air or fingers. The strip of gauze at either side of the gauze pad is folded back so that it can be opened up and the bandage compress tied in place with no disturbance of the sterile pad. The gauze of a bandage compress may be extended to twice its normal size by opening up folded gauze. Unless otherwise specified, all bandage compresses and all gauze dressings should be covered with open triangular, cravat, or roller bandages.

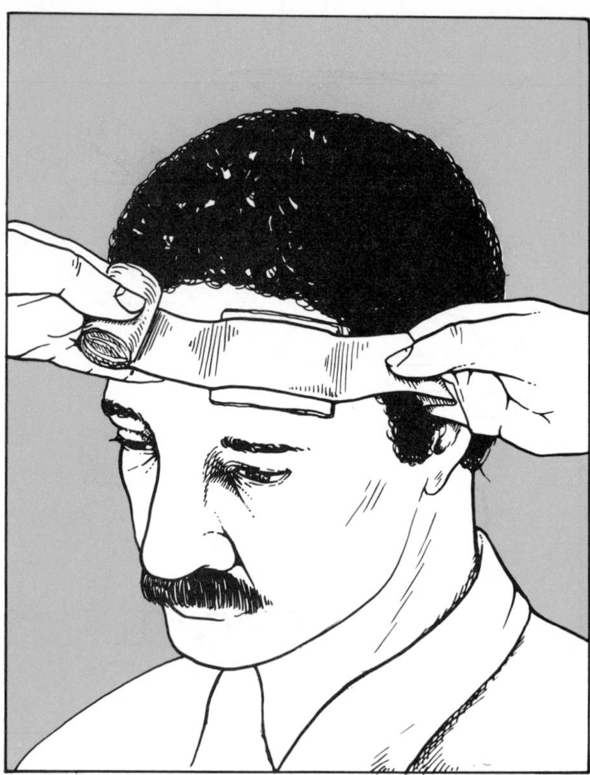

Ready-prepared bandage compresses, available in individual packages, are useful for larger wounds.

## Gauze Pads

Gauze is used several ways in applying dressings; plain gauze may be used in place of a bandage compress to cover large wounds. Plain gauze of various sizes is supplied in packets. Care should be taken not to touch the portion of the gauze that is to be placed in contact with the wound.

Sterile gauze pads, two-by-twos, four-by-fours, and four-by-eights are the most popular dressings that come individually wrapped.

## Special Pads

Large, thick-layered, bulky pads (some with an outer waterproofed surface) are available in several sizes for quick application to an extremity or to a large area of the trunk. They are used where bulk is required in cases of profuse bleeding. They are also useful for stabilizing embedded objects. These special pads are referred to as **multitrauma dressings, trauma packs, general purpose dressings,** or **burn pads.**

## SELF-ADHERING ROLLER BANDAGES

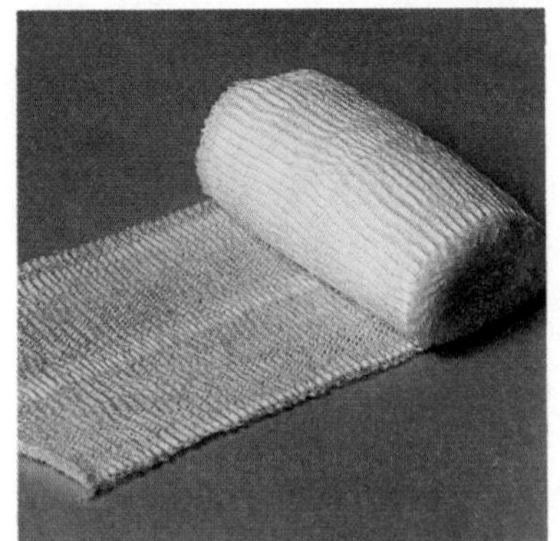

1
Self-adhering roller bandage.

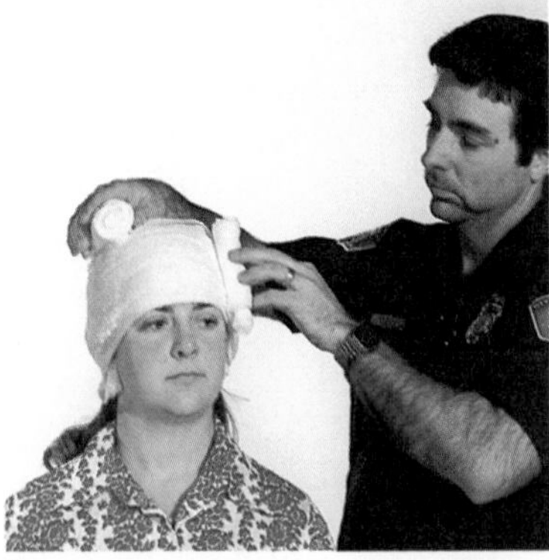

2
Head bandage.

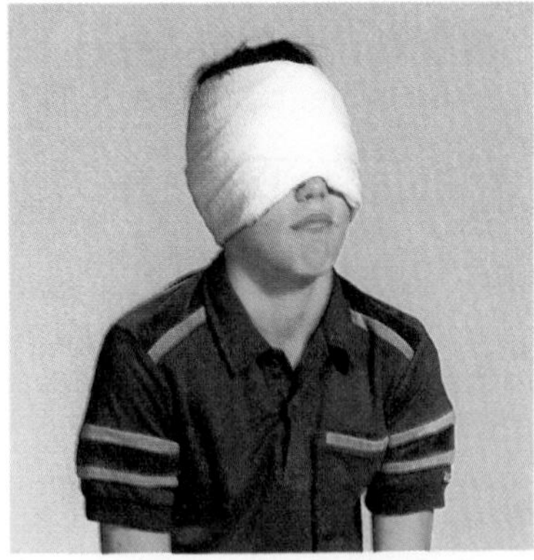

3
Head and/or eye bandage.

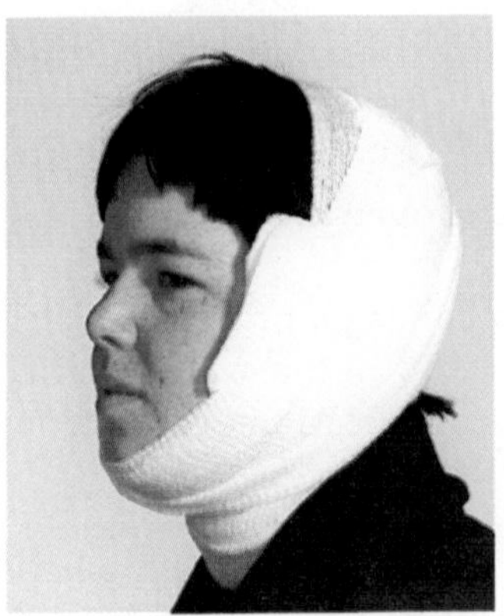

4
Cheek bandage.

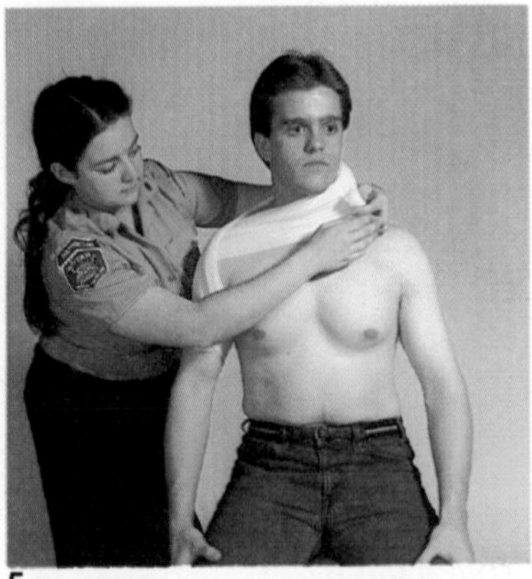

5
Bandage of neck and/or shoulder.

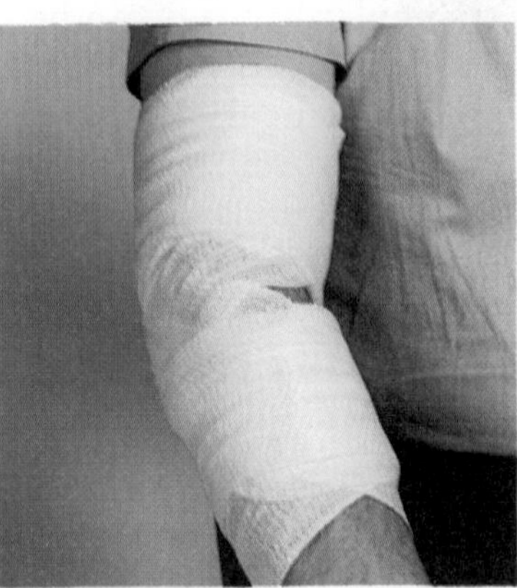

6
Elbow bandage.

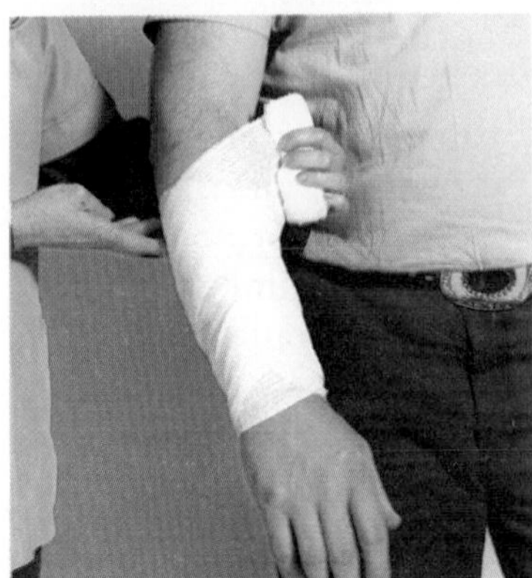

7
Lower arm bandage.

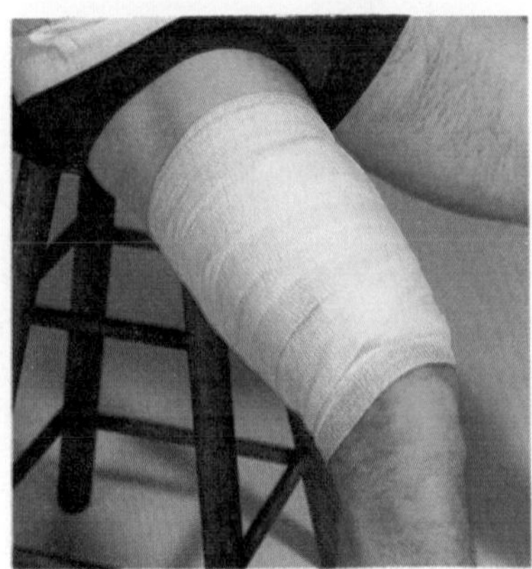

8
Thigh bandage.

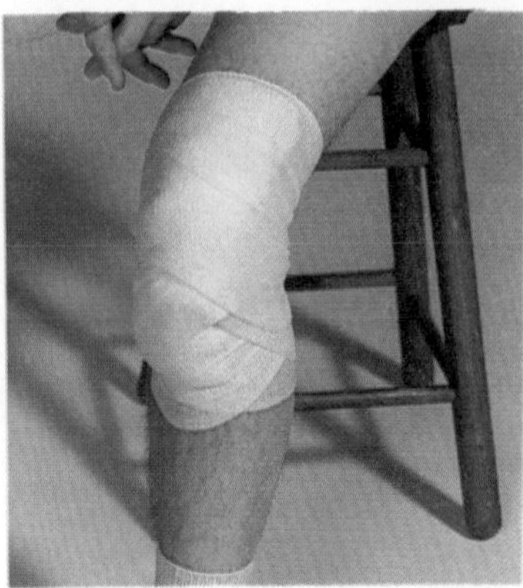

9
Knee bandage.

Because of their absorbent properties, sanitary napkins are well suited for emergency care work. Being separately wrapped, they insure a clean surface.

## Triangular Bandage

A standard triangular bandage is made from a piece of cloth approximately forty inches square by folding the square diagonally and cutting along the fold. It is easily applied and can be handled so that the part to be applied over the wound or burn dressings will not be soiled. A triangular bandage does not tend to slip off once it is correctly applied. It is usually made from unbleached cotton cloth, although any kind of cloth will do. In emergencies, a triangular bandage can be improvised from a clean handkerchief or clean piece of shirt.

The triangular bandage is used to make improvised tourniquets, to support fractures and dislocations, to apply splints, and to form slings. If a regular-size bandage is found to be too short when a dressing is applied, it can be lengthened by tying a piece of another bandage to one end.

## Roller Bandages

The self-adhering, form-fitting roller bandage is the most popular and easy to use. It eliminates the need for a lot of the complex bandaging techniques that are required with regular gauze roller bandages or cravats. This type of roller bandage is applied to hold a dressing securely in place over a wound. For this reason, it should be applied snugly, but not tightly enough to interfere with the circulation. Fingers and toes should be checked periodically for coldness, swelling, blueness, and numbness. If symptoms occur, the bandage should be loosened immediately.

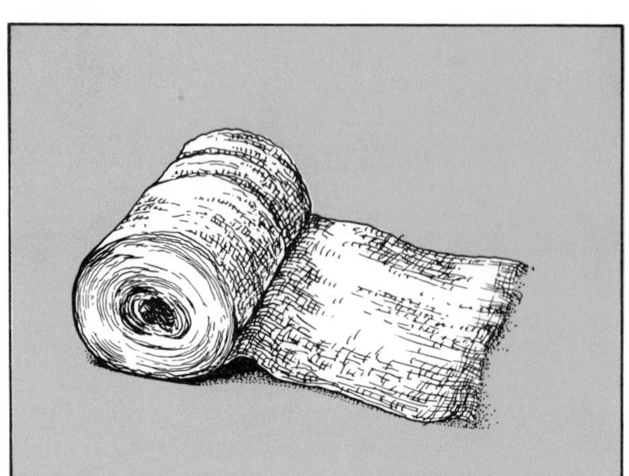

Roller bandage.

Self-adhering roller bandages are easily secured with several overlapping wraps and can then be cut and tied or taped in place.

Elastic roller bandages should **not** be used. There is too much danger of a tourniquet effect from being applied too tightly.

## Applying a Pressure Dressing

A **pressure dressing** can be applied by following these procedures:

- Cover the wound with a bulky, sterile dressing.
- Apply hand pressure over the wound until bleeding stops.
- Apply a firm roller bandage, preferably the self-adhering type. Do not use an elastic roller bandage — complications can occur from uneven distribution of pressure.
- If blood soaks through the original dressing and bandage, do not remove them — leave them in place and apply another dressing, securing it in place with another roller bandage.

## Slings

**Slings** are used to support injuries of the shoulder, upper extremities, or ribs. In an emergency, they may be improvised from belts, neckties, scarves, or similar articles. Bandages should be used if available.

### Tying a Triangular Bandage Sling

Tie a triangular bandage sling as follows:

- Place one end of the base of an open triangular bandage over the shoulder of the injured side.
- Allow the bandage to hang down in front of the chest so that the **apex** will be behind the elbow of the injured arm.
- Bend the arm at the elbow with the hand slightly elevated (four to five inches).

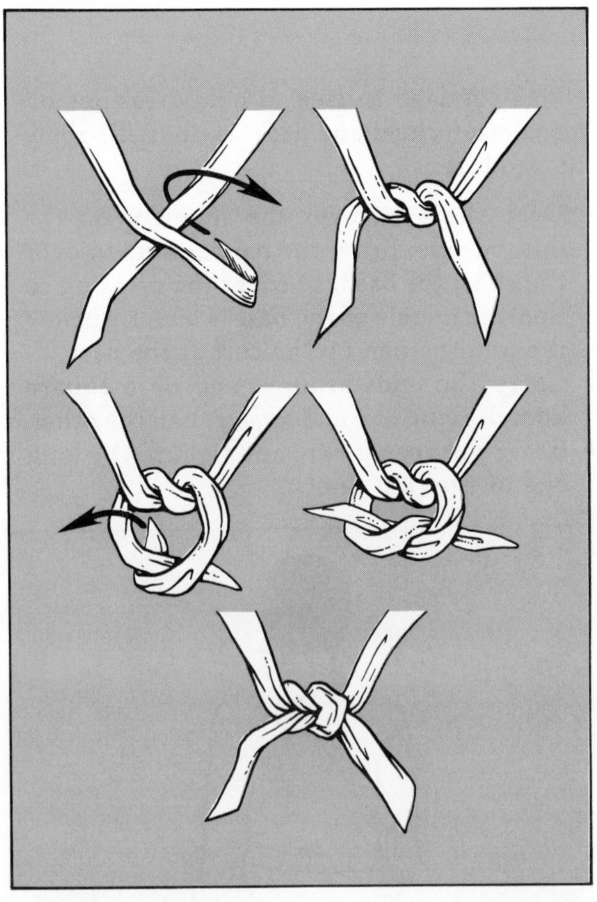

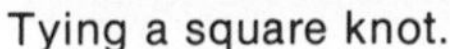

Tying a square knot.

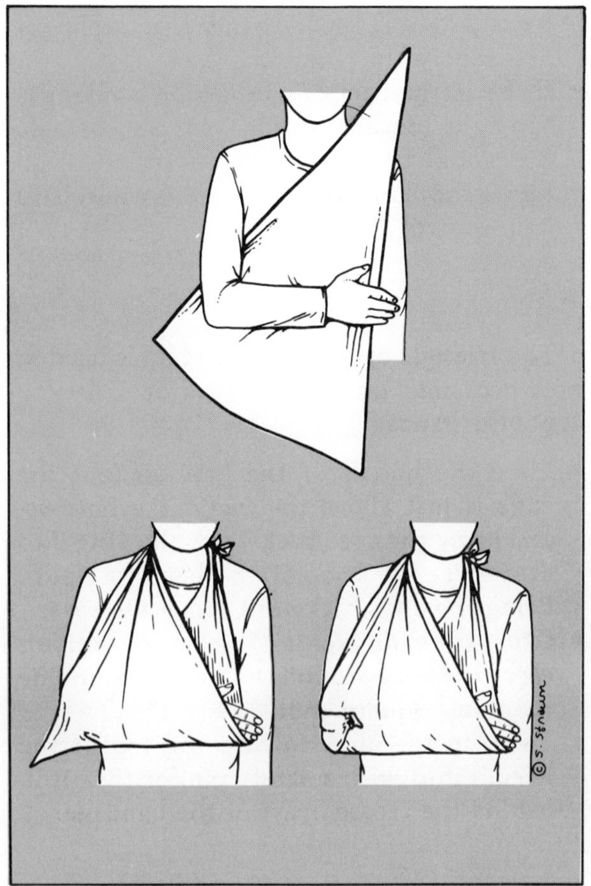

Triangle bandages as an arm sling.

- Bring the forearm across the chest and over the bandage.
- Carry the lower end of the bandage over the shoulder of the uninjured side, and tie at the uninjured side of the neck, being sure that the knot is at the side of the neck.
- Twist the apex of the bandage, and tuck it in at the elbow.

The hand should be supported with the fingertips exposed, whenever possible, to permit detection of interference with circulation.

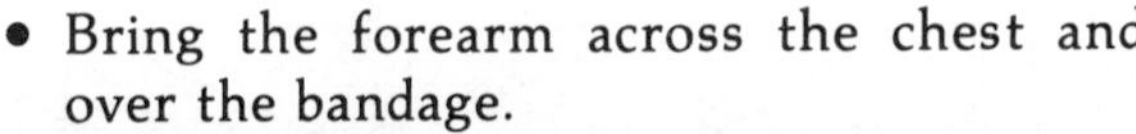

## PRINCIPLES OF BANDAGING

There are no hard and fast rules for dressing and bandaging wounds as long as the following conditions are met:

- Use sterile material or material that is as clean as possible.
- Bleeding is controlled.
- The dressing is opened carefully and handled in an aseptic manner.
- The dressing adequately covers the wound.
- Wounds are bandaged snugly, but not too tightly. Too tight a bandage may interfere with the blood supply and damage surrounding tissue.
- There are no loose ends that could get caught on other objects while the victim is being moved.
- The bandage is securely tied or fastened in a place so that it will not move.
- In bandaging the arms or the legs, leave the tips of the fingers or toes uncovered where possible so that any interference with circulation can be detected.
- Always place the body part to be bandaged in the position in which it is to be left. Because swelling frequently follows an injury, a tight bandage may cause serious interference with circulation. On the other

hand, a loosely applied bandage may slip off and expose the wound.
- If the victim complains that the bandage is too tight, loosen it and make it comfortable but snug. Unless otherwise specified, all knots should be tied over open wounds to help control bleeding.

## Triangle of Forehead or Scalp

The **triangle of forehead or scalp** is used to hold dressings on the forehead or scalp. To apply the bandage:

- Place the middle of the base so that the edge is just above the victim's eyebrows, and bring the apex backward, allowing it to drop over the back of the head **(occiput).** Bring the ends backward above the ears.
- Cross the ends over the apex at the occiput; carry the ends around the forehead, and tie them in a square knot.
- Turn up the apex toward the top of the head. Pin it with a safety pin, or tuck it in behind the crossed part of the bandage.

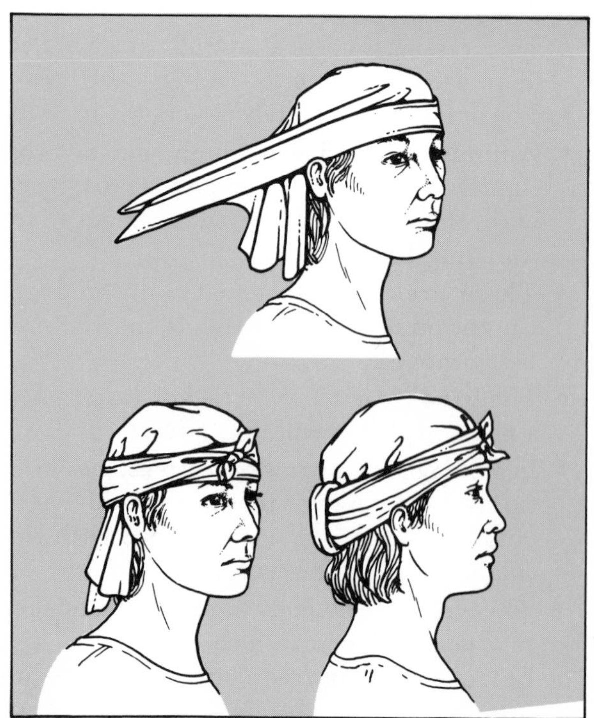

Triangle of forehead or scalp.

## Triangle of Chest or Back

This bandage is used to hold dressings on burns or on chest and back wounds. To apply the bandage:

- Drop the apex over the shoulder on the injured side. Bring the bandage down over the chest (or back) to cover the dressing so that the middle of the base is directly below the injury. Turn up the cuff at the base.
- Carry the ends around, and tie a square knot, leaving one end longer than the other.
- Bring the apex down, and tie it to the long end of the first knot.

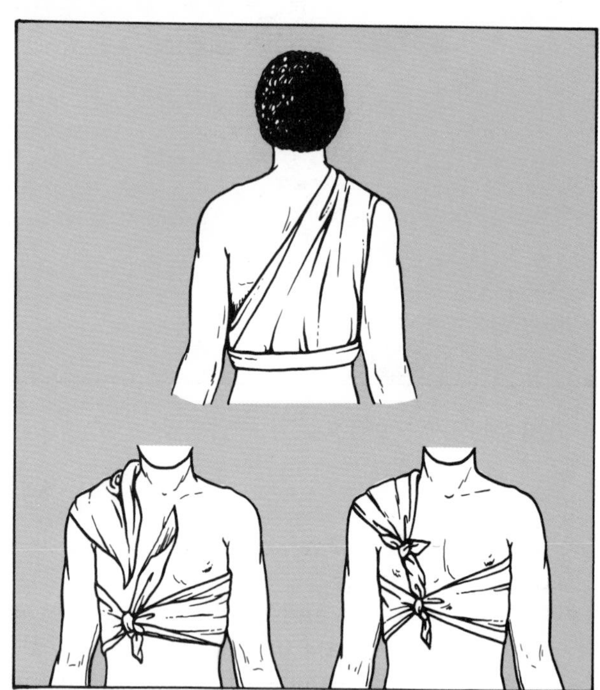

Triangle of chest or back.

## Triangle of Shoulder

This bandage is used to hold dressings on shoulder wounds. Two bandages are required: one a triangle; the other a cravat, roller bandage, or belt. To apply:

- Place the center of the cravat, roller bandage, or belt at the base of the neck on the injured side, and fasten it just forward of the opposite arm.

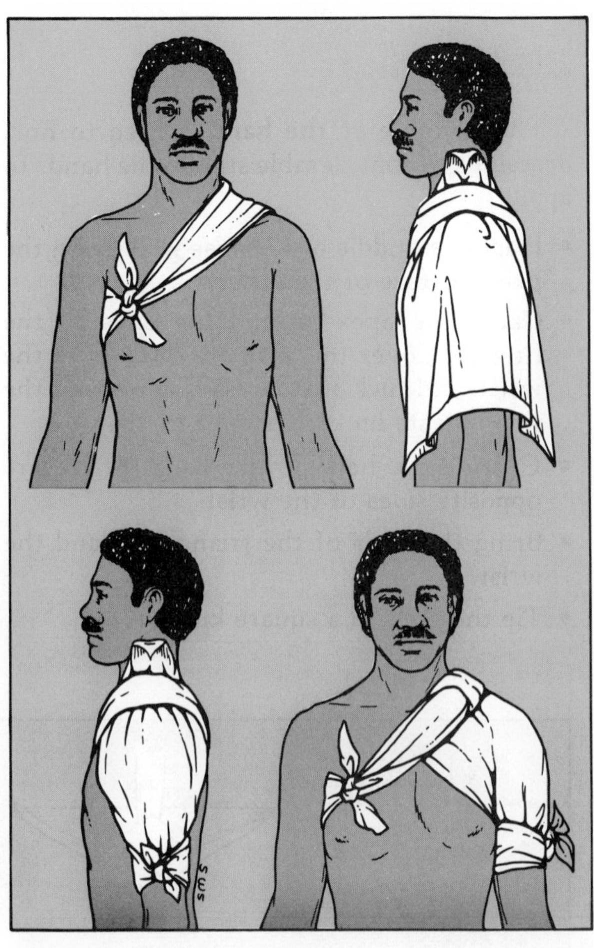

Triangle of shoulder.

- Slide the apex of the open triangle under the cravat at the back of the neck, and place it over the dressing on the injured shoulder and upper arm. Turn up the cuff at the base.
- Bring the ends around the arm, and tie them together.
- Secure the apex to the cravat at the neck by tucking it in or by using a safety pin.

## Triangle of Hip

This bandage is used to hold dressings on the buttock or hip. It requires two bandages: one a triangle; the other a cravat, roller bandage, or belt. To apply:

- Fasten the cravat, roller bandage, or belt around the waist.
- Place the base of the triangle below the buttock, and slide the apex under the cravat at the waist. Fold the base upward to form a cuff, and carry the ends of the base around the thigh.
- Tie the ends of the base with a square knot. Fasten the apex to the waist cravat with a safety pin or by tucking it under.

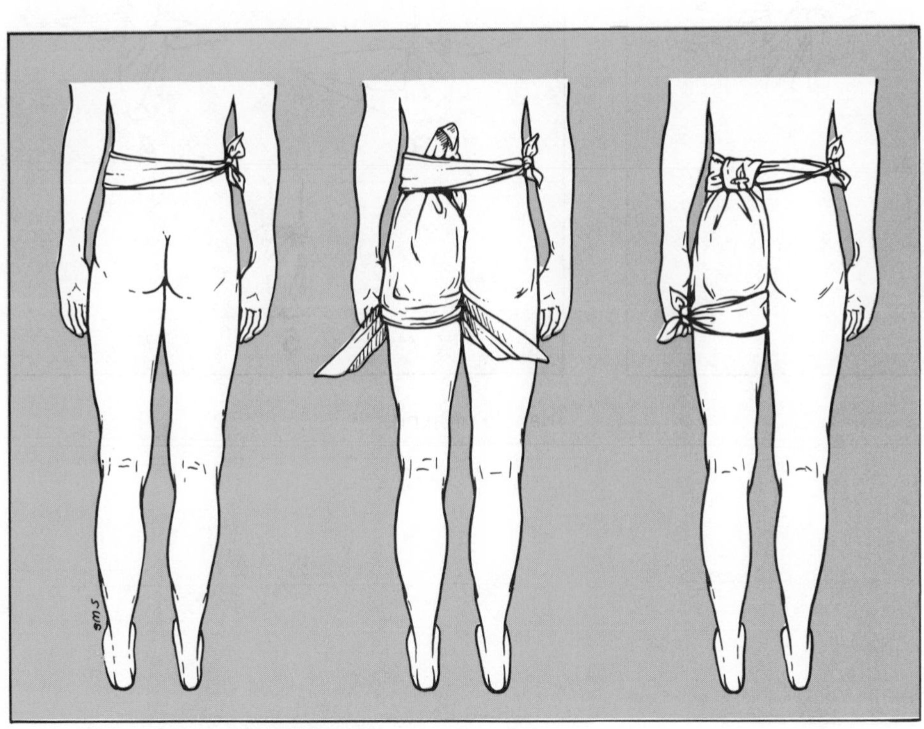

Triangle of the hip.

## Triangle of Foot

The **triangle of the foot** is used to hold dressings of considerable size on the foot. To apply:

- Center the foot on the bandage at right angles to the base, with the heel well forward of the base.
- Carry the apex of the triangle over the toes to the ankle, and tuck any excessive fullness into small pleats on each side of the foot.
- Cross each half of the bandage toward the opposite side of the ankle.
- Bring the ends of the triangle around the ankle.
- Tie the ends in a square knot.

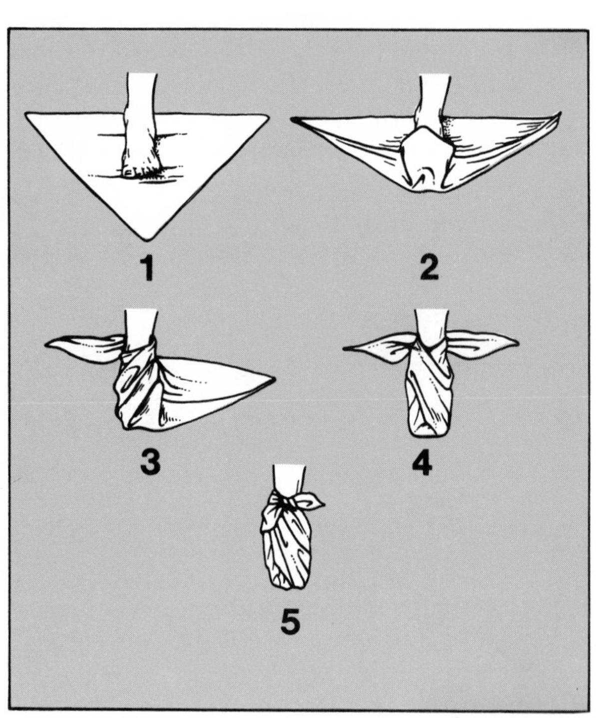


Triangle of foot.

## Triangle of Hand

The **triangle of the hand** is used to hold dressings of considerable size on the hand. To apply:

- Place the middle of the base well up on the **palm** surface of the wrist.
- Carry the apex around the ends of the fingers. Cover the back of the hand to the wrist, and tuck any excess fullness into the small pleats on each side of the hand.
- Cross each half of the bandage toward opposite sides of the wrist.
- Bring the ends of the triangle around the wrist.
- Tie the ends in a square knot.

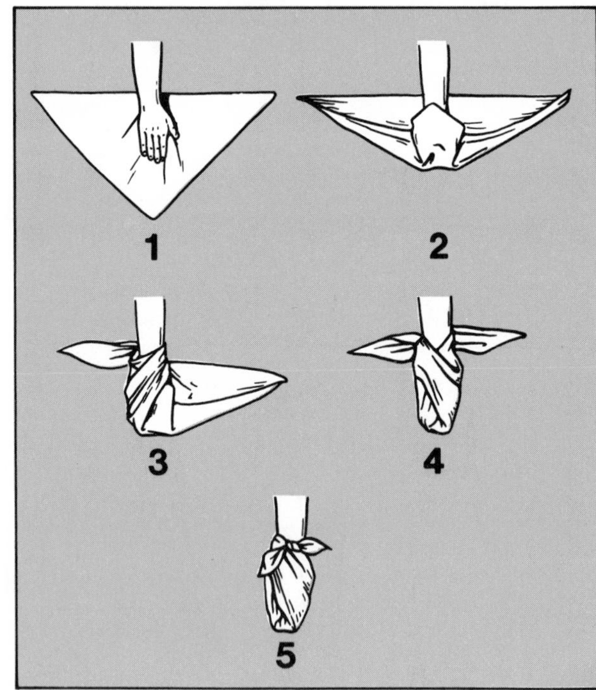


Triangle of hand.

# Work Exercises

## Care of Open Wounds

The chief duty of a First Aider in caring for an open wound is to stop bleeding and to prevent germs from entering the wound.

Indicate whether the following statements about the general care of open wounds are true or false.

| True/False | Statement |
|---|---|
| ______ 1. | Bandages should only be wide enough to cover the wound itself. |
| ______ 2. | All bandages should be loosely applied so as not to do further damage. |
| ______ 3. | Most embedded objects can be removed by the First Aider. |
| ______ 4. | Elevating a leg that has a wound would seldom help in the control of bleeding. |
| ______ 5. | All dressings should be wide enough to completely cover the wound and area around it. |
| ______ 6. | Always thoroughly clean a wound before dressing and bandaging. |
| ______ 7. | Avulsed parts or flaps of skin should not be folded back into place; this causes more contamination. |
| ______ 8. | The only protruding organ that should be put back in place after an injury is the eyeball. |

### Bites

Americans experience over ______________ dog bites a year. The most commonly bitten areas are the __________, __________, and ______________. To treat a dog bite, wash the area with ______________, __________ the area with water, and apply a __________. Do not __________ the dog. Officials will want to examine it for ______________.

### Traumatic Amputations

Rendering emergency care to an amputation victim can be traumatic for First Aider. A thorough knowledge of what to do will help immensely. Explain the proper sequence in caring for an amputation victim.

1. Establish and maintain the patient's vital functions (the ABC's).
2.
3.
4.
5.

## Impaled Objects

Impaled objects require special care. Improper care can cause additional damage to the surface wound and underlying tissues.

Decide whether the following emergency care procedures for impaled objects are correct or incorrect. Mark "T" if the treatment is correct and "F" if it is incorrect.

| True/False | Statement |
|---|---|
| ______ 1. | Break or cut off an impaled object if it is unwieldy. |
| ______ 2. | Remove an impaled object if it obstructs breathing. |
| ______ 3. | Stabilize the impaled object with bulky dressings. |
| ______ 4. | Control bleeding with direct pressure on the impaled object. |
| ______ 5. | Use a "doughnut" to stabilize an impaled object. |

There are several basic rules for giving emergency eye care. List six.

1.

2.

3.

4.

5.

6.

## Dressings and Bandages

Once bleeding has been controlled, you are ready to dress and bandage a wound. Match the type of wound dressing with its description.

| Description | Type of Dressing |
|---|---|
| ______ 1. A dressing that may not be sterile. | A. Aseptic |
| ______ 2. A dressing that forms an airtight seal. | B. Antiseptic |
| ______ 3. A sterile dressing. | C. Wet |
| ______ 4. Sterile gauze saturated with a substance to prevent the dressing from sticking to an open wound. | D. Dry sterile |
| ______ 5. A dressing that is free of moisture. | E. Petroleum gauze |
| ______ 6. A sterile dressing that contains a substance to kill bacteria. | F. Occlusive |

## SELF-TEST

### Part I: True and False

If you believe the statement is true, circle the T. If you believe the statement is false, circle F.

T F 1. After bandaging leg or foot injuries, you should frequently check the toes for signs of swelling or discoloration, indicating that the bandages are too tight.

T F 2. Abrasions are wounds that bleed freely.

T F 3. If there is an embedded or impaled object in the eye, both eyes should be bandaged.

T F 4. Closed wounds are injuries that occur without breaking the skin — the damage occurs to underlying tissue.

T F 5. Lacerations usually result from contact with a blunt, heavy object which can tear and bruise body tissues.

T F 6. The danger of infection is greater in a laceration than in any other type of wound.

T F 7. Incisions are wounds which usually pick up foreign matter (dirt, grease, or fragments) during injury, increasing the chance of infection.

T F 8. Because abrasions leave large areas of underskin tissue exposed, there is serious danger of infection.

T F 9. Dressings are applied directly over the wound, while the function of bandages is to hold them in place.

T F 10. Treat hemorrhaging of the scalp with the victim's head and shoulders raised.

T F 11. Puncture wounds usually bleed extensively, especially when the object is removed.

T F 12. An avulsion results when tissue is forcibly separated or torn from the victim's body.

T F 13. Human bites are not very dangerous and don't need any special attention.

T F 14. The best way to clean a minor wound is with soap and water.

### Part II: Multiple Choice

For each question, circle the answer that best reflects an accurate statement.

1. The first priority in wound treatment is:
   a. preventing shock
   b. preventing contamination and infection
   c. controlling bleeding

2. What is the immediate local treatment for an animal bite?
   a. wash with a mild chemical disinfectant
   b. leave it exposed to the air
   c. wash it with soap and water
   d. burn each break in the skin with a hot needle

3. In case of a suspected closed wound, your first priority should be to:
   a. monitor vital signs
   b. prevent shock
   c. determine precise location of the wound
   d. help the victim stay comfortable

4. In the case of a penetrating wound to the chest, you should:
   a. remove the penetrating object if possible
   b. apply a tight, restrictive bandage over the wound
   c. cover the wound with an airtight but nonrestrictive bandage
   d. have the victim lie flat on his/her back

5. If a foreign object is embedded in a victim's eye, you should:
   a. use a small instrument, such as a toothpick, to remove the object
   b. use a dry cotton swab to lift out the object
   c. leave the object alone, cover both eyes with a dry protective dressing, and get medical help
   d. flush the eye with water or eyewash solution until the object washes out

6. Ecchymosis means:
   a. a lump beneath the skin
   b. edema
   c. black and blue coloring
   d. external hemorrhage

7. The soft tissue injury resulting from the impact of a blunt object without breaking the skin is called:
   a. a laceration
   b. an avulsion
   c. a contusion
   d. an abrasion

8. What type of wound has as its greatest danger severe bleeding and cut tendons and nerves?
   a. an incision
   b. a laceration
   c. a contusion
   d. a puncture

9. A type of open wound characterized by jagged skin edges and free bleeding is known as:
   a. a laceration
   b. an incision
   c. a contusion
   d. a puncture

10. What type of wound has the greatest danger of infection?
    a. an incision
    b. a laceration
    c. a contusion
    d. a puncture

11. When a puncture wound is caused by an impaled object.
    a. remove the object and cover with a sterile dressing
    b. do not remove the object — stabilize it with a bulky dressing
    c. apply slight pressure on the impaled object to stop bleeding
    d. shorten the object for ease in transport

12. A serious injury in which large flaps of skin and tissue are torn loose or pulled off is called an:
    a. abrasion
    b. amputation
    c. avulsion
    d. incision

13. When an amputation has occurred, which of the following is *not* true?
    a. soak the avulsed part in sterile antiseptic solution and put it in a plastic bag
    b. place the bag with the avulsed part in a second bag filled with ice or cold water
    c. never apply a tourniquet to the severed part
    d. wrap the avulsed part in sterile material

14. The chief duties of a First Aider in caring for open wounds are:
    a. to aid in proper healing of the wound and to treat for shock
    b. to cleanse the wound and to correctly apply bandages
    c. to calm and reassure the victim and to immobilize the injured part
    d. to stop bleeding and to prevent germs from entering the wound

15. Which of the following is a general guideline for emergency care of dog bites?
    a. pack the area in ice or with a cold compress
    b. apply direct pressure to the wound to stop bleeding
    c. flush the area thoroughly with water
    d. do not cover the wound

16. A serious disease carried in the saliva of infected animals is called:
    a. lockjaw
    b. rabies
    c. tetanus
    d. convulsions

17. The danger with human bites is:
    a. infection
    b. rabies
    c. excessive bleeding
    d. lawsuit

18. To control bleeding in a victim with traumatic amputation, first use:
    a. tourniquet
    b. pressure dressing
    c. pressure points
    d. direct pressure

19. What is the first step in the sequence of care for the amputation victim?
    a. apply a dressing to the stump
    b. establish and maintain vital functions
    c. treat for shock
    d. control hemorrhage

20. If a victim has a severely lacerated or mangled limb that is not completely amputated, a First Aider should:
    a. apply a tourniquet
    b. complete the amputation
    c. wash the mangled area thoroughly with warm water and soap
    d. preserve as much as possible of the original length of the limb.

21. To prevent contamination or infection of a deep wound that has bled heavily, you should:
    a. remove foreign objects from the wound
    b. thoroughly cleanse the wound with disinfectant once the bleeding has stopped
    c. leave the initial pad or bandage in place undisturbed
    d. frequently replace pads or bandages as they become bloody or soiled

22. What should the First Aider do if a large neck vein is torn?
    a. apply pressure to both carotid arteries
    b. apply pressure above and below the point of bleeding
    c. wear sterile gloves and compress the vein with the fingers
    d. cover the wound with an airtight dressing

23. If removal of a foreign object from the eye becomes necessary, the first maneuver is to:
    a. flush the eye with clean water
    b. pull the lower lid down and use a piece of gauze to remove the foreign body
    c. turn the upper lid over a cotton swab or similar object
    d. draw the upper lid down over the lower lid

24. Eye lid injuries should be:
    a. irrigated with cool water
    b. covered with a compress and roller bandage
    c. treated with antibiotic salve
    d. covered with a light dressing

25. When a victim has a foreign object imbedded in the globe of his/her eye, a First Aider should:
    a. remove the object and then dress and bandage the eye
    b. place a loose dressing over the object
    c. prepare a thick dressing and secure a protective cone over the impaled object, leaving the uninjured eye unbandaged
    d. prepare a thick dressing and secure a protective cone over the object, bandaging the uninjured eye also.

26. If an eyeball is knocked out of the socket:
    a. do not attempt to put the eye back in the socket
    b. cover the extruded eyeball with a thick dressing moistened with sterile saline solution
    c. cover both the injured and uninjured eyes with a thick dressing
    d. gently and carefully replace the eyeball in the socket and cover with a dressing

27. Which of the following is a basic rule of giving emergency eye care?
    a. flush the injured eye with water in case of heat burns
    b. do not force the eyelid open (unless you have to wash out chemicals)
    c. administer eye drops to soothe eye injuries
    d. gently sponge blood from the injured eye

28. The first means to be used for controlling bleeding of facial injuries is:
    a. elevation
    b. flushing the wound
    c. gentle, direct pressure
    d. use of pressure points

29. An object is impaled in a victim's cheek. What is the proper emergency care procedure?
    a. leave it in and stabilize the object
    b. fill the mouth with gauze pads to control bleeding
    c. pull the object out part way to insure adequate airway
    d. remove the object.

30. A tooth can be replanted if:
    a. it is kept moist
    b. the bone structure of the mouth is not damaged
    c. a dentist is seen up to 48 hours after the tooth has been lost
    d. the dentin of the tooth is intact

31. What is the most serious problem associated with facial and jaw injuries?
    a. obstruction of the air passage
    b. loose and broken teeth
    c. permanent disfigurement
    d. potential for shock

32. One purpose of a dressing is:
    a. to prevent introduction of bacteria
    b. to hold the bandage in place
    c. to apply pressure to the wound
    d. to supply support for the injured limb

33. Which of the following is *not* a type of wound dressing?
    a. petroleum gauze
    b. aseptic
    c. bacteriostatic
    d. dry sterile

34. Bandages should never:
    a. be applied directly over the wound
    b. be applied tight enough to hinder circulation
    c. be applied loosely
    d. all of the above

35. Which of the following is *not* a principle for applying a pressure dressing?
    a. if blood soaks through the original dressing and bandage, do not remove it
    b. use an elastic roller bandage to hold the dressing in place
    c. cover the wound with a sterile dressing
    d. apply hand pressure over the wound until bleeding stops

36. What type of knot is most frequently used in bandaging?
    a. slip knot
    b. granny knot
    c. square knot
    d. half hitch

37. Which of the following is *not* a principle of bandaging?
    a. when bandaging the arm, leave the fingers uncovered
    b. place the body part to be bandaged in the position in which it is to be left
    c. leave no loose ends that could get caught on other objects
    d. if in doubt, leave a bandage tied loosely

Corresponds with:
**American Red Cross**
**Standard First Aid & Personal Safety**
Chapter 3, pages 48-57
and
**Advanced First Aid & Emergency Care**
Chapter 3, pages 49, 54-56

# 9 Specific Injuries

Injuries of the head, spine, chest, and abdomen especially those involving skull and spinal fracture, are among the most difficult and serious first aid emergencies. Your judgment, assessment, and emergency care will be essential in protecting a victim from death and/or permanent disability.

## THE ASSESSMENT

Begin with the primary survey. Correct any life-threatening problems first. A spinal injury can wait for a few minutes, but movement can cause permanent injury or death. Treat any unconscious person as if a spinal injury is present.

1. Maintain the airway. Even though the victim is not getting enough oxygen, a victim with a brain injury may never become cyanotic (turn bluish). **Do not hyperextend the neck;** use the **chin lift** or **jaw thrust** techniques. Maintaining the airway is the most important step. The brain relies on oxygen, and death can occur within a few minutes if the oxygen supply is interrupted. An injured brain is even more susceptible than a normal brain to a lack of oxygen.
2. Check the head.
   - **The skull.** Look for **lacerations, fractures,** depressions, and other deformities. Be careful not to push bone fragments into the brain during this examination. Do not remove **impaled objects.**
   - **Bruising.** Bruising behind the ears or around the eyes are indicators of a skull fracture.
   - **Ears and nose.** Is blood and/or **cerebrospinal fluid** present? Do not stop the flow from the ears or nose; dress them lightly to absorb fluid, but allow free flow of fluid to continue.
   - **Mouth.** Is blood or cerebrospinal fluid draining from the nose or ears down the back of the throat?

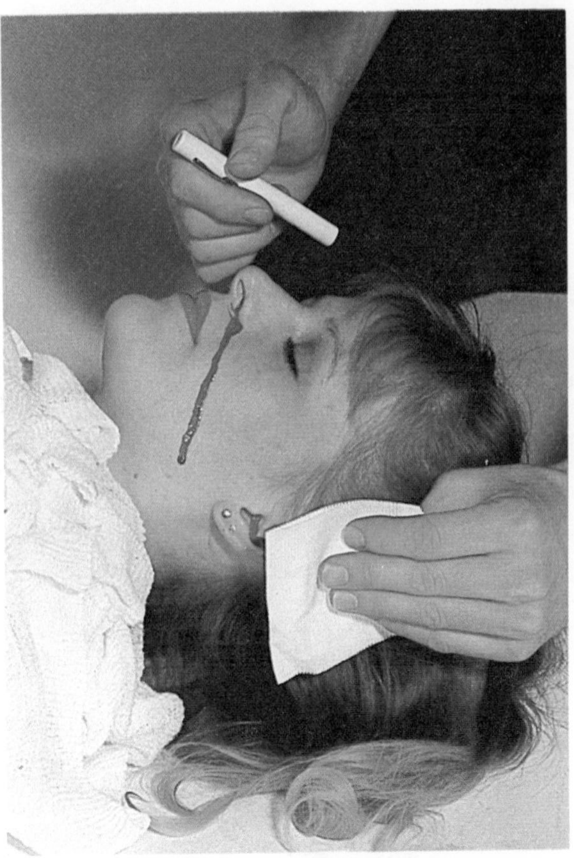

Blood and/or cerebrospinal fluid may come from the ears and/or nose of a victim of head injury. Turn victim's head to the side to allow drainage, and cover lightly with dressing. Do not block drainage.

3. Check the neck and spinal cord. Maintain traction during your assessment. Look for pain or tenderness, deformity (protrusions or spaces), lacerations, bruises, swelling, and muscle spasm. In a conscious victim, muscle spasm will frequently cause automatic immobilization and pain. A cervical collar will help relieve discomfort and prevent further injury in both the conscious and unconscious victim. The **log roll** should be used along with head traction in order to move the victim and enable you to visually inspect the spine.
4. Check the extremities for paralysis. The loss of function occurs below the point of damage to the spinal cord; therefore, examine the lower extremities first. You should check the upper extremities regardless of what you discover about the lower extremities. Remember that fractures may have occurred in paralyzed limbs.

- **Communicative victim:**
  1. Can he/she feel your touch on the feet/hands and legs/arms?
  2. Can the victim wiggle his/her toes/ fingers and raise the extremities?
  3. Can the victim determine if his/her toes/fingers are being moved up or down?
  4. Can the victim apply counterpressure with the feet?
  5. Can the victim squeeze your hand? How strong is the grip?
- **Uncommunicative victim:**
  1. Using a pointed object, lightly jab the victim on the soles of the feet and the palms of the hands. If the entire length of the spinal cord is intact, the foot will retract. No reaction indicates either spinal cord damage or a deep **coma** state. If the paralysis is only on one side, the victim may have suffered a stroke.

## HEAD AND BRAIN INJURIES

Head injury is exceeded only by stroke as a cause of major **neurological trauma.** In one recent year, 114,000 accident deaths occurred in the United States, and head injury was primarily responsible for most of these deaths.

A **direct blow** may fracture the skull. A fracture may go undetected or may cause gross bleeding due to laceration of surface vessels from bone fragments. However, with a fracture, brain tissue damage may be less severe since more of the impact is absorbed

### EXAMPLES OF CERVICAL COLLARS

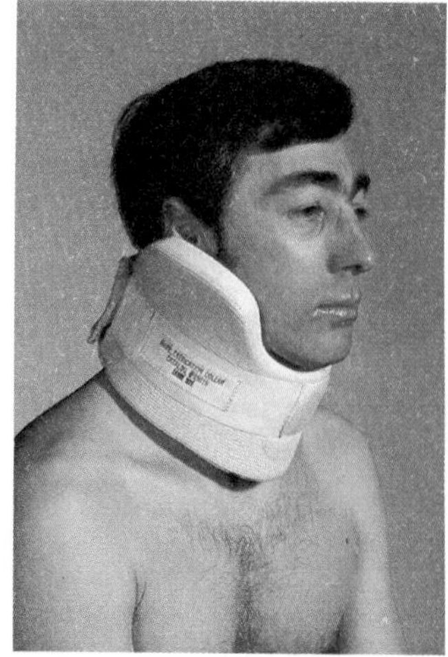

Hare extrication collar.

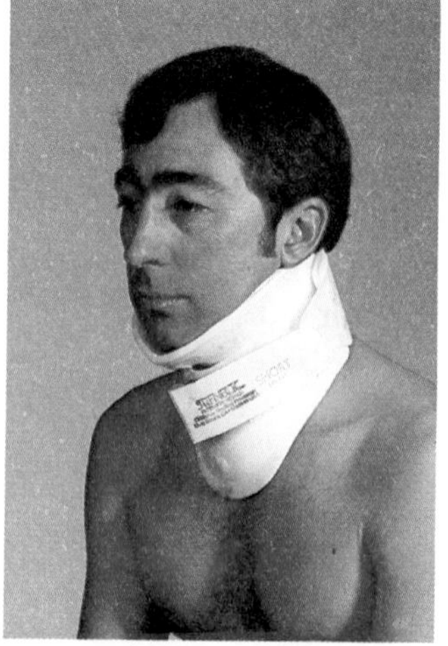

STIFNECK® cervical collar.

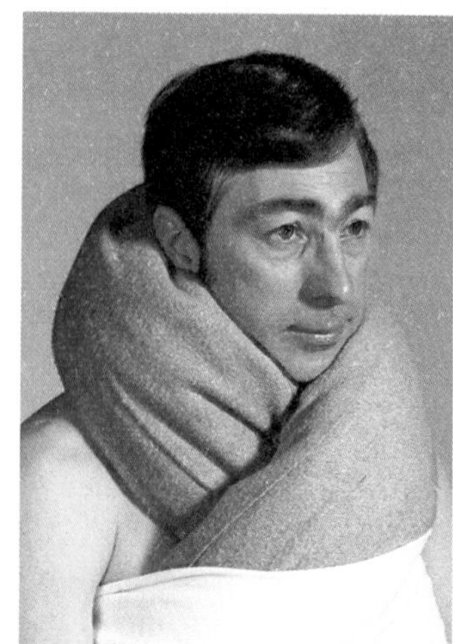

Improvised cervical collar.

than with no fracture. Fractures of the skull are common in accident victims. The seriousness of the fracture depends on the amount of injury to the brain. Serious brain injury is much more common when there is *no* skull fracture.

Rule of care — do *not* attempt to stop bleeding and cerebrospinal fluid from draining from the nose or ears when a skull fracture is suspected. Doing so may cause increased pressure on the brain.

## Skull Fractures

The most common injury to the skull is fracture — and the presence of a skull fracture does not necessarily mean that the brain has been damaged. In fact, serious brain injury occurs much more often when the skull has **not** been fractured.

There are two basic kinds of skull fracture: **open head injuries** and **closed head injuries.** An open head injury is one in which the skull and/or brain are exposed as a result of laceration of the scalp and destruction of the underlying tissues. In some cases, the scalp will be lacerated, the skull will be fractured, the membranes protecting the brain will be lacerated, and the brain itself may be extensively damaged. In other cases, the brain will be untouched. The severity of the injury depends on the mechanism and force of the injury.

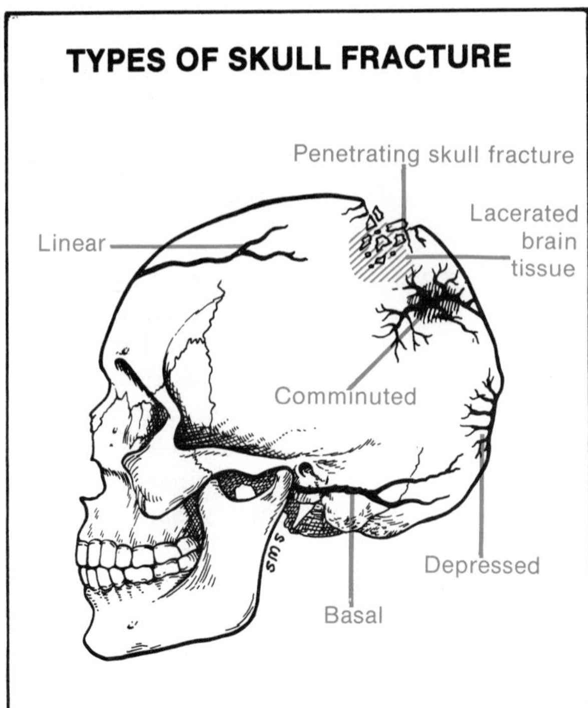


In a closed head injury, the scalp may be lacerated, but the skull remains intact. In other words, the injury results in no opening to the brain. While closed head injuries may *appear* to be uncomplicated, the brain damage is usually far more extensive than in an open head injury, because the force of the injury usually reverberates to the depths of the brain, causing hemorrhage.

Other categories of skull fractures include:

1. Linear. A thin-line crack in the skull is referred to as a **linear fracture.**
2. Comminuted. A **comminuted fracture** looks like a cracked egg or like the cracks that develop in a windshield when it is hit with a rock: a fracture appears at the point of impact, and multiple cracks radiate from the center of impact.
3. Depressed. A **depressed skull fracture,** caused by the impact of an object striking the head, causes fragments of bone to be driven into the membrane surrounding the brain or into the brain itself. A depressed skull fracture leaves an obvious deformity in the shape of the head. Depending on the force behind the injury, the bone fragments may simply lie against the brain, or they may lacerate the brain and penetrate deeply, causing extensive damage. Bullets almost always cause considerable damage, driving fragments of the skull deep into the brain.
4. Basal. A **basal skull fracture** — a break in the bed of the cranium — is extremely difficult to detect, even by X-ray. The damage from this type of fracture is usually extremely serious.

### Signs and Symptoms of Skull Fracture

Some skull fractures are obvious — the scalp has been lacerated, affording a view of the skull underneath, or the mechanism of injury strongly suggests the possibility. Most of the time, however, you will not be able to *see* a fracture. You should suspect skull fracture in a victim of head injury if any of the signs or symptoms shown in the illustration on the next page are present.

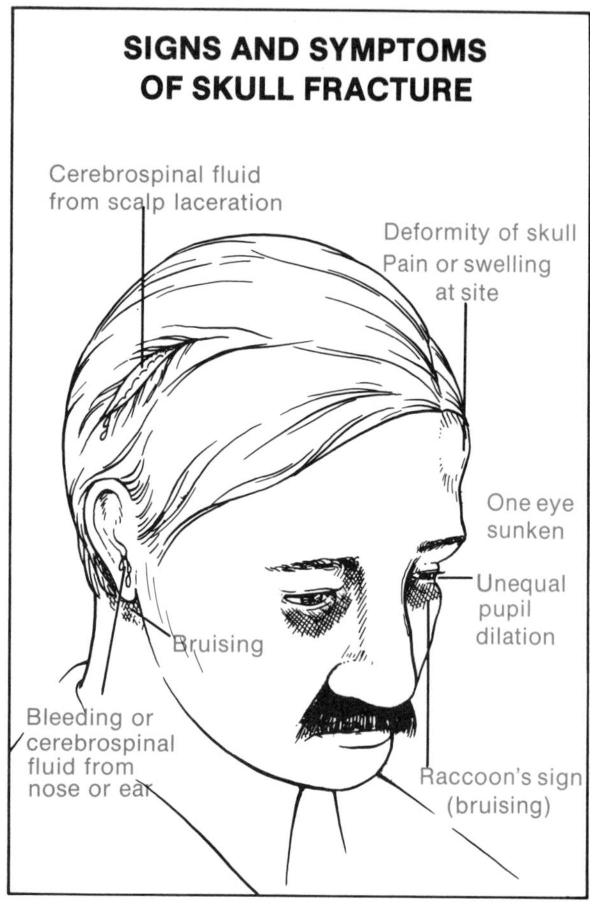


## Injuries to the Brain

Injuries to the brain are relatively common, because the brain tissue is extremely delicate and prone to injury from forces that are not extreme. Like all other body tissues, the brain is susceptible to injury from bruises, laceration, or pressure.

### Concussion

A temporary loss of the brain's ability to function, **concussion** is the most common but least serious head injury. Manifest by a brief loss of consciousness with following confusion and loss of memory, concussion can result from a strike on the head or face. Usually the brain has no observable damage. Victims may become verbally abusive and physically restless; many times, confusion prompts the victim to struggle against First Aiders and attempt to escape. Sometimes the victim will be totally unconscious, but this episode is almost always brief and usually does not recur.

In most cases of concussion, signs and symptoms disappear within forty-eight hours, and recovery is complete. The victim will usually experience **amnesia** (loss of memory) about the accident. If the victim cannot remember the events that *preceded* the accident, the injury is more serious. In rare cases, victims may suffer prolonged periods of unconsciousness, and some may die. In any concussion case, you should always be on the alert for signs and symptoms of more serious injury.

## Helmet Removal

In the event of an emergency situation where the victim is wearing some type of helmet and there is the possibility of head, neck, or cervical spine injury, attention must be paid to whether or not the helmet should be removed. If the victim is unconscious, it is a difficult task to remove the helmet; if the victim complains of increased pain when you are attempting to remove the helmet, it should be left on and the victim's head immobilized.

The various sizes, shapes, and configurations of helmets require some understanding of proper removal technique, for improper removal may aggravate head and cervical spine injury. The steps for removing a full face helmet are illustrated in this chapter.

## Emergency Care for Head Injuries

1. The first priority is to establish and maintain an adequate airway, because oxygen deficiency in the brain is the most frequent cause of death in a head injury.
    - Remove false teeth or bridges; assist drainage of any blood or mucous from the nose and mouth. If breathing is absent, shallow, or gasping, initiate mouth-to-mouth resuscitation. You may have to replace the false teeth to do this. If you suspect that spinal injury may have occurred, take great care when administering mouth-to-mouth ventilations; do not **hyperextend** the neck in the usual way. If the victim is not conscious and you are unable to determine the extent of injury to the spinal column, keep the head stationary. Fasten

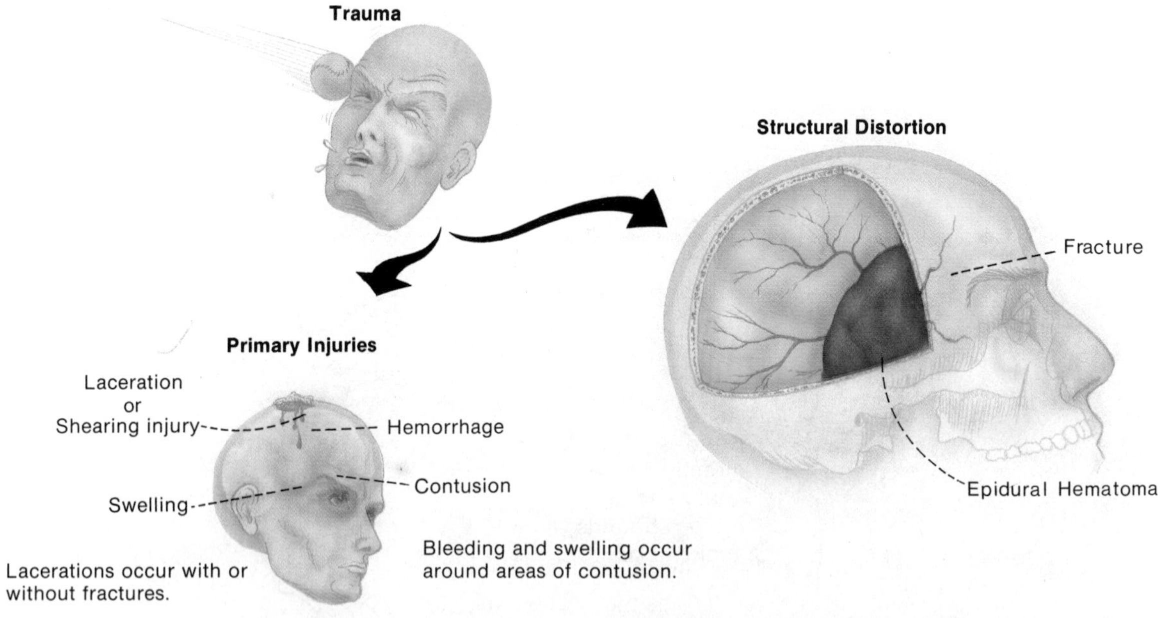


Lacerations occur with or without fractures.

Bleeding and swelling occur around areas of contusion.

**Secondary Factors**

Contusions with pressure may result in loss of consciousness.

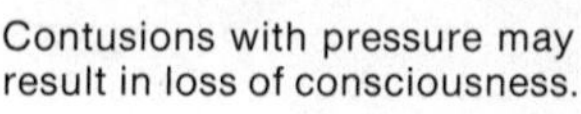

Respiratory and circulatory changes may result from primary brain injury.

Shock and low blood pressure can develop.

**Brain Damage**

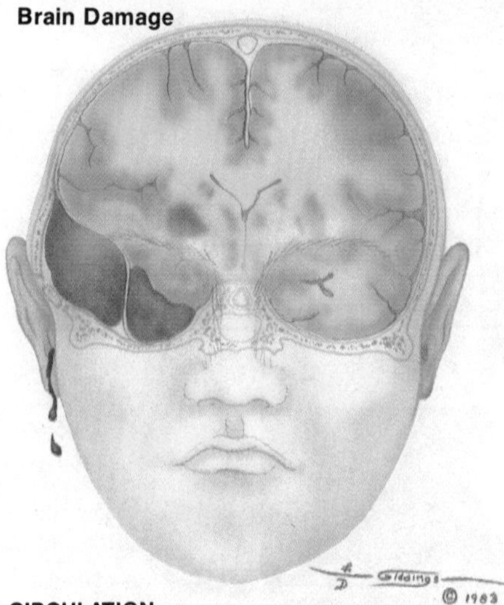

**Signs & Symptoms**

- -Deformity of the skull.
- -Drainage of spinal fluid or blood from nose and ears.
- -Black eyes.
- -Disorientation or confusion.
- -Unconsciousness or coma.
- -Unequal pupils or pupils that don't respond to light.
- -Partial or total paralysis.

Subdural and/or epidural hematomas and brain swelling lead to increased pressure on the brain.

**EMERGENCY CARE**

- **MAINTAIN OPEN AIRWAY AND CIRCULATION**
- **SUSPECT CERVICAL SPINAL INJURY AND USE CARE (MODIFIED JAW THRUST TECHNIQUE) FOR AIRWAY MAINTENANCE**
- **CONTROL BLEEDING BUT NOT DRAINAGE FROM NOSE AND/OR EARS**
- **DRESS AND BANDAGE OPEN WOUNDS — MINIMIZE PRESSURE**
- **POSITION VICTIM ACCORDING TO INJURY**
- **BE PREPARED FOR VOMITING**
- **IMMOBILIZE ON SPINEBOARD IF SPINAL DAMAGE LIKELY**
- **TREAT FOR SHOCK — AVOID OVERHEATING**
- **CALM AND REASSURE VICTIM**
- **MONITOR VITAL SIGNS**
- **CALL FOR EMERGENCY MEDICAL AID**

## HEAD INJURY & BRAIN DAMAGE

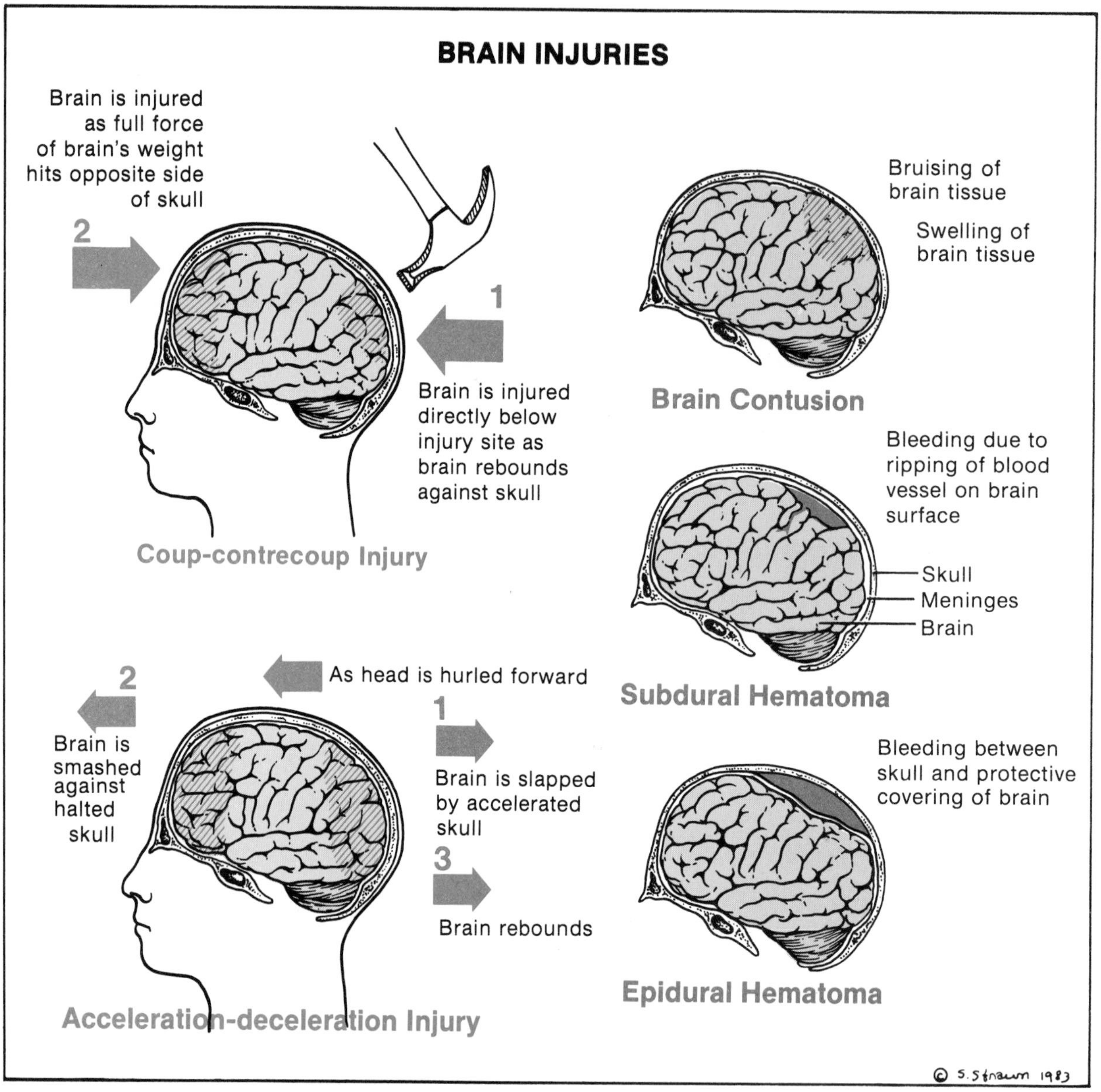

## BRAIN INJURIES

Brain is injured as full force of brain's weight hits opposite side of skull

2

1

Brain is injured directly below injury site as brain rebounds against skull

Coup-contrecoup Injury

2

As head is hurled forward

1

Brain is smashed against halted skull

Brain is slapped by accelerated skull

3

Brain rebounds

Acceleration-deceleration Injury

Bruising of brain tissue

Swelling of brain tissue

Brain Contusion

Bleeding due to ripping of blood vessel on brain surface

Skull

Meninges

Brain

Subdural Hematoma

Bleeding between skull and protective covering of brain

Epidural Hematoma



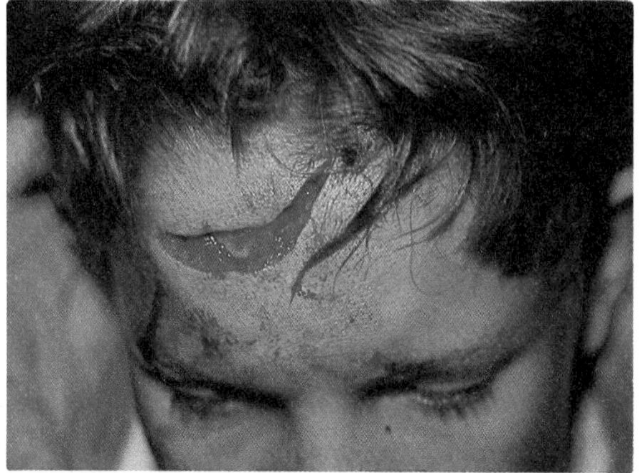

Always suspect and assess for spinal injury in a head-injured patient.

the victim to a spineboard, and support the head with sandbags.

2. The secondary priority is to control any external hemorrhage resulting from scalp or forehead lacerations.
   - Apply direct pressure over the wound with a sterile cloth to stop bleeding.
   - Secure the dressing with a roller bandage. The dressing *must* be as **sterile** as possible.
   - If evidence indicates a depressed fracture, apply pressure only at the edges of the fracture, over intact bone.

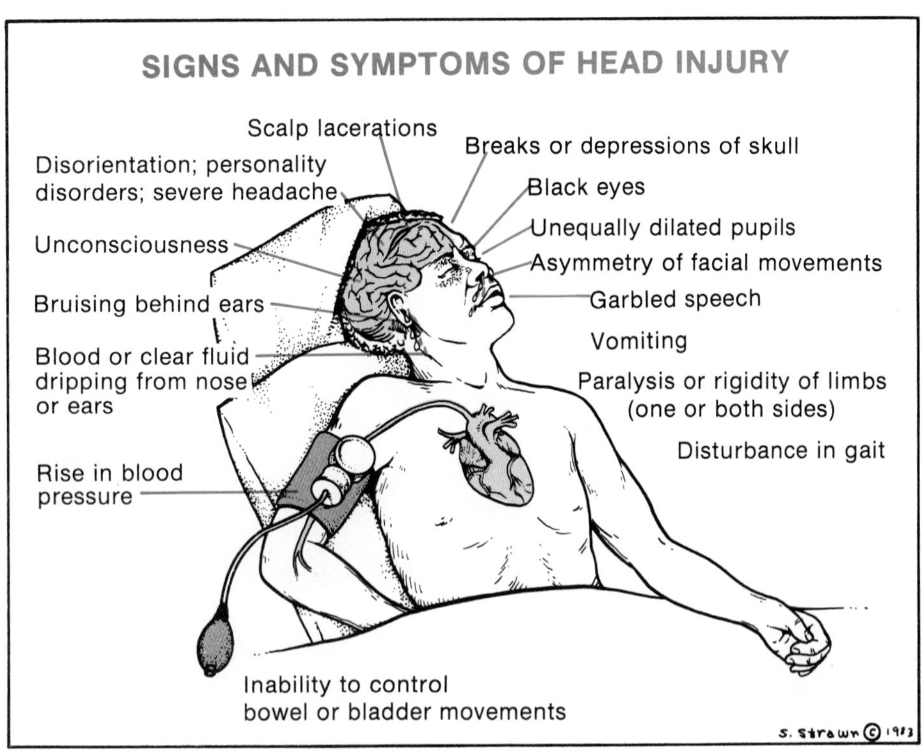


- When you apply pressure or dressings to control bleeding, avoid moving the victim's neck or back.
- If the victim has an open skull fracture, place a sterile dressing loosely over the wound; it will aid in clotting but will not obstruct drainage and create pressure. Never apply direct pressure if there is evidence of bone fragments, and never attempt to stop the flow of cerebrospinal fluid or blood from the nose or ears.

3. Keep the victim in a supine position, and give the victim care for shock. **Shock is rarely caused by the head injury itself,** but it can complicate the situation and lead to severe illness or death. Assist ventilations if necessary.
4. Victims with head injuries may become violent and/or combative. The victim may even have signs of intoxication and/or drug use that can be attributed to a head injury. The victim may require restraint, necessitating the aid of other rescuers. Even in the combative victim, proper consideration for spinal injuries must be exercised.
5. Any unconscious victim with a brain injury should also be suspected of having a cervical spinal injury. About 10 percent of those who are unconscious after a fall or automobile accident have sustained an injury that causes damage to the spinal cord.
6. Maintain gentle traction on the head and neck, and apply a cervical collar or support whenever spinal cord damage is a possibility. If in doubt always immobilize.
7. Avoid overheating the victim — brain damage causes the body temperature to rise, and increased temperature leads to additional brain damage. If you are in a warm climate, strip away as many of the victim's clothes as you can, and place the victim where air currents will blow over his/her body. If the temperature increases, sponge the victim off with cool water or place a cool compress on the forehead.
8. Send for emergency medical assistance as soon as possible.

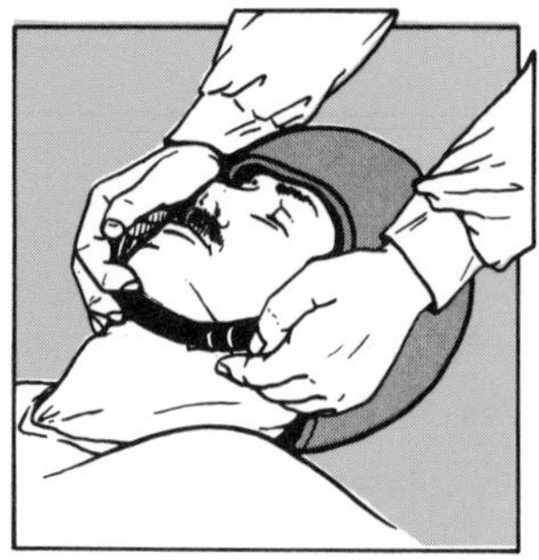
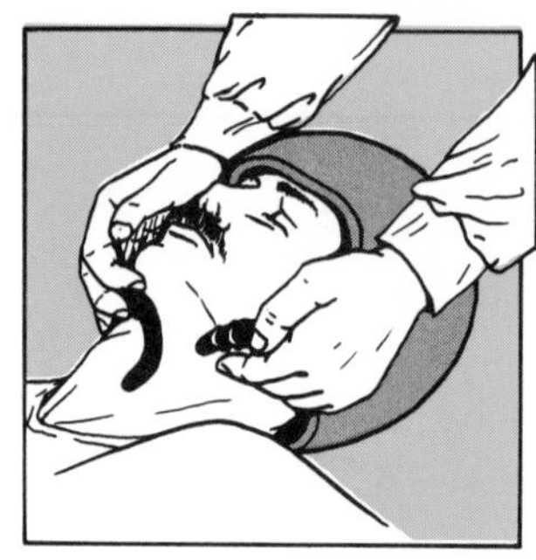
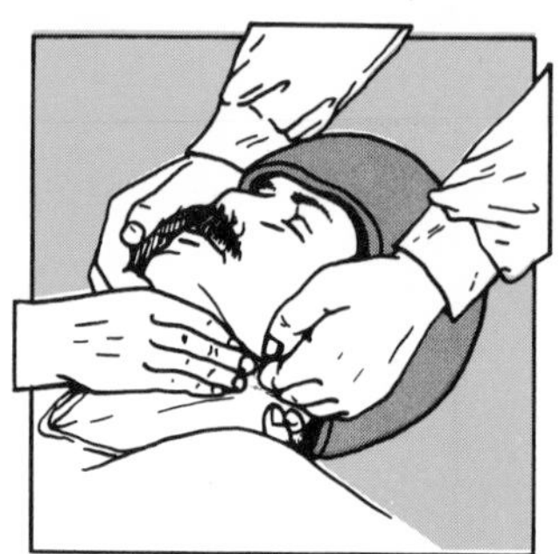
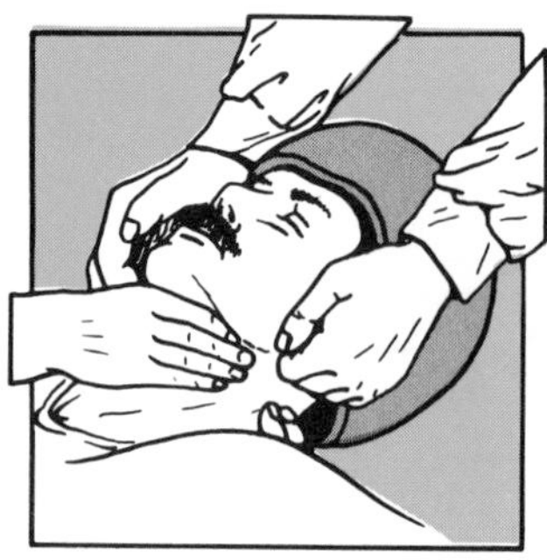
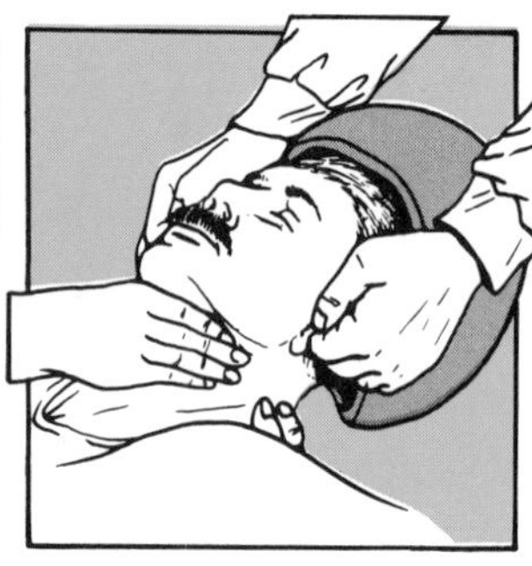
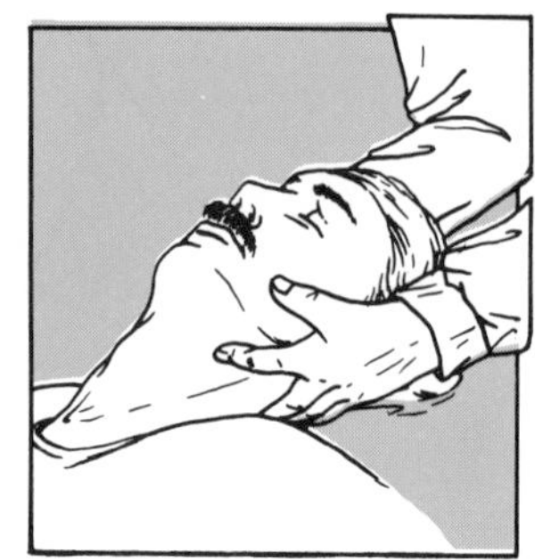
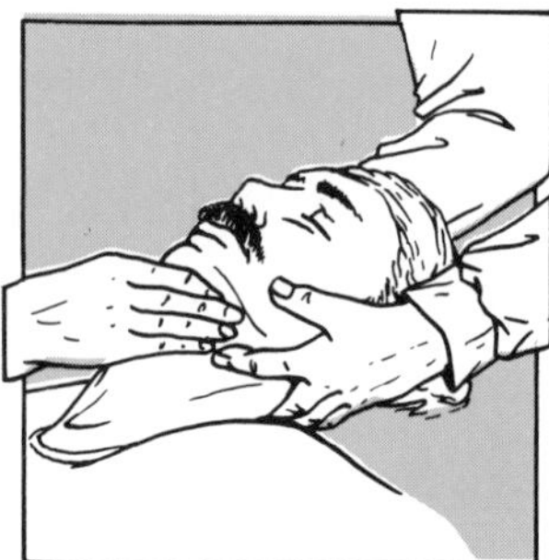

**Removing a helmet from injured victim.**
Beginning at upper left: (1) One rescuer applies in-line traction by placing the hands on each side of the helmet with the fingers on the victim's mandible. This position prevents slippage if the chin strap is loose. (2) The rescuer cuts or loosens the chin strap while maintaining in-line traction. (3) A second rescuer places one hand on the victim's mandible, with the thumb on one side and the long and index fingers on the other. Pressure is applied from behind the neck with the other hand. (4) The rescuer at the top of the victim's head removes the helmet, keeping the following in mind: The helmet may have to be expanded to clear the ears; the victim's glasses should be removed if the helmet is the full-face type. (5) The second rescuer continues to maintain in-line traction from the neck and jawbone area to prevent head tilt. (6) When the helmet is removed, the rescuer at the top of the victim's head replaces the hands on either side of th victim's head with the palms over the victim's ears. (7) In-line traction is maintained from above the victim's head until a backboard and head and neck supports are in place.
**Helmet removal can be dangerous and should not be performed by a First Aider unless absolutely necessary.**

## SPINAL CORD INJURIES

The spinal column may be damaged by disease or by injury. If any of the vertebrae are crushed or displaced, the spinal cord at that point may be squeezed, stretched, torn, or severed. Movement of the disabled part by the injured person, or careless handling by well-meaning but uninformed persons, may result in displacement of sections of the spinal column, causing further injury to the cord and possibly resulting in permanent paralysis.

### Emergency Care for Spinal Cord Injuries

1. The first priority is to establish and maintain an adequate airway. Do not straighten the victim's neck if it is twisted unless it obstructs the breathing. Then, extend the neck only to the degree necessary to maintain an airway.
2. Assist ventilations as needed.
3. Use gentle traction on the head. If you encounter any resistance, stabilize the neck in position; lift the tongue forward by the modified jaw thrust technique. Immobilize the victim's head and neck with a cervical collar or with heavy, rolled cloths. Sandbags can help limit neck motion.
4. Check the victim's pulse and circulation. Take measures to maintain or establish the heartbeat if necessary, but do not move the victim. Keep the victim covered to avoid heat loss, but do not overheat.

## SIGNS OF POSSIBLE SPINAL CORD INJURY

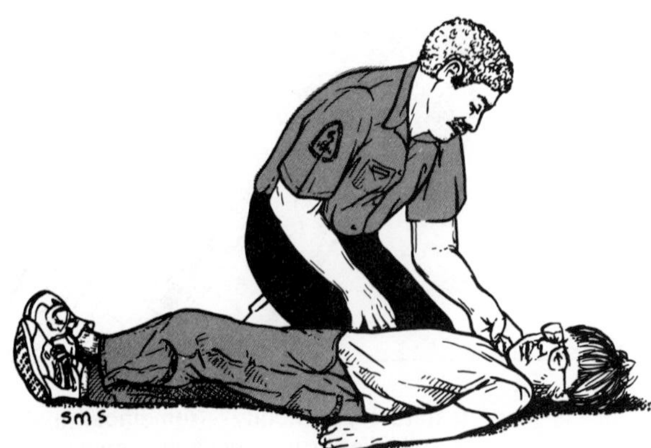


**Pain.** The victim may be aware of pain in the area of injury.

**Tenderness.** Gently touching the suspected area may result in increased pain.

**Deformity.** Deformity is rare although there may be an abnormal bend or bony prominence.

**Cuts and bruises.** Victims with neck fractures will have cuts and bruises on the head or face. Victims with injuries in other spine areas will have bruises on the shoulders, back or abdomen.

**Paralysis.** If the victim is unable to move or feels no sensation in some part of his body, he may have a spinal fracture.

**Painful movement.** If the victim tries to move, the pain may increase - never try to move the injured area for the victim.

STEPS FOR CHECKING SIGNS AND SYMPTOMS

| CONSCIOUS VICTIMS | UNCONSCIOUS VICTIMS |
|---|---|
| • Ask: what happened? where does it hurt? can you move your hands and feet? can you feel me touching your hands (feet)? can you raise your legs and arms?<br>• Look: for bruises, cuts, deformities.<br>• Feel: for areas of tenderness, deformities, sensation.<br>• Have victim move, if he can do so comfortably.<br>• The victim's strength can be determined by having him squeeze the First Aider's hand or by checking pressure against the foot. | • Assess for breathing.<br>• Look: for cuts, bruises, deformities.<br>• Feel: for deformities, sensation.<br>• Ask others: what happened?<br>• Probe the soles of the feet, then the palms of the hands with a sharp object to check for response. |

**See Photos in Victim Assessment chapter on assessing conscious and unconscious victims for possible spinal cord injury.**

5. When helping prepare for transport, immobilize the victim. If he/she must be turned, turn the body as a unit — preferably in a log roll using at least three people. Immediately prior to transport and as soon as possible in the course of the emergency rescue, immobilize the victim with a long spineboard. Make sure that any additional method used to render the victim immobile — such as sandbags — does not interfere with breathing. If you have no equipment at all, maintain immobility of the victim's head with your hands, and elicit help from others trained in emergency rescue. **If possible it is best to leave spinal cord immobilization to professional rescue personnel.**

## CHEST INJURIES

The two general categories of chest injury are **closed injuries** and **open injuries.** In closed chest injuries, the skin is not broken. This type of injury commonly occurs from the blunt trauma of being struck by a falling object, being buried in a cave-in, or being thrown against a steering wheel in an automobile accident. Although the skin may not sustain any lacerations, serious underlying damage can occur, especially lacerations to the tissues of the heart and lungs caused by broken ribs.

In an open chest injury, the skin is broken, usually by a bullet or knife or by the end of a

## EMERGENCY CARE FOR SUSPECTED SPINAL INJURY

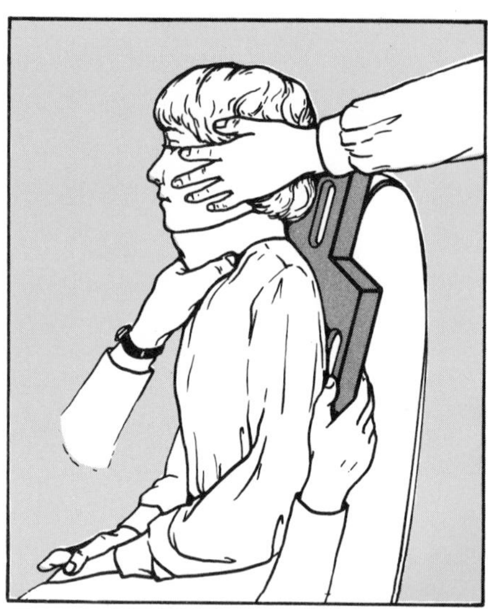

Take every precaution against converting a **spine injury** into **cord damage.** In vehicular accidents, immobilize cervical spine before removing victim (spine board, cervical collar, rolled blanket, etc.). Advise the conscious victim **not to move the head.** A helmet should be removed unless there is difficulty in removing it, increased pain, or the victim is unconscious. In such cases, immobilize on spine board with helmet in place.

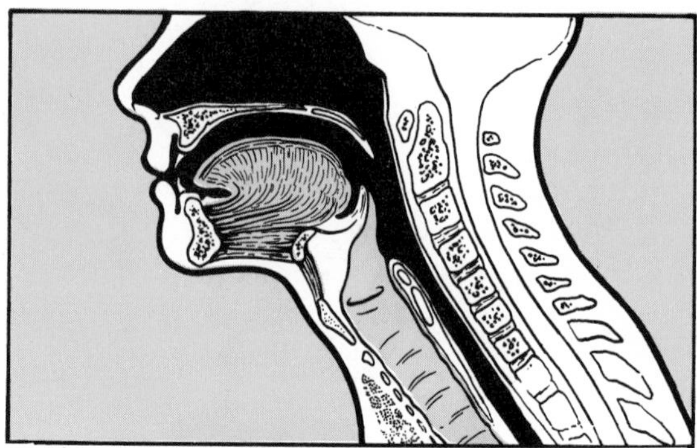

Is there respiratory difficulty? Remember that the airway has first priority. If resuscitative measures are indicated, support the head, immobilize the neck, and move the victim to a flat surface **with help.** Check the mouth for obstruction (dentures, tongue, etc.), and begin mouth-to-mouth breathing giving all care to minimize motion of the neck. Check for severe bleeding and control by direct pressure. If necessary, initiate CPR.

Keep in mind that respiratory paralysis may occur with cervical spine injury and that death may rapidly occur if respiratory assistance is delayed. Unless it is necessary to change a victim's position to maintain an open airway or there is some other compelling reason, it is best to splint the neck or back in the original position of deformity.

Be alert for shock.

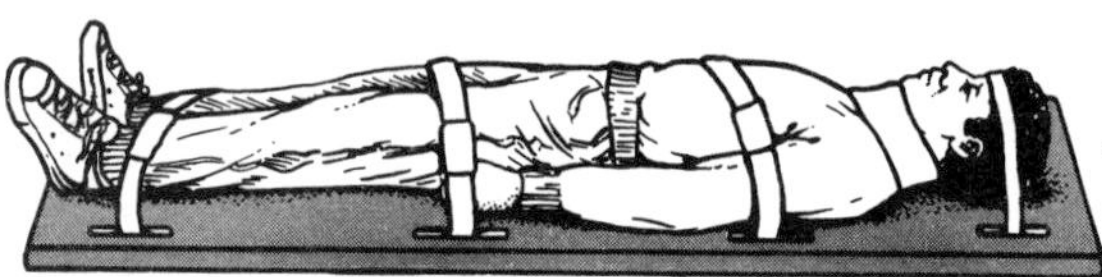

Immobilize victim before moving. As soon as possible, transfer to a firm stretcher or spine board and restrict head mobility with tape, sandbags, collar, rolled towels, and/or blankets.

Provide emotional support, and get emergency medical assistance as soon as possible.

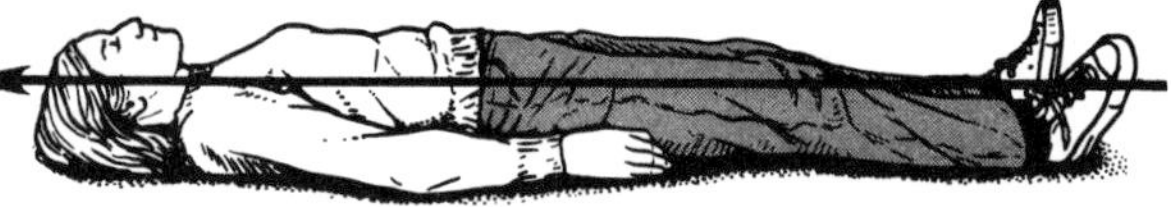

Always support the head in neutral alignment with body. Avoid flexion and rotation.

broken rib protruding through the skin. Although the skin is broken, the same injuries may be present as if the injury were closed (that is, lacerations to the heart and lung tissues).

### Flail Chest

Flail chest results when the chest wall becomes unstable due to fractures of the **sternum** (breastbone), cartilage connecting the

## THREE-RESCUER LOG ROLL FOR SPINAL INJURY

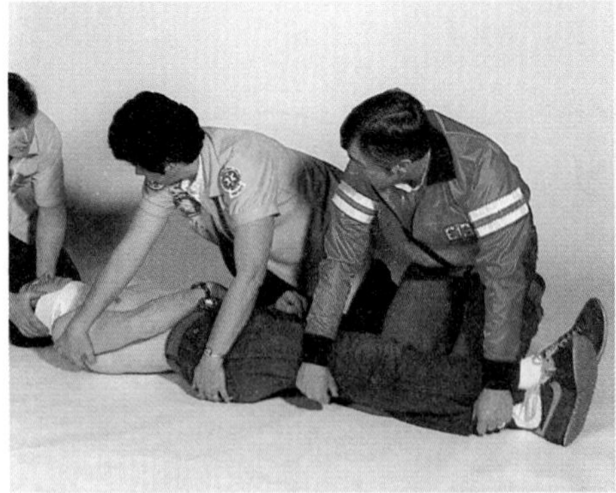
1
Maintain head and neck traction while preparing for log roll.

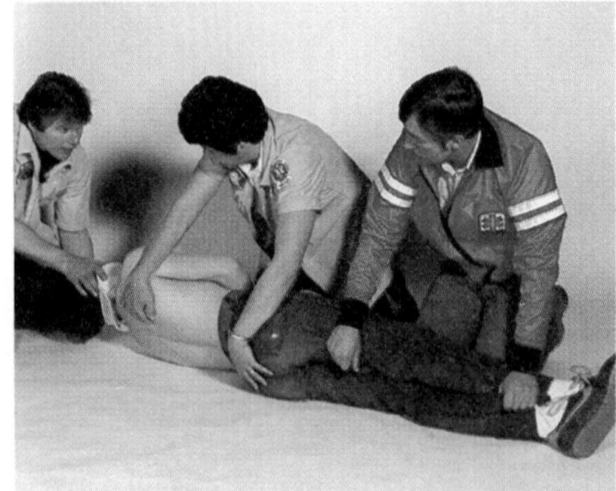
2
Roll victim onto side at command of rescuer maintaining traction.

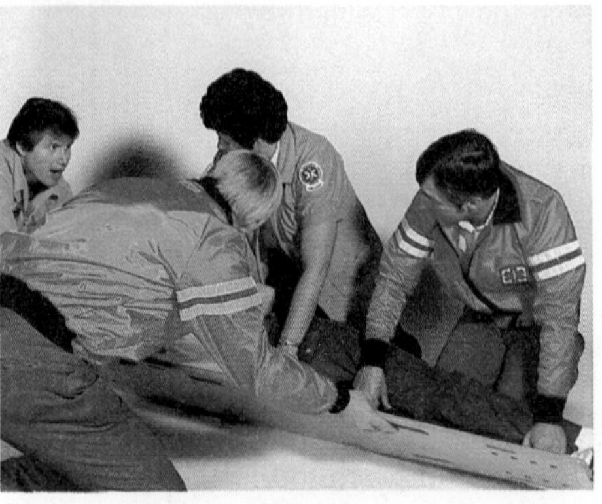
3
Move spineboard into place.

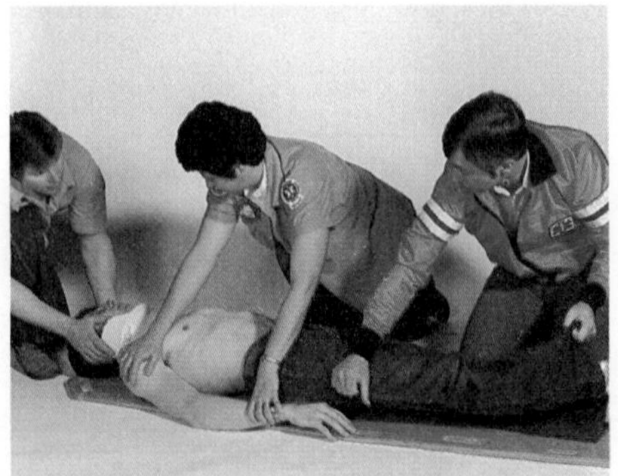
4
Lower victim onto spineboard at command of rescuer maintaining in-line traction.

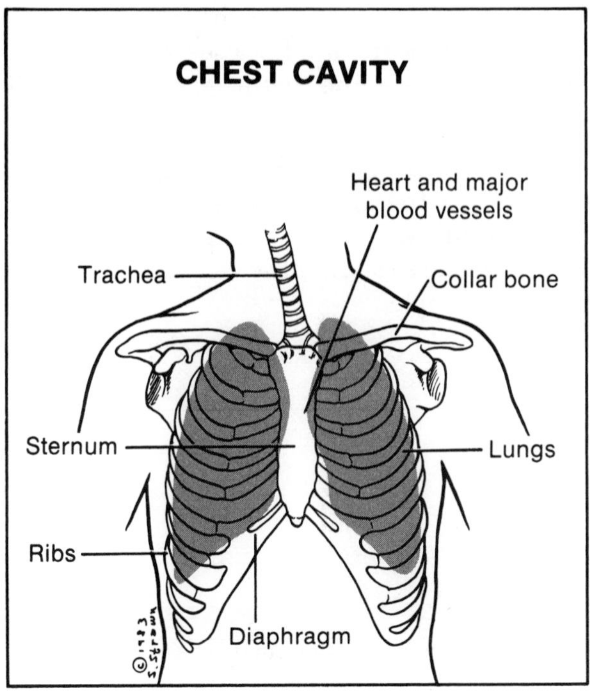


The rib cage encloses the lungs and heart, and damage to the ribs can result in damage to these organs, as can penetrating injuries that do not injure the ribs.

ribs to the sternum, and/or the ribs. It can affect the front, back, or sides of the rib cage.

Flail chest is a result of blunt trauma to the chest. Three or more ribs break, and the part of the chest wall that lies over the break area collapses (called the "flail area"). The motion of that area is opposite the motion of the remainder of the chest. When the victim inhales, the area does not expand; when exhaling, it protrudes while the rest of the chest wall contracts **(paradoxical breathing).**

## FLAIL CHEST: PARADOXICAL BREATHING

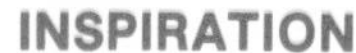

EXPIRATION

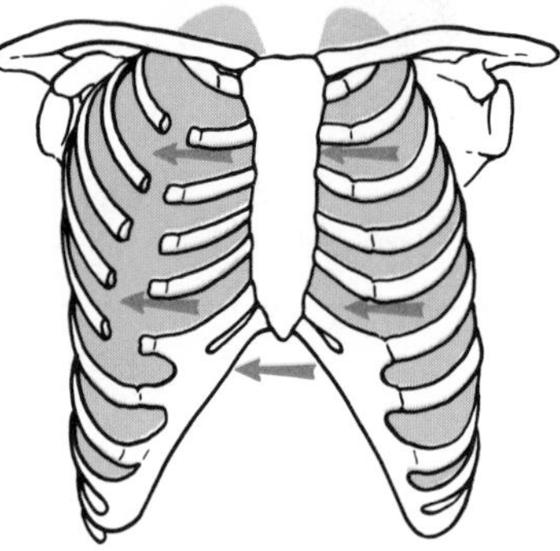

Injured chest wall moves out
Uninjured chest wall moves in

INSPIRATION

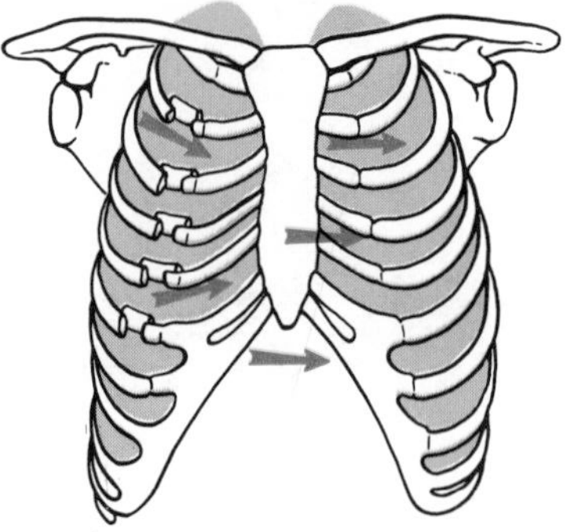

Injured chest wall collapses in
Uninjured chest wall moves out

### EMERGENCY CARE

Have victim lie on back.

Remove clothing from chest area.

Tape a small pillow, sandbag or thick, heavy dressing over the injury site.

Maintain open airway and assist ventilations as needed.

Treat for shock.

Regularly monitor vital signs.

Victim should be in semi-sitting position if you suspect internal bleeding, or if the victim has increased pain and discomfort in semi-sitting position keep victim lying on the injured side.

Send for emergency medical aid as soon as possible.

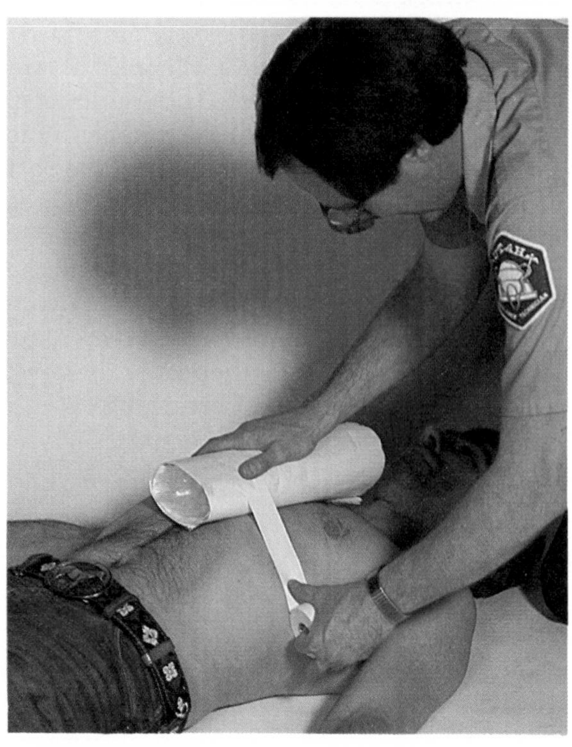

Stabilize flail chest by applying sandbag and taping in place.

To check for flail chest, have the victim lie on his/her back. Bare the chest and stand at his/her feet, watching for a seesaw motion of the chest while the victim breathes. If flail chest has occurred:

1. Maintain an open airway.
2. Stabilize the chest with a sandbag or pillow secured with tape and placed over the injured area so that the victim will be more comfortable.

## COMMON SIGNS AND SYMPTOMS OF CHEST INJURY

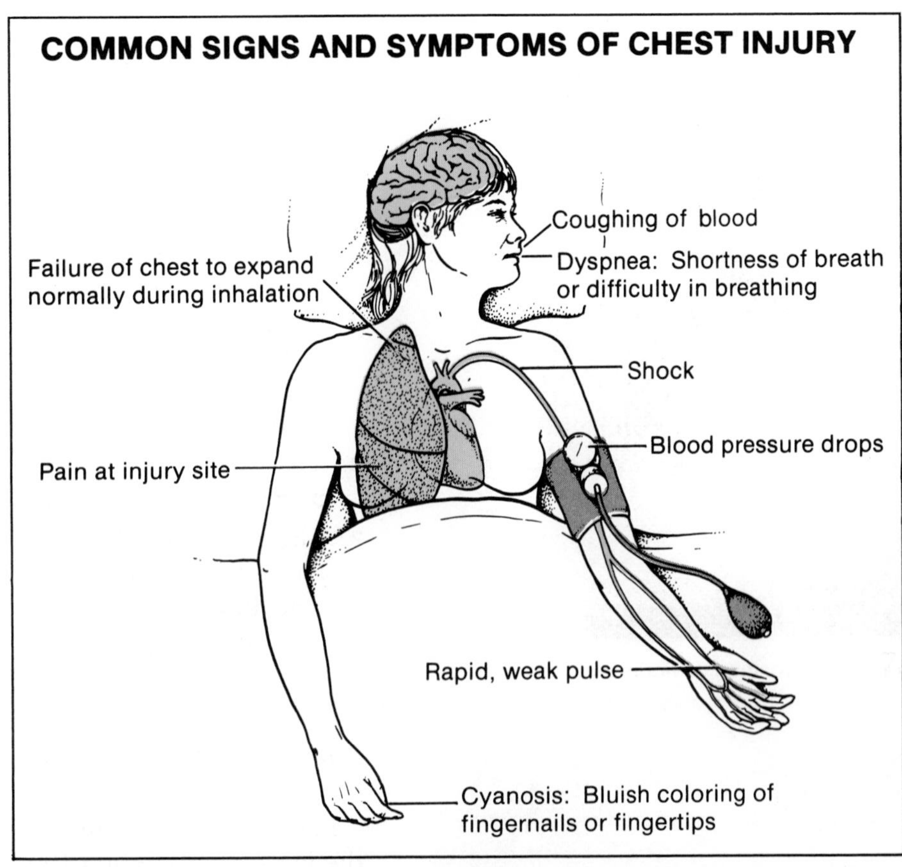


### BROKEN RIBS

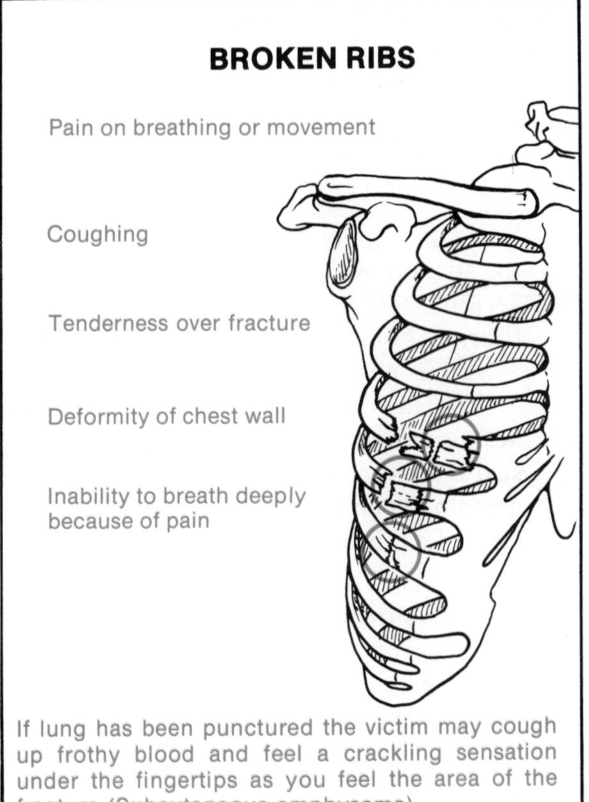


If lung has been punctured the victim may cough up frothy blood and feel a crackling sensation under the fingertips as you feel the area of the fracture (Subcutaneous emphysema).

## Broken Ribs

Direct blows or blunt trauma to the chest often result in fractured ribs — usually those in the middle of the rib cage. The upper ribs are difficult to fracture, because they are protected by the bony shoulder girdle, and the lower ribs are not attached to the breastbone and can withstand greater impact.

The most common symptom of rib fracture is pain at the fracture site. It usually hurts the victim to move suddenly, to cough, or to breathe deeply. The victim may want to hold a hand over the area, since immobilization sometimes offers pain relief. Deformity may or may not be present.

If only one rib has been fractured, and if no danger exists of the simple fracture lacerating the lung or heart, the chest is usually not bound. For cases of more serious or a multiple fracture:

1. Apply three cravat bandages or one elastic bandage around the chest to support the ribs. Center the first bandage immediately below the site of the pain. Place the second

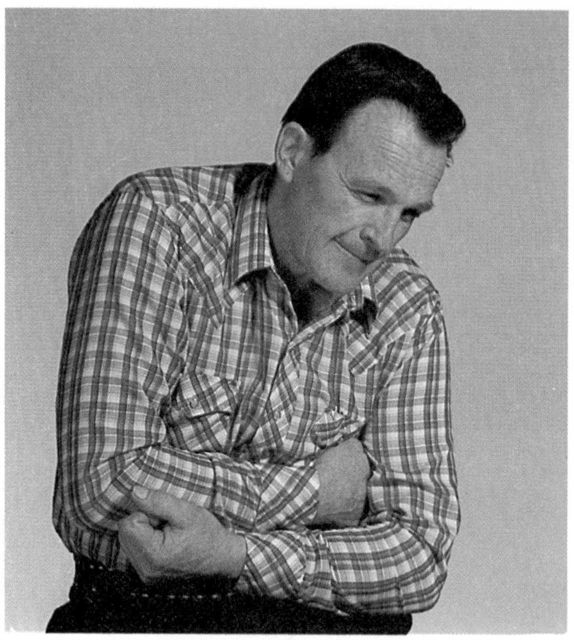

Typical "guarded" position of victim with rib fractures.

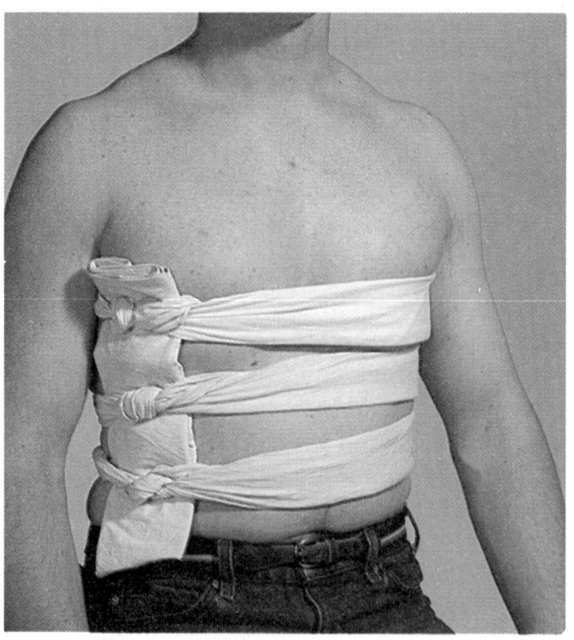

Immobilizing fractured ribs.

bandage above the site of the pain. Place the third bandage around the lower half of the victim's chest to restrict movements and relieve pain.

2. Have the victim exhale.
3. Tie the two bandages over a pad on the uninjured side before allowing the victim to inhale. This will reduce the movement of the ribs caused by breathing.
4. Make sure that the bandages are snug but that they do not interfere with breáthing.

**OR**

1. The chest should not be wrapped when the ribs are depressed and/or frothy blood comes from the victim's mouth. These may be indications of a punctured lung. An open wound from the outside to the lung should be covered immediately with a nonporous material.
2. The victim should be given a pillow or blanket to hold against the fractured ribs.
3. The victim should be placed in a semiprone position with the injured side down. This will allow more room for expansion of the uninjured lung.

## Sucking Chest Wounds

In open chest wounds, air sometimes enters the chest cavity when the chest is expanded during the victim's normal breathing and moves through the wound as the victim inhales, since the air remains in the chest cavity outside the lungs. When the victim exhales, the air is forced back out of the wound. Each time the victim breathes, a sucking sound is produced as the air passes.

1. You **must** apply an airtight dressing over the sucking wound immediately to prevent serious respiratory problems (pneumothorax). You can use any material available — gauze, aluminum foil, plastic wrap, etc. — held in place with a pressure dressing. Your goal should be to create an airtight seal over the wound. Make sure that the dressing is large enough so that it will not be sucked into the wound.
2. If you seal the sucking chest wound and the pressure continues to increase (indicated by continued breathing problems), try releasing the dressing for a few seconds to see if the pressure is released.
3. Place the victim in a sitting up or "lying on the injured side" position.
4. Call for emergency aid immediately.

## SUCKING CHEST WOUND

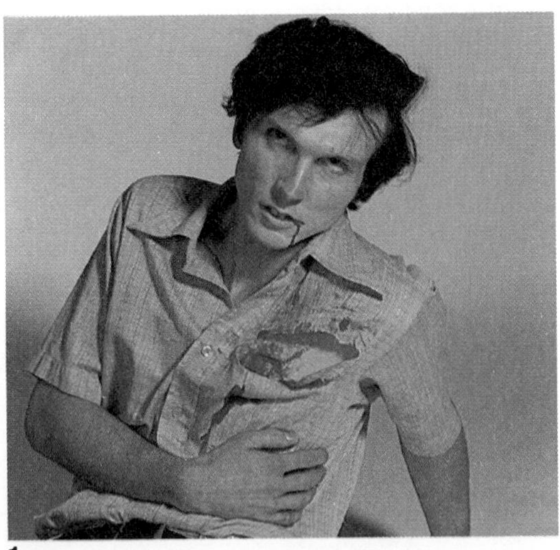

1
Sucking chest wound and possible pneumothorax.

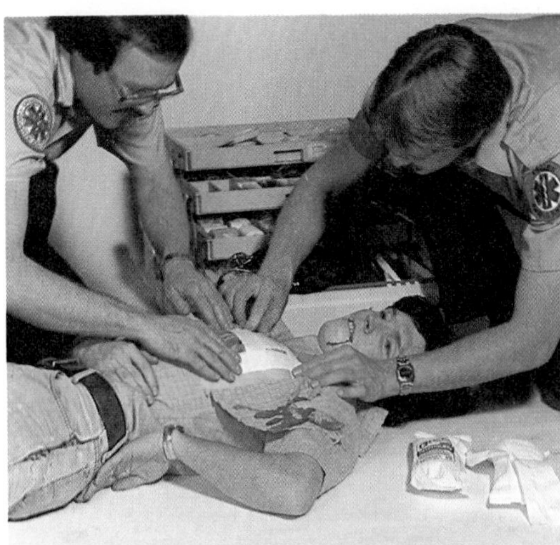

2
Position occlusive covering over dressing.

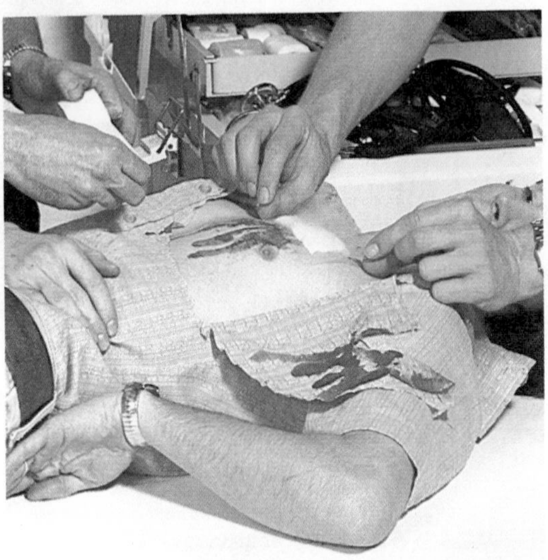

3
Tape dressing and occlusive covering in place.

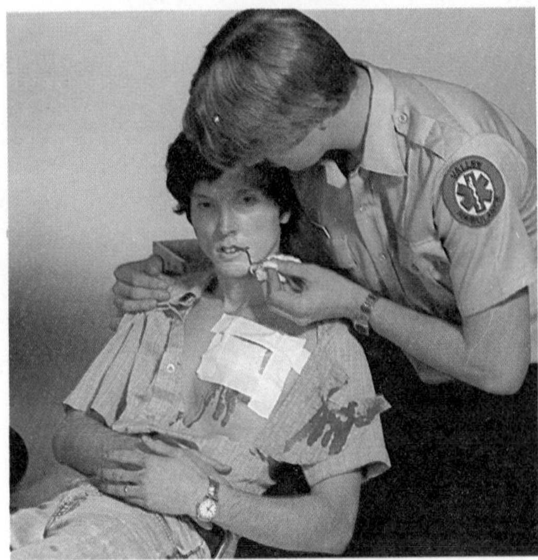

4
Position victim to ease breathing.

### Sucking Chest Wounds

**Pneumothorax results when air enters the chest cavity but does not enter the lung from the wound site. The pressure of the air in the chest cavity presses against the lung, causing it to collapse.**

**Air can enter the chest cavity in two ways: (1) from a sucking wound that allows air to enter from outside; or (2) from air that leaks out of the opposite lung due to laceration. Once the lung is compressed, it does not expand properly with breathing, and within minutes the victim suffers from a lack of oxygen. (In some cases, called spontaneous pneumothorax, the lung does not collapse because of injury, but because a weak area on the surface of the lung ruptures. The weakened lung loses its ability to expand, and the victim experiences sharp chest pain and breathing difficulty.)**

**If you seal the sucking chest wound and the pressure continues to increase, indicated by continued breathing problems, try releasing the dressing for a few seconds to see if the pressure is released. Then reseal.**

## Abdominal Eviscerations

An **evisceration bandage** is used when an abdominal laceration wound has resulted in a protrusion of the abdominal contents. In such cases:

1. For all abdominal injuries, suspect shock and work to prevent it.
2. Constantly monitor vital signs.
3. Do **not** touch protruding organs.
4. Do **not** try to replace organs within the abdomen.
5. Cover the organs with a moist, clean, sterile dressing. Use sterile gauze compresses if available, and moisten them with clear water or saline.
6. Cover the compresses with clean aluminum foil (to retain moisture and warmth).
7. Gently wrap the compresses in place with a bandage or clean sheet, and have the victim transported in a lying down position with knees up.
8. Call for emergency medical aid immediately.

### ABDOMINAL EVISCERATION

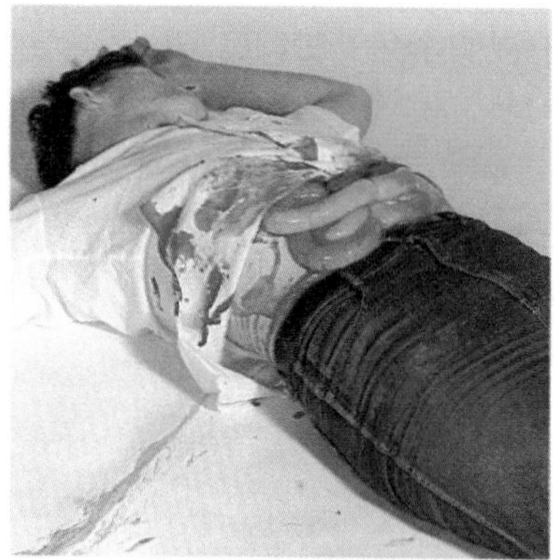

1
Abdominal evisceration — an open wound resulting in protrusion of intestines.

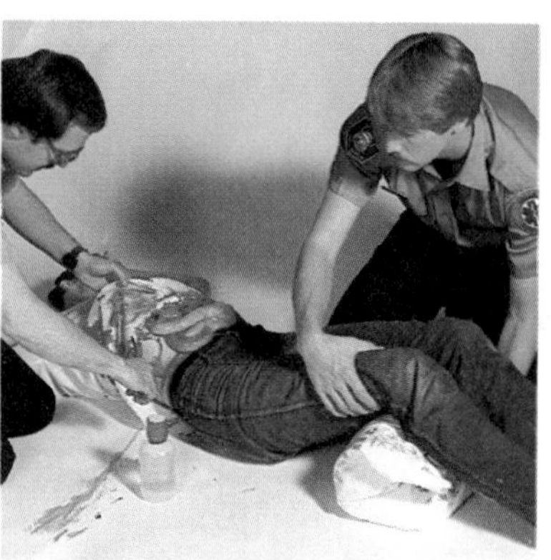

2
Cut away clothing from wound and support knees in a flexed position.

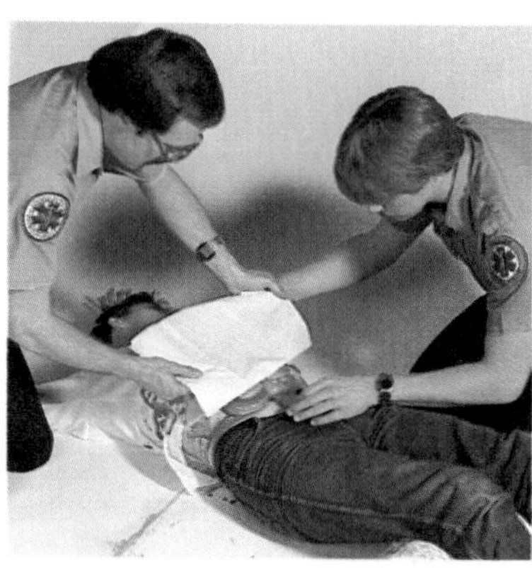

3
Place dressing over wound. **Do not attempt to replace intestines within abdomen.**

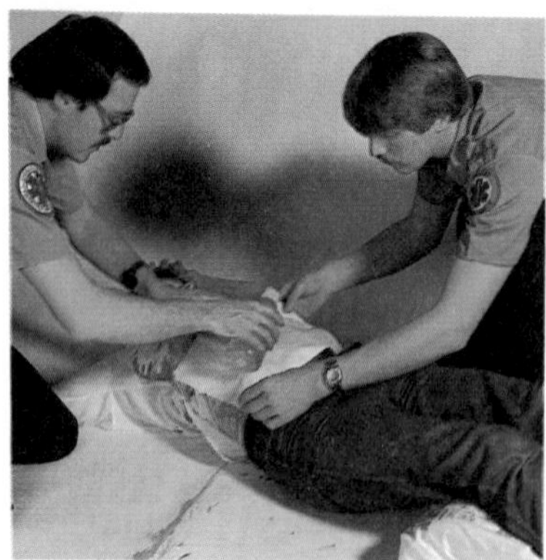

4
Moisten dressing with clean water.

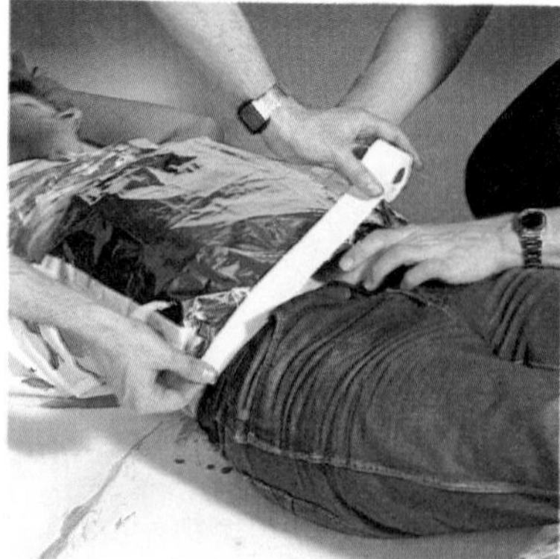

5
Gently and loosely tape the dressing in place, then apply an occlusive material such as aluminum foil or plastic wrap. Tape loosely over dressing to keep dressing moist.

## SUMMARY — GENERAL SIGNS AND SYMPTOMS OF CHEST WOUNDS

- Obvious trauma
- Chest or back pain at injury site
- Dyspnea: shortness of breath and difficulty in breathing
- Cough, with or without frothy blood
- Failure of chest to expand normally during respiration
- Marked cyanosis of fingernails and tips and/or tongue and lips
- Rapid weak pulse
- Low blood pressure
- Shock
- Sudden sharp pain which may be referred to shoulder, across chest and to abdomen
- Deviation of larynx and trachea from midline
- Distended neck veins
- Sucking sound when victim breathes
- Bloodshot and bulging eyes
- Purplish blue color of the head, neck and shoulders
- These signs may be indicative of serious emergency, however usually only few of the signs will be manifested at any one time.

## SUMMARY — EMERGENCY CARE FOR CHEST WOUNDS

- Remove clothing to assess for open wounds; always check for an exit wound on back.
- Maintain an open airway and assist with ventilation.
- Seal any open sucking wounds with an airtight dressing (plastic wrap, aluminum foil, vaseline, gauze, etc.). Tape all edges snugly. If necessary, seal the wound with your bare hands until proper dressing can be prepared.
- Be alert for tension pneumothorax. If it develops unseal the dressing for a few seconds to release pressure, then reseal.
- Do not remove impaled objects; stabilize with bulky dressings and bandage in place.
- Care for other bleeding and wounds with direct pressure and appropriate dressings, bandaged in place.
- Treat for shock.
- Continually monitor vital signs.
- Calm and reassure victim.
- Be alert for vomiting, secretions of blood from the mouth. Prevent aspiration and allow proper drainage.
- Put the victim in semi-reclining positions or lying on his injured side if breathing is easier and/or you suspect internal bleeding.
- Call for emergency medical aid immediately.

# Work Exercises

## Head and Spine Injuries

The assessment should begin with the primary survey. Treat any unconscious person as if a spinal injury is present.

Complete the following table by indicating what procedures, cautions and signs you would look for in each phase of the survey.

### The Assessment

| Phase of Survey | Procedures, Cautions and Signs |
|---|---|
| Maintain Airway | |
| Examine Head<br>Skull<br>Bruising<br>Eyes & Pupils<br>Ears & Nose<br>Face<br>Mouth | |
| Examine Neck and Spinal Cord | |
| Examine Extremities for Paralysis | |

### Helmet Removal

In the event of an emergency situation where the victim is wearing a helmet of some type, attention must be paid to whether or not the helmet should be removed.

When do you leave a helmet on?

List four guidelines for removal of a helmet:

1.

2.

3.

4.

## Skull Fractures and Brain Injuries

Match the correct definition with each of the terms.

| Terms | Definition or Care |
|---|---|
| ______ 1. Linear fracture | A. Bruising of the brain |
| ______ 2. Comminuted fracture | B. Break in the bed of the cranium |
| ______ 3. Depressed fracture | C. Temporary loss of the brain's ability to function |
| ______ 4. Basal fracture | D. Impact of an object striking the head |
| ______ 5. Concussion | E. Thin-line crack in the skull |
| ______ 6. Contusion | F. Looks like a cracked egg or like the cracks that develop in a windshield |
| ______ 7. Subdural hematoma | |
| ______ 8. Epidural hematoma | G. Injury involves bruising of the brain just beneath the site of trauma as the skull rebounds against it from a blow. |
| ______ 9. Coup-contrecoup | |
| ______ 10. Acceleration-deceleration | H. When the head is hurled forward or stopped abruptly. |
| | I. Bleeding between the brain and its protective covering. |
| | J. Blood from the arteries pools between the skull and protective covering of the brain. |

## Signs and Symptoms that Manifest Head Injury

Match the signs and symptoms with the correct descriptive terms.

| Signs & Symptoms | Descriptive Terms that may Indicate Head Injury |
|---|---|
| ______ 1. Pulse | A. In an adult, usually begins an hour or more after head injury. |
| ______ 2. Temperature | B. Inability to control |
| ______ 3. Limbs | C. Asymmetry |
| ______ 4. Blood Pressure | D. Slowing |
| ______ 5. Vomiting | E. Slowing and increase |
| ______ 6. Bowel and bladder | F. Slow or rapid |
| ______ 7. Facial movements | G. Severe |
| ______ 8. Headache | H. Rigid |
| ______ 9. Pupils | I. Rise |
| ______ 10. Battle's sign | J. Unequal size |
| | K. Bluish tinge of skin surrounding ear |

## Signs/Symptoms and Assessing Spinal Cord Injuries

Describe the steps in testing conscious and unconscious victims for possible spinal cord injuries.

| Signs and Symptoms | Testing the Conscious Victim |
|---|---|
| 1. Weaknesses or paralysis below the level of injury | 1. |
| 2. Absolute loss of function in either the lower or upper extremities | 2. |
| 3. Absence of bowel or bladder control | |
| 4. Loss of response to pain or other stimuli | 3. |
| 5. Pain | |
| 6. Tenderness | 4. |
| 7. Painful movement | |
| 8. Lacerations or bruising | 5. |
| 9. Spinal deformity | |
| 10. Impaired breathing | **Testing an Unconscious Victim** |
| 11. Position of the arms. A victim with arms across chest or raised above head may have a spinal cord injury. | 1. |
| | 2. |
| 12. Loss of bladder or bowel control. | 3. |
| | 4. |
| | 5. |

## Chest Injuries

The two general categories of chest injury are open and closed injuries. Both categories of injuries have similar symptoms. Label the following diagram that illustrates common signs and symptoms associated with chest injury.

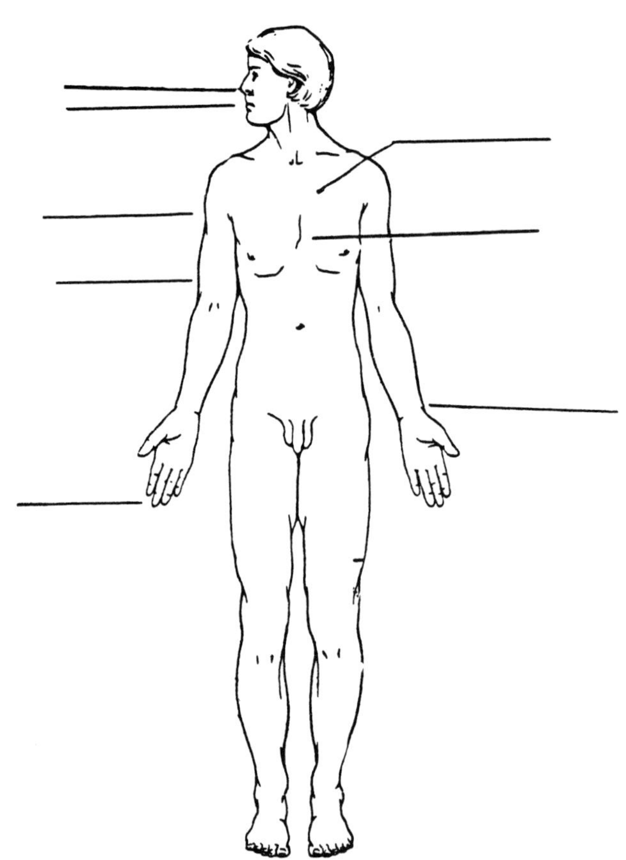

## SELF-TEST

### Part I: True and False

If you believe the statement is true, circle the T. If you believe the statement is false, circle F.

T F 1. Clear or blood-tinged cerebrospinal fluid may drain from the nose or ears for several days after a skull fracture.

T F 2. If cerebrospinal fluid is draining from the nose or ears, they should be packed with dressings to prevent further fluid loss.

T F 3. Constricted pupils of the same size is a common symptom of head injury.

T F 4. It is not uncommon for a head-injury victim to have a loss of bowel and bladder control.

T F 5. A linear skull fracture is one in which pieces of bone are pushed inward, pressing on brain tissue.

T F 6. If cerebrospinal fluid from a skull fracture is draining from an ear, you should turn the victim on his/her injured side and let the fluid run freely from the ear.

T F 7. If you suspect that a victim has sustained brain injury, have him/her lie on his/her back with the head lower than the rest of the body.

T F 8. A spinal injury should be suspected in vehicular accidents or falls.

T F 9. Stimulants, such as coffee or amphetamines, should be given to a head injury victim to prevent him/her from going into a coma.

T F 10. The First Aider should not remove foreign objects in the brain.

T F 11. It is better to do nothing than to mishandle victims of possible spinal injuries.

### Part II: Multiple Choice

For each question, circle the answer that best reflects an accurate statement.

1. To maintain an airway for a person you suspect has a spinal injury:
   a. have a trained professional perform a tracheotomy
   b. use the chin lift or jaw thrust technique
   c. hyperextend the neck
   d. administer oxygen

2. What is one way the First Aider can test the conscious victim for spinal cord damage?
   a. help the victim get up to see if he/she can walk
   b. ask the victim to wiggle his/her fingers
   c. hold a burning match close to the victim's foot to see if he/she moves it
   d. ask the victim to read something (a billboard, newspaper headline, etc.)

3. To examine the extremities for paralysis in an unconscious victim, you would:
   a. lightly jab the soles of the feet and palms of the hands with a pointed object and watch for retraction
   b. hold an ice cube or lit match close to the extremity and watch for retraction
   c. test reflexes at the knee or elbow
   d. there is no way to test for paralysis in an unconscious victim

4. Brain damage is usually far more severe in a/an ________________ than in a/an ________________.
   a. closed head injury, open head injury
   b. open head injury, closed head injury
   c. basal skull fracture, depressed skull fracture
   d. stroke, comminuted fracture

5. A comminuted skull fracture is one where:
   a. the fracture is not in the area of impact or injury
   b. the skull is depressed
   c. scalp laceration and brain laceration are present
   d. multiple cracks radiate from the center of impact.

6. A sure sign of brain damage is:
   a. pain and swelling
   b. bruises, especially on the face beneath the eyes
   c. unequal pupils
   d. none of the above are sure signs of brain damage

7. A contusion of the brain resulting from a blow to the skull is called:
   a. coup-contrecoup
   b. acceleration-deceleration
   c. concussion
   d. none of the above

8. When a foreign object is impaled in the skull, the First Aider should:
   a. not remove the object, but carefully stabilize it in place
   b. remove the object and apply a loose sterile dressing
   c. not remove the object unless it will hinder transportation
   d. remove the object and pack the wound carefully with sterile pads

9. In a head laceration where the injury causes an opening to the brain, you should:
   a. apply direct pressure to the laceration to stop the bleeding
   b. lightly cover the laceration but do not pack it to restrict bleeding or fluid flow
   c. apply direct pressure to the laceration but release it periodically to reduce pressure in the brain
   d. cover with an occlusive dressing to prevent contamination

10. If the clear, water-like cerebrospinal fluid is coming from the ears and nose, the First Aider should:
    a. pack all openings firmly so that no fluid is lost.
    b. pack the ears, and allow the nose to drain
    c. keep victim's head low to help drainage
    d. cover the openings with a loose dressing

11. Which of the following is out of order with respect to helmet removal?
    a. in-line traction is applied from above the victim's head
    b. the helmet is removed
    c. in-line traction is reestablished from above the victim's head
    d. in-line traction is transferred below the victim's head with pressure on the jaw and neck area

12. When a victim has a bleeding, open head wound, the First Aider should:
    a. apply a snug pressure bandage
    b. apply a loose sterile dressing to aid the clotting process
    c. apply pressure to the carotid artery
    d. lightly apply pressure to the wound with sterile dressings

13. Two general categories of chest wounds are:
    a. open and closed
    b. simple and compound
    c. fracture and puncture
    d. lung-related and heart-related

14. Which of the following is *not* a sign or symptom of chest injury?
    a. shortness of breath
    b. cyanosis of the lips and nails
    c. coughing up blood with coffee grounds appearance
    d. failure of one or both sides of the chest to expand

15. A flail chest is a result of:
    a. a broken rib
    b. a perforated lung
    c. a broken sternum or three or more broken ribs
    d. a sharp, penetrating puncture wound to the chest

16. Paradoxical breathing occurs when:
    a. compression injuries cause gasping breaths interspersed with extremely shallow breathing
    b. lack of oxygen from a compressed lung
    c. air remains in the chest cavity outside the lungs
    d. the motion of the injured chest area is opposite the motion of the remainder of the chest

17. To stabilize flail chest:

    a. apply an airtight dressing over the flail area
    b. place a sandbag or pillow over the flail area and secure with tape
    c. put sandbags on either side of the patient's chest and bandage in place
    d. maintain the victim in a semireclining position

18. With multiple rib fracture, a First Aider should:

    a. not bind the chest as a general rule
    b. put the arm over the injured rib in a sling and bind it to the chest
    c. bind the chest with swaths to prevent unnecessary movement
    d. strap the victim's arm (or arms) to his/her chest with a swathe to immobilize the area

19. You have bandaged a sucking chest wound. The victim then manifests such symptoms as bulging neck veins, bulging chest wall above the collarbone and between the ribs, and low blood pressure, you would:

    a. lie the victim flat and raise the feet
    b. release the dressing for a few seconds to see if pressure is released
    c. suspect internal hemorrhage of other organs
    d. give positive pressure ventilations

20. The primary consideration in treating a sucking chest wound is:

    a. stopping the air leak
    b. controlling the bleeding
    c. treating for shock
    d. preventing infection

21. Which of the following is *not* an appropriate material to use for treatment of a sucking chest wound?

    a. plastic wrap
    b. aluminum foil
    c. Vaseline, gauze pads
    d. single layer gauze

22. Eviscerated organs should be:

    a. replaced within the abdomen
    b. covered with a dry cloth
    c. covered with a moist sterile dressing
    d. rinsed thoroughly with copious amounts of water and replaced within the abdomen

Corresponds with:
**American Red Cross**
**Standard First Aid & Personal Safety**
Chapter 14, pages 195-224
and
**Advanced First Aid & Emergency Care**
Chapter 13, pages 155-201

# 10
# Bone and Joint Injuries

Injuries to muscles, joints, and bones are some of the most common situations that First Aiders encounter. These injuries can range from the simple and non-life-threatening — such as a broken finger or sprained ankle — to the critical and life-threatening — such as a multiple break of the femur or a fracture of the neck or spine. Whether the injury is mild or severe, your ability to provide first aid efficiently and quickly may prevent further painful and damaging injury and may even keep the victim from suffering permanent deformity or death.

First aid for **fractures, dislocations,** and **soft tissue injuries** within the first four hours following injury is critical in preventing permanent disabilities. An immediate assessment of the victim is essential so that concealed injury is not overlooked.

## TENDONS AND LIGAMENTS

A tendon is connective tissue that attaches muscle to bone. Ligaments connect bone to bone.

## THE SKELETAL SYSTEM

The skeletal system has four major functions:

- It gives shape or form to the body.
- It supports the body, allowing it to stand erect.
- It provides the basis for locomotion, or movement, by giving muscles a place to attach, and it contains joints that allow movement (where bones are joined together by ligaments).
- It forms protection for major body organs, such as the brain (skull), the heart and lungs (rib cage), pelvic organs, and the spinal cord (vertebrae).

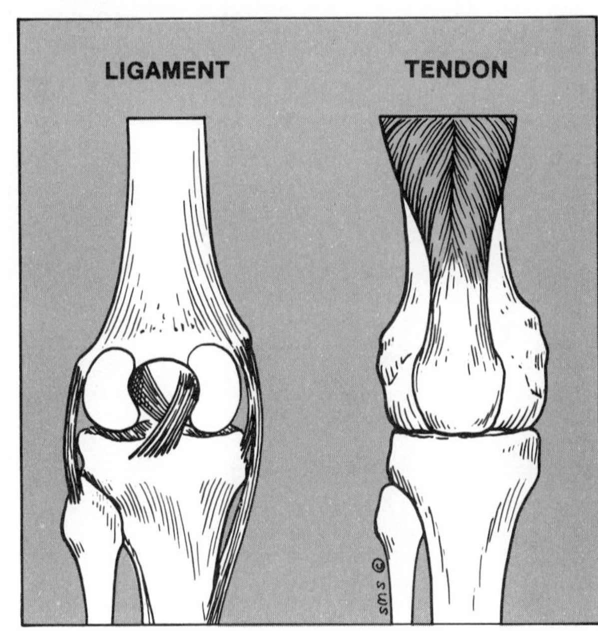


Comparison of a ligament and a tendon

## TYPES AND MECHANISMS OF INJURY TO MUSCLES, JOINTS, AND BONES

The four major types of injuries that occur to the musculoskeletal system are:

1. **Sprains** — injuries in which ligaments are stretched and partially torn, usually due to

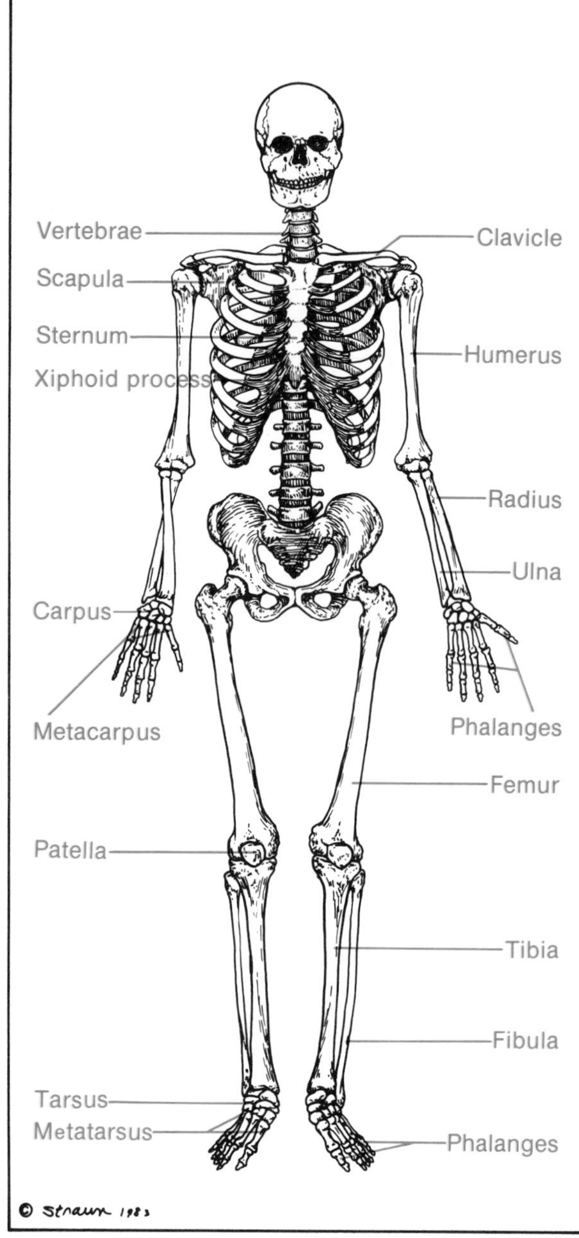


The skeletal system.

sudden twisting of a joint beyond its normal range of motion.

2. **Strains** — soft tissue injuries or muscle spasms around a joint.
3. **Dislocations** — displacement of a bone end from a joint.
4. **Fractures** — one or more breaks in a bone.

## Emergency Care For Sprains

1. Place the joint at absolute rest in an elevated position. If the sprain is at the ankle or knee, do not allow the victim to walk or stand on the injury. Do not remove the victim's shoe until ice is available, but loosen the shoelaces.
2. Pack the sprained area in ice to reduce swelling, control internal bleeding, and reduce pain. Do **not** apply heat. Remember to cover the affected joint with a towel, etc., to avoid **frostbite.**
3. Apply a **pillow** or **blanket splint,** then transport.

## Emergency Care For Strains

1. Place the victim in a comfortable position, such as in a reclining position with the knees drawn up to take pressure off of the back muscles.
2. If the victim does not have to be moved, apply heat directly to the strained area.
3. Have the victim get plenty of rest on a firm mattress, possibly with a board support beneath it.

## Emergency Care For Dislocations

1. DO NOT try to straighten, or reduce, the dislocation.
2. Splint above and below the dislocated joint to maintain stability.
3. Place a cold pack of some type on the dislocation, and transport carefully to a medical facility.

## Emergency Care For Fractures

1. Quiet the victim as much as possible. Have the victim sit or lie down.
2. Control any possible bleeding.
3. Carefully splint the fracture with the appropriate splint, considering the materials you may have on hand. Guard against causing a closed fracture to become an open fracture.
4. Treat for shock and either carefully transport or call for an ambulance

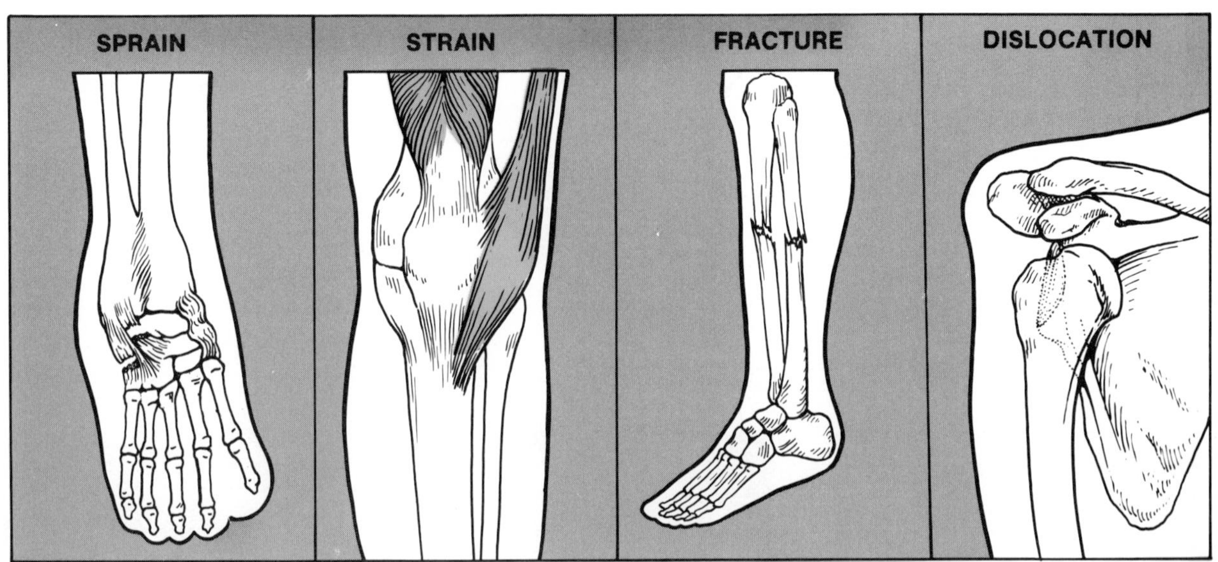


## Signs and Symptoms of Common Orthopedic Injuries

| Sprain | Strain | Fracture | Dislocation |
|---|---|---|---|
| pain on movement<br>tenderness<br>painful movement<br>swelling<br>redness | - acute,<br>tearing<br>radiating pain<br>- stiffness and<br>pain when affected<br>part is moved.<br>- spasm and pain in<br>the strain area. | pain, tenderness<br>deformity<br>loss of use<br>swelling<br>bruising<br>grating<br>exposed bone ends | pain<br>deformity<br>loss of movement |

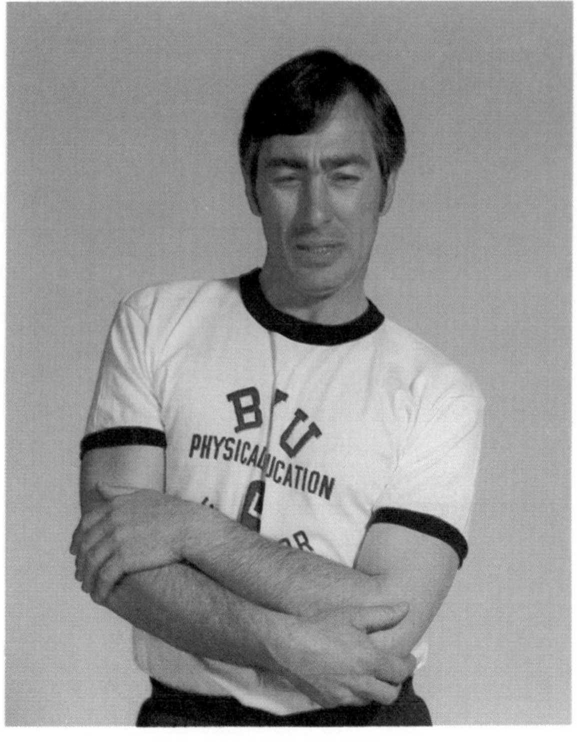

A victim manifesting the signs of a dislocated shoulder.

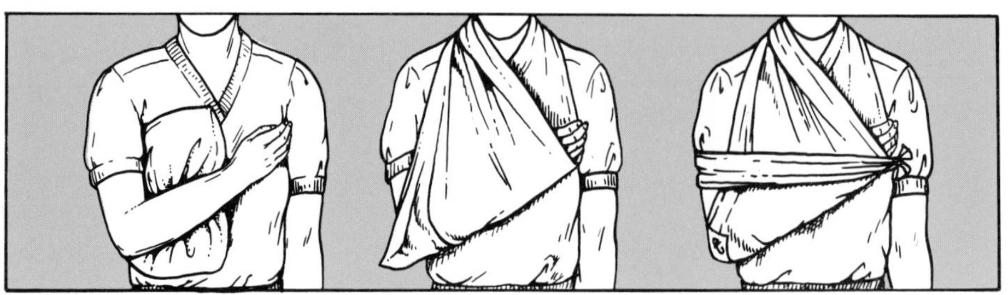

Immobilizing dislocation of shoulder. *Left:* position of cravat with pad; *Right:* position with sling. Cravat can be positioned over sling if desired.

## CLOSED AND OPEN FRACTURES

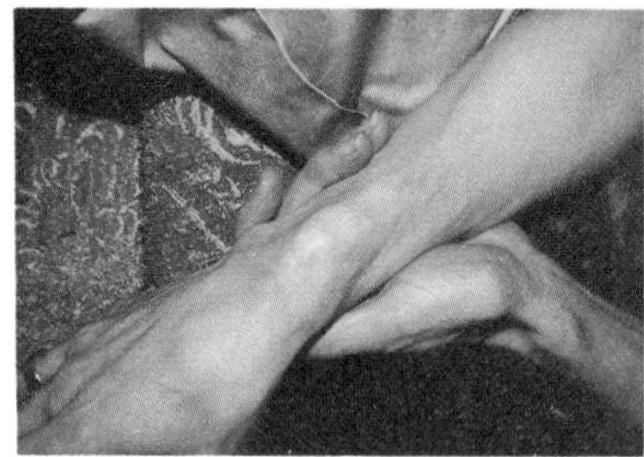

Closed fracture of the radius.

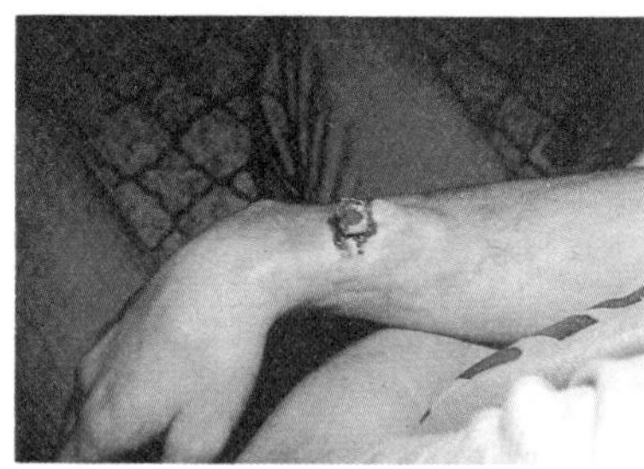

Open fracture of the radius.

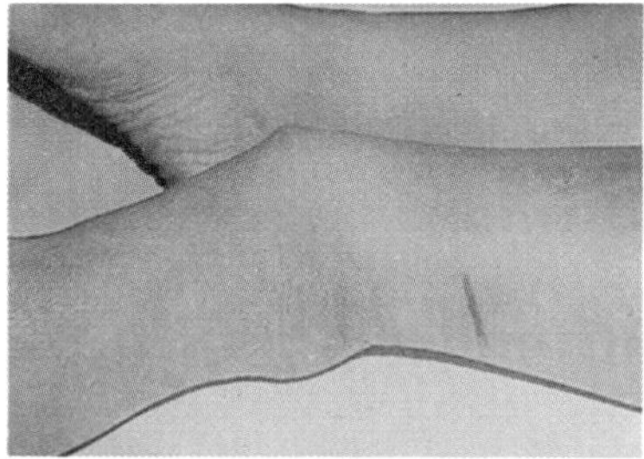

Closed ankle fracture. Observe the deformity.

## OPEN FRACTURES NEED SPECIAL CARE

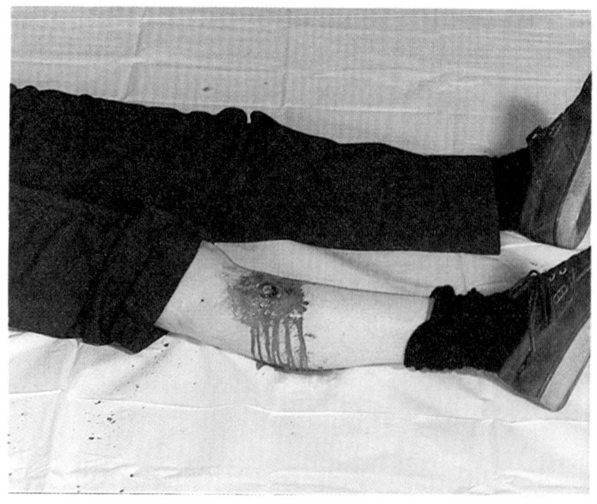

An open tibia fracture.

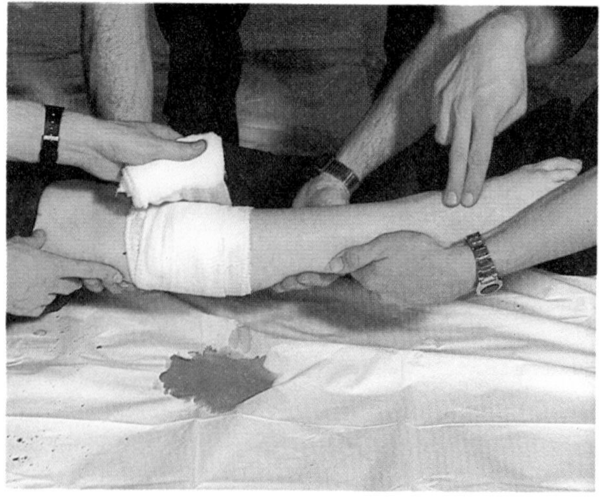

Support the limb, control bleeding, apply traction, locate a distal pulse, and splint.

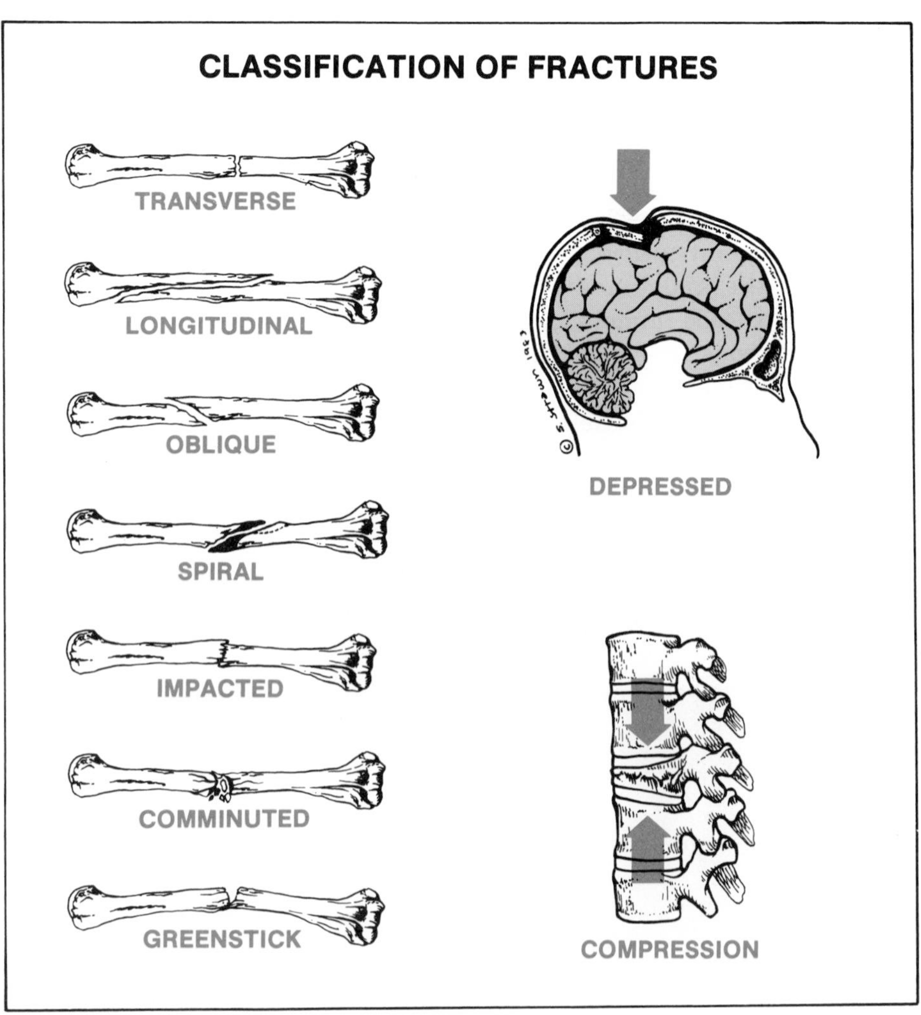
CLASSIFICATION OF FRACTURES
TRANSVERSE
LONGITUDINAL
OBLIQUE
SPIRAL
IMPACTED
COMMINUTED
GREENSTICK
DEPRESSED
COMPRESSION

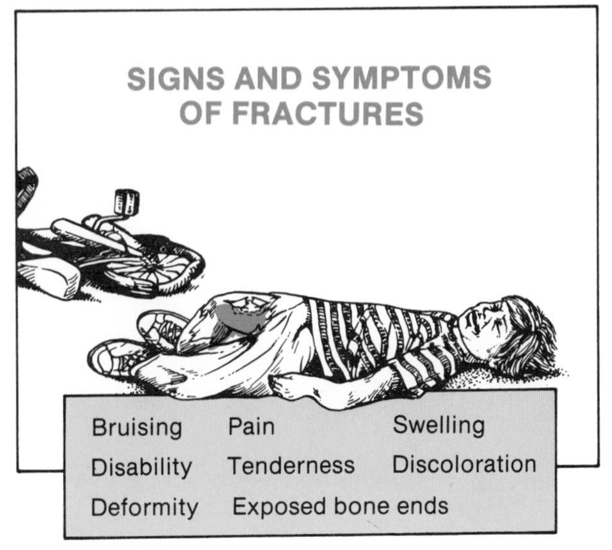
SIGNS AND SYMPTOMS OF FRACTURES
Bruising
Pain
Swelling
Disability
Tenderness
Discoloration
Deformity
Exposed bone ends

## SPLINTS

Splints are used to support, immobilize, and protect parts with injuries such as known or suspected fractures, dislocations, or severe sprains. When in doubt, treat the injury as a fracture and splint it. Splints prevent movement at the area of the injury and at the nearest joints. Splints should immobilize and support the joints or bones above and below the break.

Many types of splints are available commercially. Plastic inflatable splints can be easily applied and quickly inflated, require a minimum of dressing, and give rigid support to injured limbs. Improvised splints may be made from pieces of wood, broom handles, heavy cardboard, newspapers, magazines, or similar firm materials.

Certain guidelines should be followed when splinting:

- Gently remove all clothing from any suspected fracture or dislocation.
- Do not attempt to push bones back through an open wound.
- Do not attempt to straighten any fracture.
- Cover open wounds with a sterile dressing before splinting.
- Pad splints with soft material to prevent excessive pressure on the affected area and to aid in supporting the injured part.
- Pad under all natural arches of the body such as the knee and wrist.
- Support the injured part while the splint is being applied.
- Splint firmly, but not so tightly as to interfere with circulation or cause undue pain.
- Tie all knots on or near the splint.
- Do not transport the victim until the fracture or dislocation has been supported.
- Elevate the injured part and apply ice packs when possible.

Improvised self-splint.

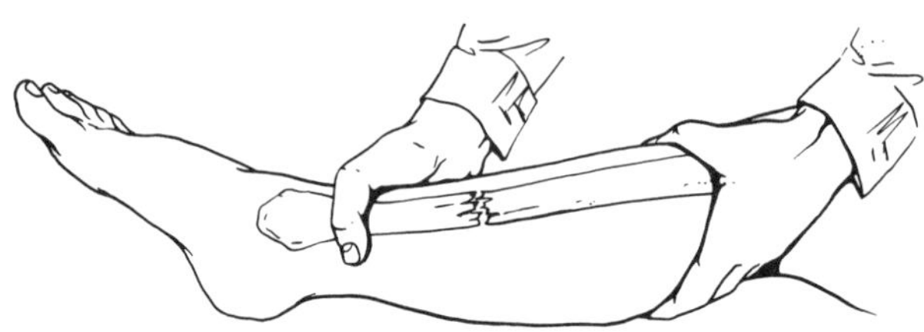

Grasp limb above and below break and apply slight traction.

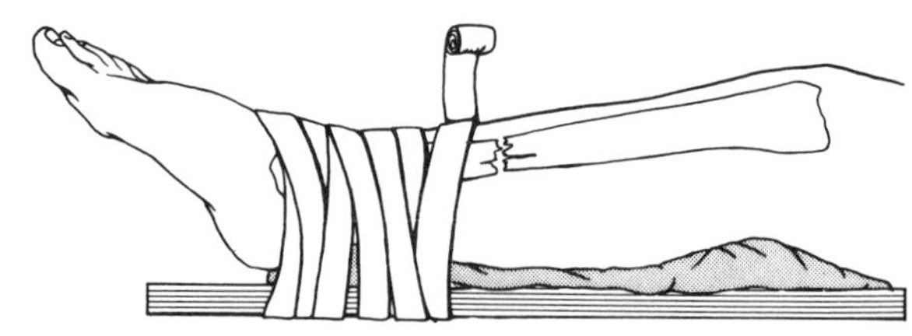

Place padded splint in position and secure limb to splint with bandage.

Applying a fixation splint.

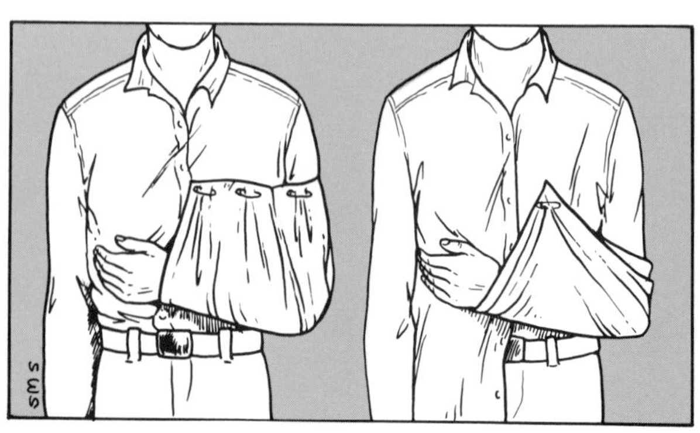

Improvised forearm sling.

## SPLINTING A FRACTURED FOREARM

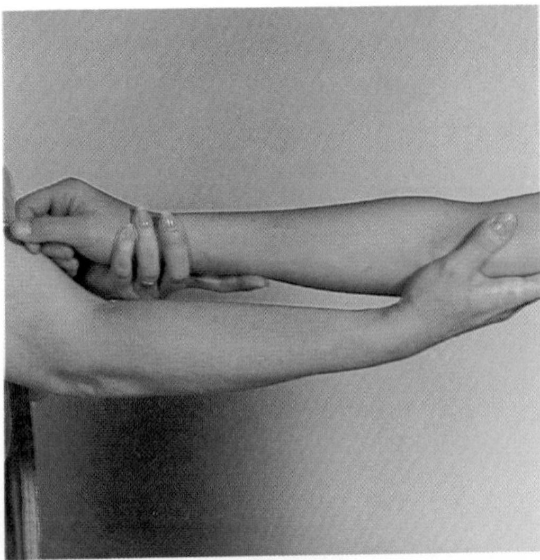

1
A fractured, angulated forearm may be straightened by gently pulling in opposite directions on the long axis of the arm.

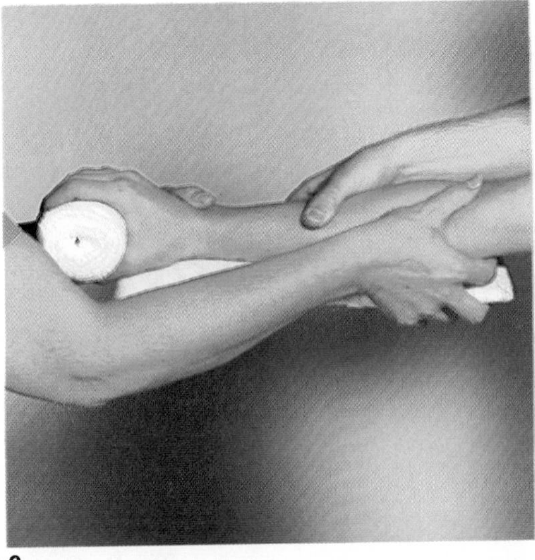

2
A well-padded splint that extends beyond both joints is positioned into place. Continue traction.

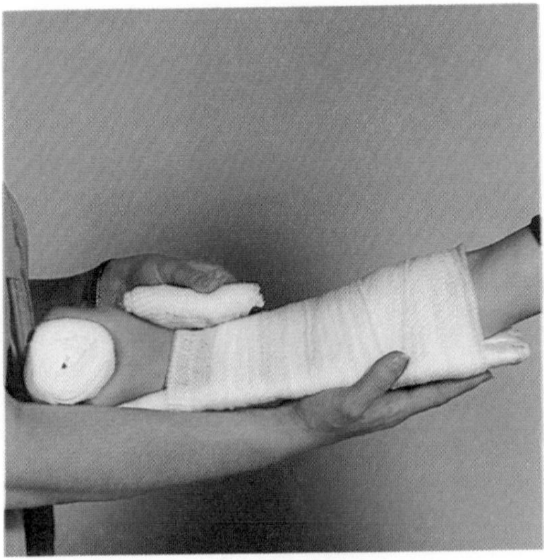

3
Splint is securely bandaged into place.

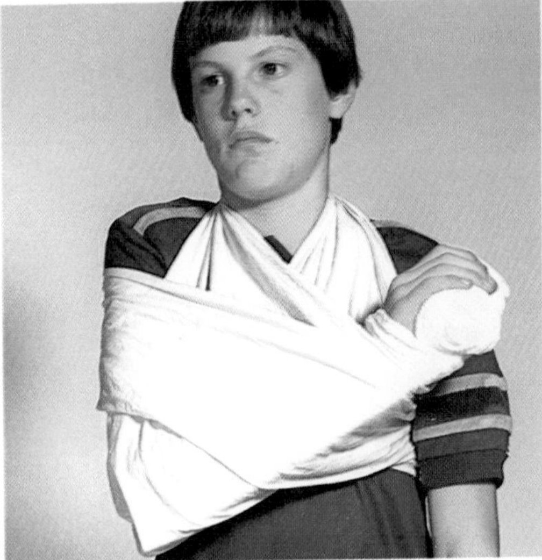

4
Sling and swathe binds fractured arm to chest.

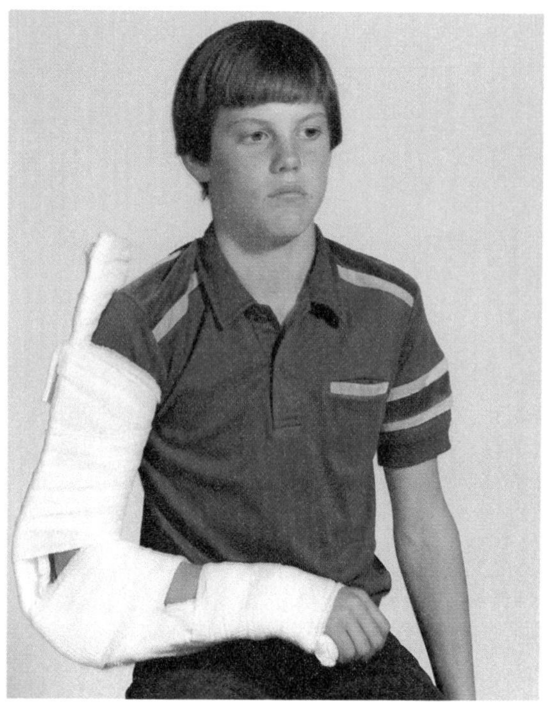

A ladder splint is formed to the injured limb, well padded, and secured with gauze rolls.

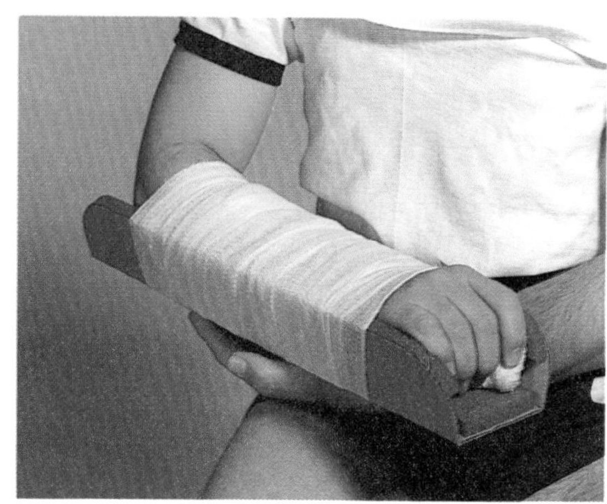

Cardboard splint of the lower arm.

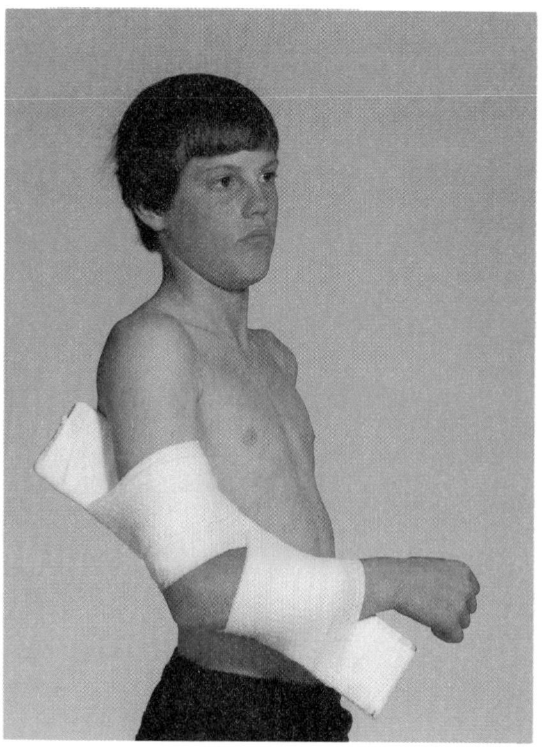

Immobilizing a fractured elbow.

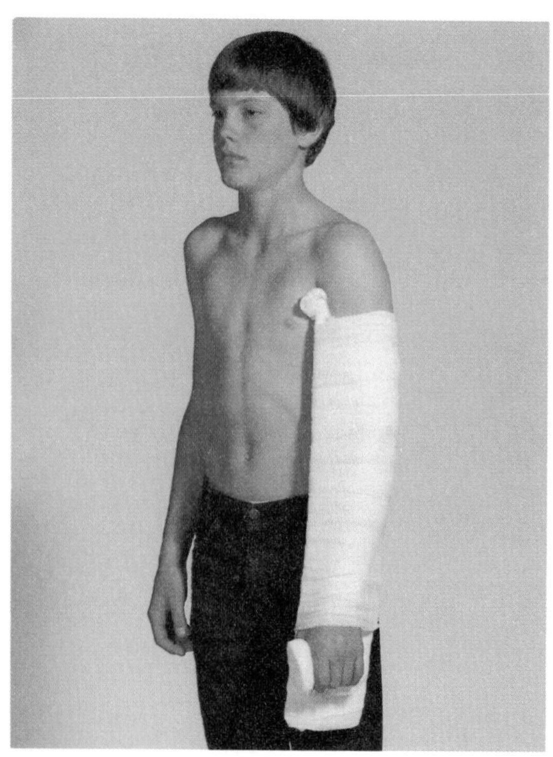

Splint a dislocated or fractured elbow in the position found.

## APPLYING AN AIR SPLINT

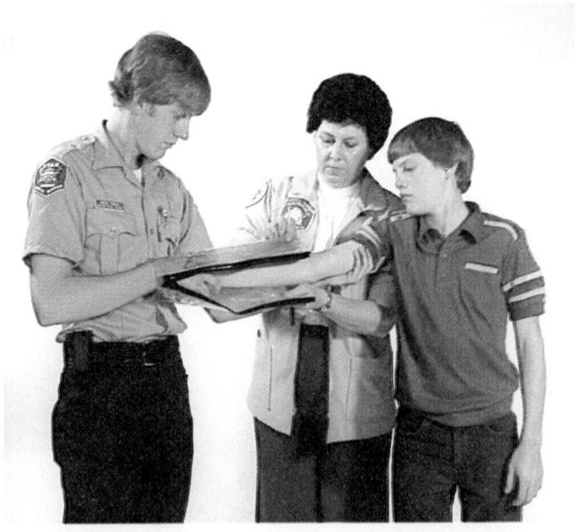

1
Slide closed end up your arm; grasp victim in a handlock and apply traction to the arm.

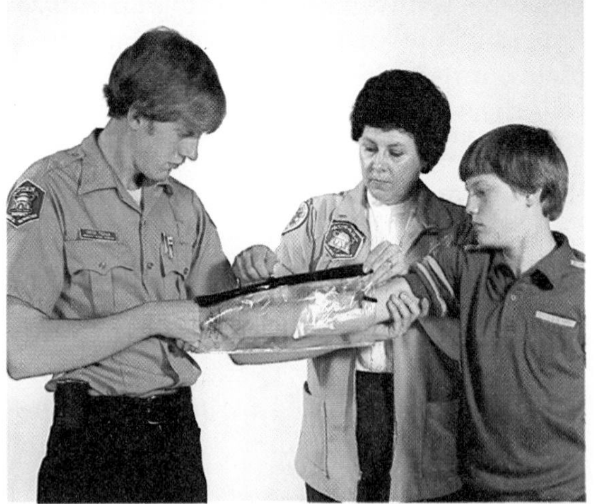

2
Position lower end of splint just above victim's knuckles. Make sure splint is free of wrinkles, then zip up.

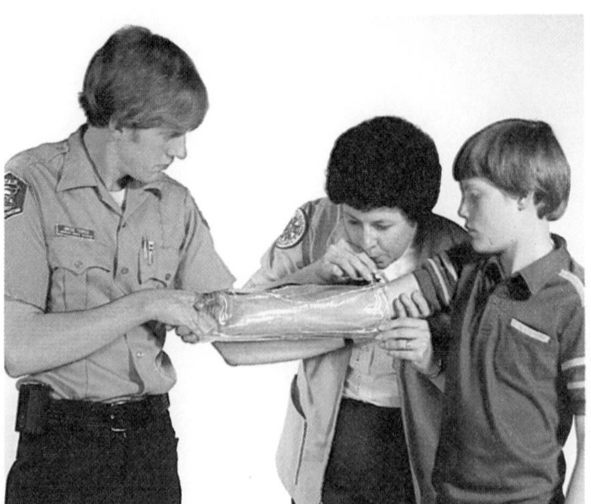

3
While one First Aider maintains traction, other First Aider inflates splint until thumb can only make a slight dent in plastic.

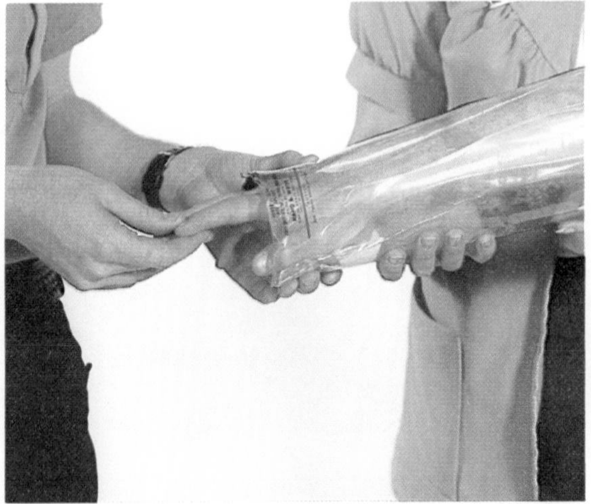

4
Monitor victim's fingernail beds, fingertips, and distal pulse.

## Inflatable Splints

Inflatable splints can be used to immobilize fractures of the lower leg or forearm. When applying inflatable splints (nonzipper type), follow these guidelines:

- Gather the splint on your own arm so that the bottom edge is above your wrist.
- Help support the victim's limb or have someone else hold it.
- Take hold of the injured limb, and slide the splint from your forearm over the limb.
- Inflate by mouth only to the desired pressure. The splint should be inflated to the point where your thumb would make a slight indentation.

For a zipper-type air splint, lay the victim's limb in the unzippered air splint, zip it and inflate. Traction cannot be maintained when applying this type of splint. Change in temperature can effect air splints. Going from a cold area to a warm area will cause the splint to become overinflated because the air expands. Constantly monitor the splint and limb.

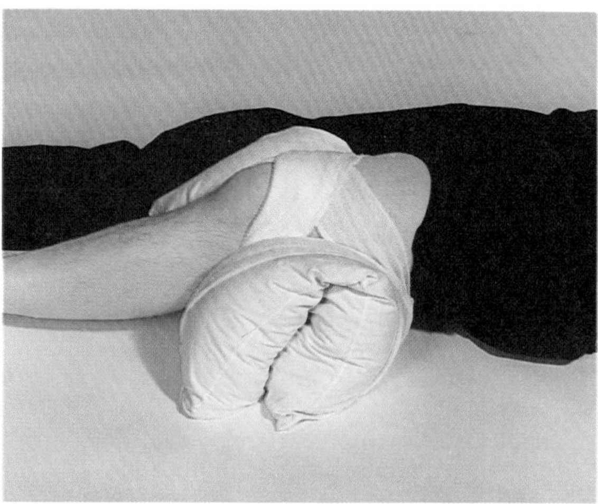

A pillow splint for a fractured patella or a dislocated knee.

## Work Exercises

Tendons and ligaments are specialized connective tissue composed of collagen. Tendons connect __________ to __________. Ligaments connect __________ to __________.

What are the four major functions of the skeletal system?

1.

2.

3.

4.

Muscle, joint and bone injuries are among the most common types of injuries that First Aiders care for.

There are four major types of muscle, joint, and bone injuries. In the chart below, provide the emergency care for each.

| | DEFINITION | CAUSES OF INJURY | SIGNS AND SYMPTOMS | BASIC FIRST AID |
|---|---|---|---|---|
| **Strains** | Overstraining of muscles and/or tendons, causing muscle bundles and tendons to stretch and possibly rupture. | Usually in back area due to lifting improperly or lifting something that is too heavy. | Acute tearing pain when injured, possibly radiating down to leg muscles. Stiffness when moving back and leg muscles. Spasm and terrible pain in low back region. | |
| **Sprains** | Injury to ligaments around joint or joint covering, producing undue stretching or tearing of these tissues. | Sudden twisting or wrenching of joint; direct blow or fall; whiplash in auto accident. | Pain around joint. Inability to use joint. Rapid and marked swelling. Discoloration of area around joint. | |
| **Dislocations** | Displacement of bone ends that form the joint. | Area caught or trapped; rest of body can move, but it can-not. Blow to joint causing displacement. | Rigidity and loss of function. Deformity or irregularity of joint. Pain at joint. Moderate or severe joint swelling. | |
| **Fractures** | Crack or break in skeletal bone, either an open or closed fractures. | Falling, direct impact, crushing injuries such as multiple trauma, falling down stairs, heavy object falling on bone. | Pain; loss of function; deformity or irregularity (crookedness, limb rotation, angulation, open wound over bone, different bone shape; swelling and discoloration; victim may have heard bone snap, may feel broken bones grating. | |

## Dislocations

Match the following dislocations with their correct emergency care procedure:

| Emergency Care | Anatomical Area |
|---|---|
| ________ 1. Immobilize arm with ladder splint. | A. Shoulder |
| ________ 2. Immobilize the leg with a ladder splint. | B. Elbow |
| ________ 3. Immobilize with air splint. | C. Wrist |
| ________ 4. Allow victim to hold injured limb in a comfortable position. | D. Hip |
| ________ 5. Difficult to splint. | E. Knee |
| | F. Ankle |

What two classifications of fractures are there? Describe them.

1.

2.

## Fractures

A fracture is a crack or break in a skeletal bone. In the table below, label the diagrams with the correct description from the left-hand column.

A. Greenstick
B. Transverse
C. Spiral
D. Oblique
E. Comminuted
F. Impacted

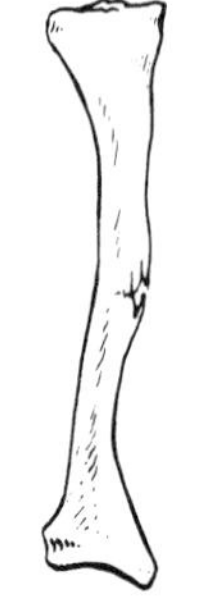
______

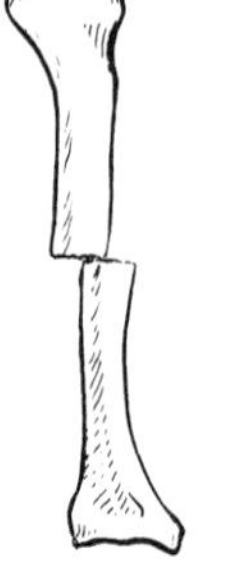
______

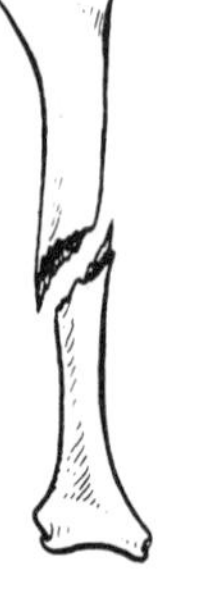
______

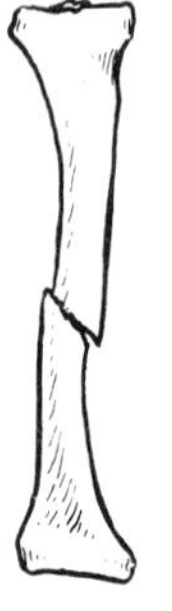
______

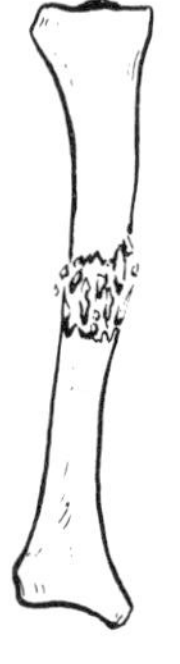
______

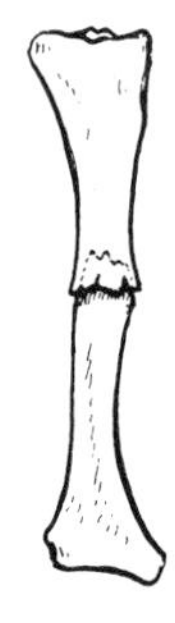
______

1. Label the two fractures illustrated below.

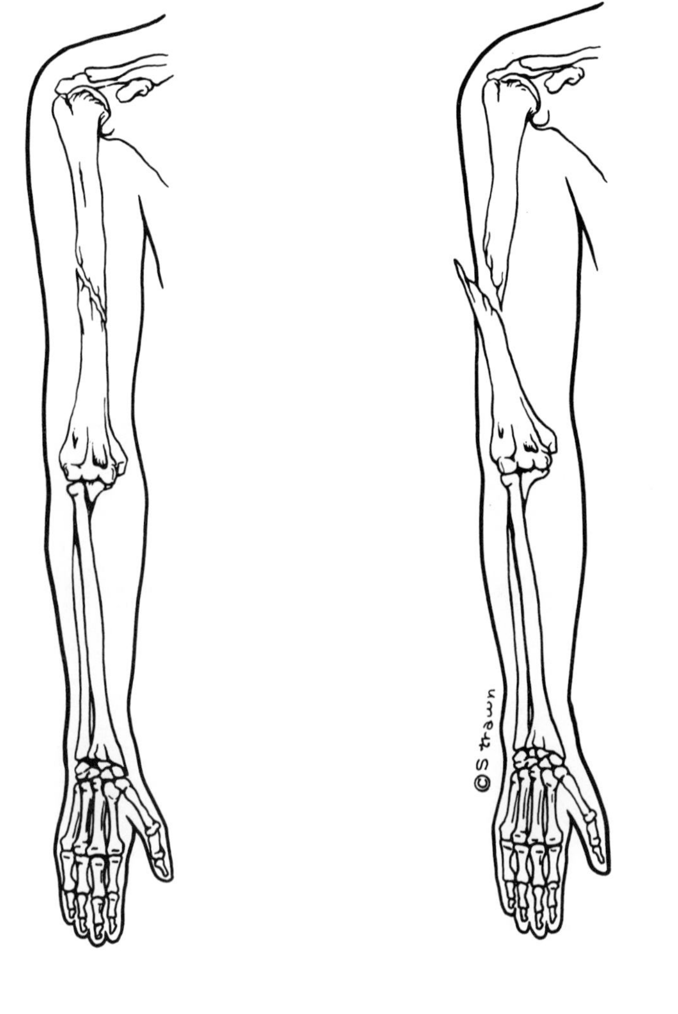


______________________ ______________________

2. Describe briefly how a sprain differs from a strain.

There are three major types of splints. Complete the following table by giving a description of each splint.

### Splint Description

| Type of Splint | Description |
|---|---|
| 1. Self-Splint | |
| 2. Fixation Splint | |
| 3. Traction Splint | |

Occasionally, the First Aider will not have commercial or already-made splints available and will have to create splints from available materials at the accident scene. Give below five examples of splinting materials the First Aider can probably find at an accident scene.

1.

2.

3.

4.

5.

There are many variations of splints. The type of splint that the First Aider will use will depend upon the fracture site and available splinting materials. In the table below, choose the best splint for each body area involved by placing a check in the appropriate box.

### Choose Appropriate Splint

| | Triangular Bandage | Air Splint | Pillow Blanket | Traction Splint | Wire Ladder Splint | Straight Board |
|---|---|---|---|---|---|---|
| Clavicle | | | | | | |
| Humerus | | | | | | |
| Elbow | | | | | | |
| Forearm and Wrist | | | | | | |
| Hand | | | | | | |
| Hip | | | | | | |
| Femur | | | | | | |
| Knee | | | | | | |
| Lower Leg | | | | | | |
| Ankle and Foot | | | | | | |

## SELF-TEST

### Part I: True and False

If you believe the statement is true, circle the T. If you believe the statement is false, circle F.

T F 1. It is usually impossible to tell the difference between a sprain and a closed fracture without X-ray.

T F 2. For a fractured leg, a simple substitute for a splint is to tape or tie the injured leg to the uninjured one.

T F 3. To test for fracture, you should ask the victim to try to move the injured part or walk on the injured leg.

T F 4. In an open fracture, the wound is always contaminated.

T F 5. In cases of ankle and/or foot fracture, you should leave the victim's shoe and stocking on to provide support and lessen the chance of further injury.

T F 6. A fracture is a crack or splinter in a bone that is not broken.

T F 7. A closed fracture may become an open fracture through mishandling or motion during transport.

T F 8. In suspected neck or back fracture, you should avoid moving the victim unless environmental hazards (such as fire or noxious fumes) threaten his/her life.

T F 9. In cases of suspected dislocation, you should correct the deformity before splinting it.

T F 10. The only accurate diagnosis of closed fracture is made by X-ray, but if you suspect that a fracture is present, you should treat it accordingly, even without X-ray confirmation.

T F 11. If you suspect a fracture of the lower arm, you should immobilize the wrist and lower arm, but not the elbow.

T F 12. In fracture of the upper leg, the affected leg will be longer than the uninjured leg.

T F 13. If a fracture victim is unconscious, you should always assume that he/she has sustained spinal injury and take appropriate precautions.

T F 14. A splint should be placed directly against the skin without padding or dressings for maximum effectiveness.

T F 15. A splint should not extend to joints above and below the suspected fracture.

T F 16. Permanent nerve damage can result from a splint that is too tight; you should watch carefully for signs of discoloration or swelling, and loosen the splint if necessary.

T F 17. Heat should be applied to a sprained joint for the first twenty-four hours.

T F 18. A sign of strain is immediate and profuse swelling.

T F 19. A First Aider should try to relocate a dislocation.

T F 20. A fractured elbow should always be immobilized in the position in which it is found.

T F 21. The First Aider should never attempt to straighten a deformity that involves a joint.

### Part II: Multiple Choice

For each question, circle the answer that best reflects an accurate statement.

1. A sprain differs from a strain in that a strain:
   a. results from overstretching a muscle
   b. involves partial tearing of a muscle
   c. is primarily a joint injury
   d. involves extensive damage to blood vessels

2. Signs and symptoms of fracture include:
   a. obvious deformity
   b. discoloration
   c. swelling
   d. any of the above

3. The primary objective in first aid care for fracture is to:
   a. set the bone
   b. immobilize the fracture
   c. push a protruding bone end back into its original position
   d. all of the above

4. To treat an open fracture, do the following:
   a. wash the wound thoroughly with either disinfectant or clear running water
   b. control bleeding with pressure through a dressing
   c. if bone is protruding, do not cover the wound
   d. replace bone fragments before covering the wound with a dressing

5. To treat a sprain, you should:
   a. soak the sprained area in hot water to relieve pain
   b. pack the sprain in ice to reduce swelling
   c. apply cold packs to the sprain
   d. soak the sprained area in ice water

6. When splinting for fracture of the upper leg, the outer side splint should:
   a. extend from the armpit to the knee
   b. extend from the armpit to below the heel
   c. extend from the waist to the knee
   d. extend from the waist to below the heel

7. In cases of fracture, the purpose of a splint is to:
   a. reduce the chance of shock
   b. decrease pain
   c. prevent motion of the injured limb
   d. prevent further injury
   e. all of the above

8. To treat an open fracture of the upper arm:
   a. cover the wound with a compression dressing that will control bleeding
   b. cleanse the wound as thoroughly as possible
   c. apply a splint that does not press against the wound
   d. all of the above

9. If you suspect a fracture of the upper arm, you should immobilize:
   a. the elbow
   b. the upper arm
   c. the shoulder
   d. all of the above

10. When splinting for a fractured kneecap, you should position the splint:
    a. along the outside of the leg
    b. along the inside of the leg
    c. along the back of the leg, behind the knee
    d. along the front of the leg, over the kneecap

11. Tendons attach:
    a. muscle to ligaments
    b. muscle to bone
    c. bone to bone
    d. muscle to muscle

12. The best emergency care measure for a sprain is to immediately:
    a. apply ice or cold treatment
    b. apply heat
    c. get the victim to use the joint to prevent the joint from "freezing"
    d. massage the area.

13. What is a sign or symptom of a strain?
    a. immediate swelling
    b. inability to move
    c. sharp pain which lasts for prolonged periods
    d. a sudden burning sensation

14. Ligaments connect:
    a. muscle to tendon
    b. muscle to bone
    c. bone to bone
    d. muscle to muscle

15. What type of fracture results when a break passes only part way through the bone?
    a. compression
    b. depressed
    c. greenstick
    d. comminuted

16. A dislocated elbow should be immobilized with a/an:
    a. sling and swathe
    b. air splint
    c. blanket, pillow, or towel
    d. ladder splint

17. The lower extremity consists of all *but one* of the following:
    a. metacarpals
    b. patella
    c. ilium
    d. femur

18. An injury in which ligaments are partially torn is called a:
    a. sprain
    b. strain
    c. tendonitis
    d. dislocation

19. Displacement of a bone end from a joint with associated ligament damage is called:
    a. strain
    b. sprain
    c. dislocation
    d. fracture

20. The principal signs/symptoms of a dislocation are:
    a. pain and a feeling of pressure over the joint
    b. loss of motion and deformity
    c. deformity and loss of pulse
    d. numbness and pain

21. All of the following are principal signs of fractures except:
    a. deformity or shortening of a limb
    b. pulselessness in the extremity
    c. grating or crepitus
    d. swelling and discoloration

22. A fracture in which the break is straight across the shaft of the bone is called:
    a. an oblique fracture
    b. a transverse fracture
    c. an impacted fracture
    d. a comminuted fracture

Corresponds with:
**American Red Cross**
**Standard First Aid & Personal Safety**
Chapter 7, pages 99-125
and
**Advanced First Aid & Emergency Care**
Chapter 7, pages 95-117

# 11 Poisoning Emergencies

Each year in the United States, thousands of people die from suicidal or accidental poisonings. In addition to the fatalities, approximately one million cases of nonfatal poisonings occur because of exposure to substances such as medicines, industrial chemicals, cleaning agents, and plant and insect sprays. Approximately 90 percent of all poisoning cases involve children.

A poison is any liquid, solid, or gas that impairs health or causes death when it is introduced into the body or onto the skin surface. Some substances, otherwise harmless, become deadly if used incorrectly.

There are numerous ways in which poisons may enter the body:

- **Ingestion** (mouth).
- **Inhalation** in the form of noxious dusts, gases, fumes, or mists.
- **Injection** into the body tissues or bloodstream by hypodermic needles or the bites of poisonous snakes, insects, or **rabid** animals.
- **Absorption** through the skin (mercury or certain other poisonous liquids) or contact by the skin (poisonous plants and certain fungi).

## INGESTED POISONS

The chief causes of poisoning by ingestion are:

- Overdose of medicine (intentional or accidental).
- Medicines, household cleaners, and chemicals within the reach of children.
- Combining drugs and alcohol.
- Poisons transferred from the original container to a food container.
- Carelessness on the part of those who should know better.

### Signs and Symptoms

The signs and symptoms of poisoning by ingestion are variable depending on the substances involved. The common ones are:

- Nausea, vomiting, and diarrhea.
- Severe abdominal pain and cramps.
- Slowed respiration and circulation.
- Excessive salivation or sweating.
- Corrosive poisons (strong acids and alkalis) may corrode, burn, or destroy the tissues of the mouth, throat, and stomach.
- Contents of a drug bottle spilled out, and not all of the contents accounted for.
- Liquids such as kerosene or turpentine may leave characteristic odors on the breath.

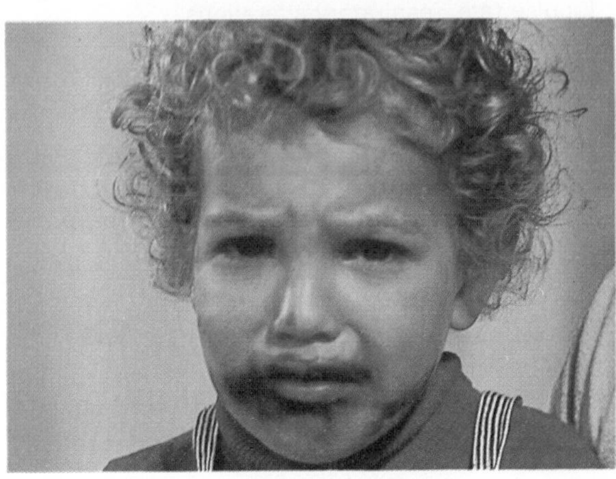

Skin discoloration — possible poisoning.

- Certain poisons may stain the mouth.
- Unconsciousness.
- Convulsions.

## Victim Assessment

In addition to the standard procedures for primary and secondary survey, you should be especially alert for certain signs:

- Observe the victim's skin color for unusual hues.
- Smell the victim's breath for the characteristic odor of petroleum products, alcohols, or other suggestive odors.
- Assess level of consciousness.
- Assess pupillary reaction.
- Assess respirations.
- Assess condition of mouth and lips and appearance of vomiting and/or diarrhea.

## Emergency Care

1. **Maintain the airway.** This cannot be overemphasized. The sleepy or comatose victim is in constant danger of aspiration, and it is the First Aider's primary responsibility to prevent this from happening.
2. **When to not induce vomiting.** As a general rule, if the victim has ingested a poisonous substance within the past three to six hours, **the stomach should be emptied.** However, there are several important exceptions. **Never induce vomiting in:**

- The stuporous or unconscious victim. The vomitus may be aspirated into the lungs, causing pneumonia.
- The victim with seizures.
- The victim with possible heart attack.

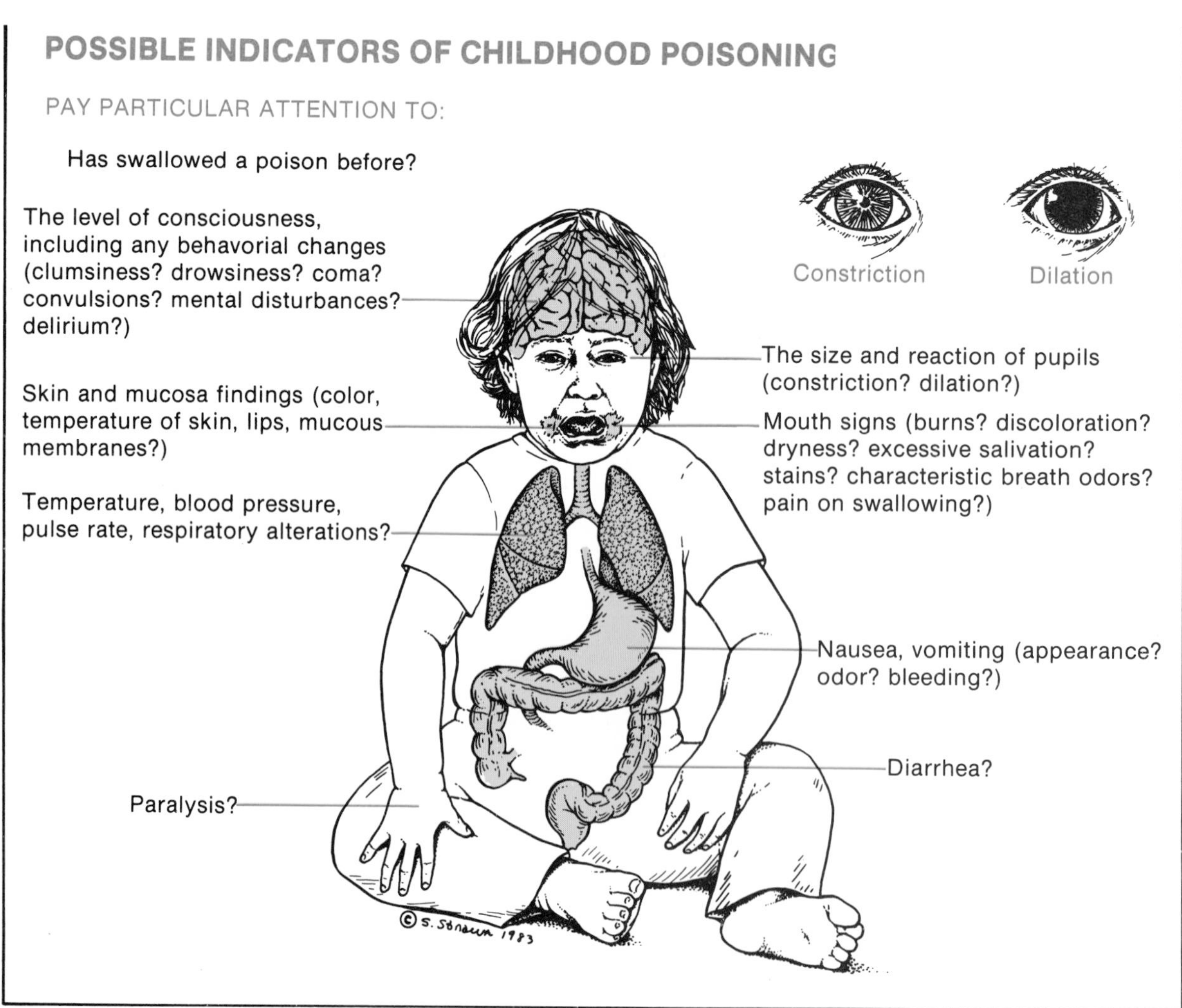

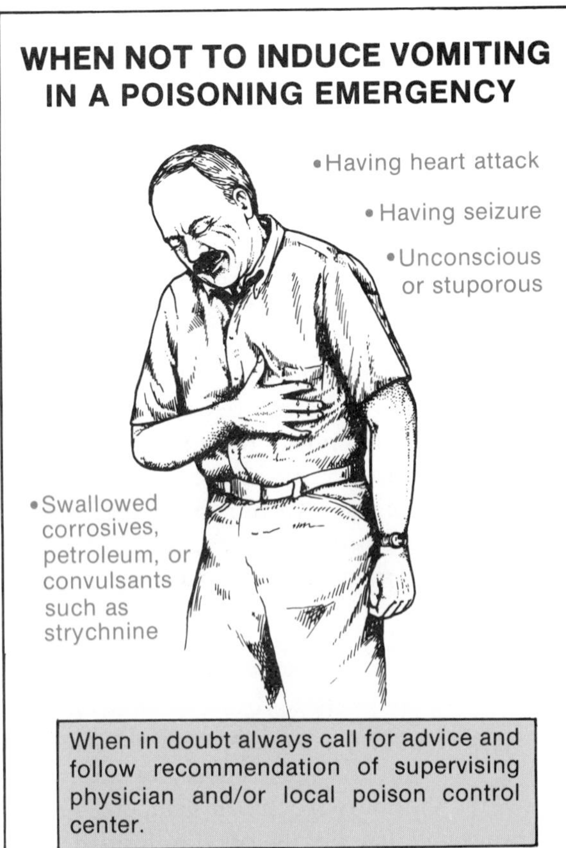


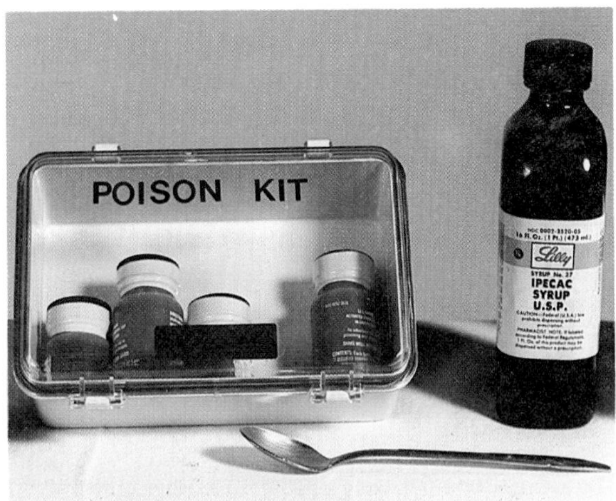


Emergency care kit for poisoning includes syrup of ipecac and activated charcoal.

- The victim who has ingested corrosives (strong acids or alkalis). These include many household cleaners that can damage the esophagus and lining of the mouth as it is vomited.
- The victim who has ingested petroleum products (kerosene, gasoline, lighter fluid, furniture polish). Generally, vomiting should not be induced in these cases; however, sometimes an exception is made if the amount is excessive or if the victim has swallowed an extremely toxic product such as a pesticide or one containing heavy metals. Check with a poison control center.
- The victim who has ingested a convulsant such as strychnine often found in mouse poisons. Vomiting may induce convulsions.

3. For practically all other cases of ingested poisons, **prompt emptying of the stomach is of great importance.** The method of choice is:

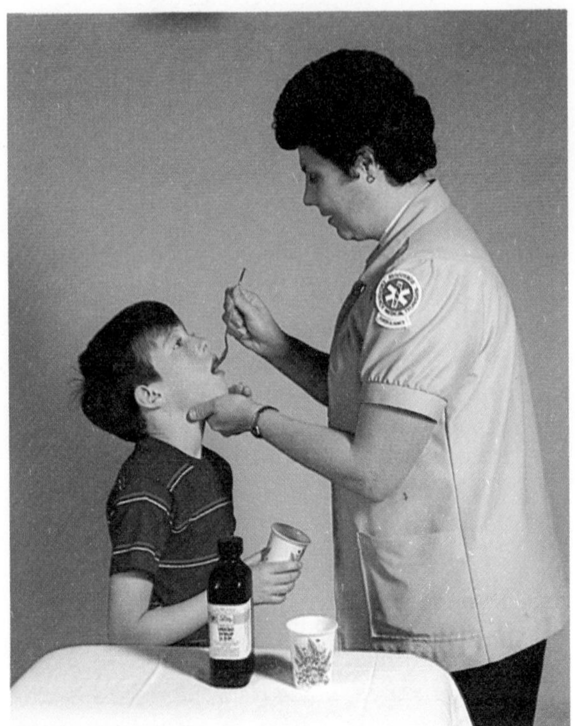

Administering syrup of ipecac after possible poisoning.

- Give syrup of ipecac: fifteen milliliters (one tablespoon) with one to two glasses of water for a child over one year of age, and thirty milliliters (two tablespoons) with two to three glasses of water for an adult.

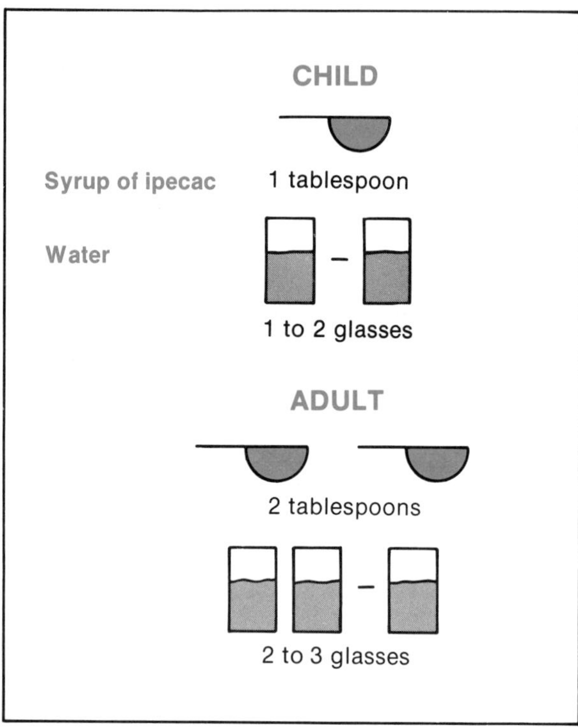


How to induce vomiting.

- The victim should be sitting and leaning forward to prevent vomitus from being aspirated into the lungs. Keep the victim's face down with the head lower than the rest of the body. Place a small child on his/her stomach with head down and feet elevated to cause vomiting and prevent aspiration.
- If vomiting does not occur within twenty minutes, the dose of ipecac may be repeated, once.
- After vomiting has ceased, give activated charcoal (at least two tablespoons mixed in tap water) to make a slurry. Children may require some persuasion to drink this mixture, since its appearance is uninviting. But a firm, positive approach generally works. **Do not give activated charcoal before or together with syrup of ipecac,** because the charcoal will inactivate the ipecac and render it ineffective.

4. **Be prepared to manage shock, coma, seizures, and cardiac arrest** as detailed in other chapters of this book.
5. **Do not use milk or carbonated beverages with syrup of ipecac.**
6. **Do not give mustard or salt to induce vomiting.**
7. If syrup of ipecac is not available, **vomiting can be induced by using the end of a napkin or handkerchief-padded spoon to tickle the back of the throat** and stimulate the gag reflex. This should only be used as a last resort because it is not very effective. Using your finger to tickle the throat may result in a bite. If the victim is a child, administer a cup of water and place him/her in "spanking position" — across the First Aider's knees — before tickling the throat.
8. The ingestion of poisonous plants can cause severe reactions ranging from gastrointestinal disturbances to nervous system disorders and circulatory collapse. Basic life support and medical assistance are essential.

### Strong Alkalis & Acids

Strong alkalis include drain cleaner, washing soda, ammonia, and household bleach. Strong acids include toilet bowl cleaners, rust removers, phenolhydrochloric acid, etc. These substances cause burns of the mouth and esophagus, producing pain and difficulty in swallowing. Emergency care consists of the following:

1. Do not attempt to neutralize.
2. Do not induce vomiting.
3. Dilute with water and transport immediately.
4. If a child has handled or been poisoned by a corrosive substance, always wash his/her hands and fingers thoroughly to prevent any damage to the eyes from rubbing.

## INHALED POISONS

About 1,400 deaths each year in the United States are attributed to persons having inhaled poisonous vapors and fumes, some of which can be present without any sign. It is critical that care be immediate, because the body absorbs inhaled poisons rapidly.

The most common gas that causes poisoning is carbon monoxide. It is completely tasteless and odorless. If the victim is not removed from the source quickly, he/she will become

## Emergency Aid for Poisonings

It is a MEDICAL EMERGENCY when anyone swallows a poison! Every *non-food substance* should be considered a potential poison!

### What To Do First

1. Try to determine the probable poison and the amount swallowed. Carefully assess the victim's condition.
2. If the poison container is available, read the label for **ingredients** of the poison.
3. Call poison control center.
4. Provide the emergency care stated below.
5. Keep the victim warm.

### Swallowed Poisons

Make the victim vomit (if instructed to do so by base hospital) . . . but **remember** there are conditions in which the patient should NOT be made to vomit.

**1. Do NOT make the victim vomit when:**

- The patient is unconscious or convulsing.
- The poison swallowed is a strong corrosive, such as acid or lye.
- The swallowed poison contains kerosene, gasoline, lighter fluid, furniture polish, or other petroleum distillates, unless instructed to do so by poison control center.

(Exception: If these are mixed with dangerous insecticides, then the poison must be removed.)

**2. Directions for making the victim vomit:**

- Give two tablespoonfuls (30 ml) syrup of ipecac for an adult. Follow this with two to three glasses of water. For a child, give one tablespoonful (15 ml), followed by one to two glasses of water. Transport. If no vomiting occurs after twenty minutes and medical help is still not available, this dose may be repeated one time only. To stimulate vomiting, gently tickle the back of the throat with a spoon or similar blunt object.

**3. Administration of activated charcoal:**

- Activated charcoal (two to four tablespoonfuls in a glass of water) may be given after vomiting has occurred or if ipecac has failed to cause vomiting within an hour (if you are still in transit). Do **not** give activated charcoal before ipecac has had an opportunity to cause vomiting.

**4. Do not wait at the scene to accomplish any of the above. Have victim transported immediately.**

**Important**

- Under no circumstances should liquids be given to a victim who is unconscious or convulsing!
- Transport whatever was ingested to the hospital, i.e., plant, pills, pesticide, unknown poison, etc. Also bring any containers, bottles, etc., that may have contained the ingested drug or unknown poison. Also collect a sample of any vomitus and deliver to the emergency room.

unconscious and will have trouble breathing. It takes only a few minutes to die from carbon monoxide poisoning.

Signs and symptoms of carbon monoxide poisoning are:

- Headache.
- Dizziness.
- Yawning.
- Faintness.
- Lethargy and stupor.
- Mucous membranes becoming bright cherry red in color. (Late stage with high levels.)
- Lips and earlobes possibly turning bluish in color. (Not a consistent sign.)
- Nausea or vomiting.

Assessment of the victim will reveal a bounding pulse, dilated pupils, and cyanosis or pallor.

## Emergency Care

1. Get the victim into fresh air immediately. Watch out for yourself! If the victim is in a closed garage or room or some other small or closed space, take a deep breath and hold it while you enter. If you cannot get the victim into fresh air, call a rescue squad or the fire department. Remember — the presence of carbon monoxide is difficult to detect. Do not delay unnecessarily in an area that may be contaminated.
2. Loosen all tight-fitting clothing, especially around the neck and over the chest.
3. If the victim is not breathing, start artificial ventilation immediately. Do not interrupt the artificial ventilation for any reason. If necessary, administer CPR.

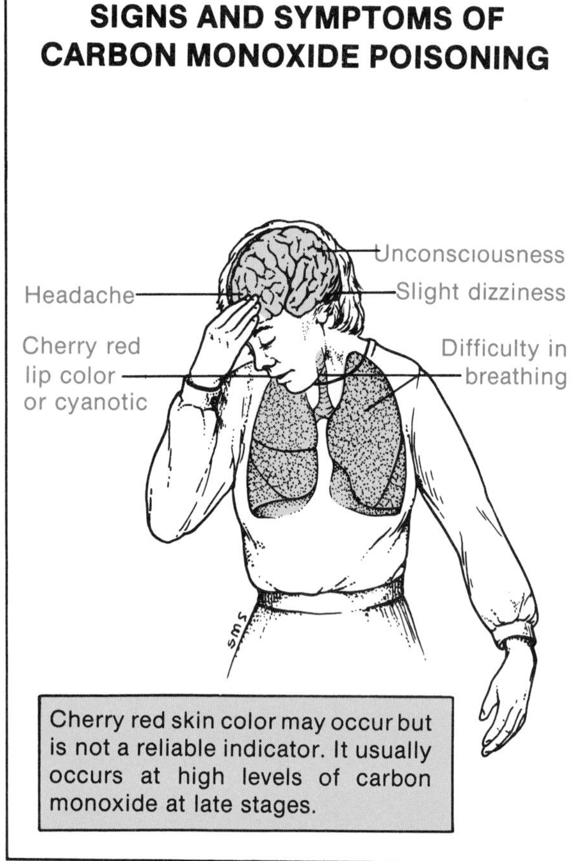


4. Keep the victim completely inactive and quiet.
5. Call for medical assistance immediately, even if the victim seems to have recovered (awakening or seeming alertness can be false signs of recovery).
6. Contact a poison control center for further instructions.

## SNAKEBITE

About 45,000 people every year are bitten by snakes in the United States; 7,000 of those involve poisonous snakes. About 20 of the 120 species of snakes in the United States are poisonous; they include **rattlesnakes, coral snakes, water moccasins,** and **copperheads.**

Signs and symptoms indicating that a snakebite is poisonous include:

1. The bite consists of one or two distinct puncture wounds. Nonpoisonous snakes usually leave a series of small, shallow puncture wounds (because they have teeth instead of fangs).
2. The victim experiences severe pain and burning almost immediately, but always within four hours of the incident.
3. The wound begins to swell and discolor within four hours.

The characteristics of most poisonous snakes include the following:

1. Kind of teeth. Poisonous snakes have large fangs; nonpoisonous snakes have small teeth. The two fangs of a poisonous snake are hollow and work like a hypodermic needle.
2. Shape of the pupil. **Venomous** (poisonous) snakes have elliptical pupils (vertical slits, much like those of a cat); nonvenomous snakes have round pupils.
3. Absence or presence of a pit. Poisonous snakes (often called "pit vipers") have a telltale pit between the eye and the mouth.

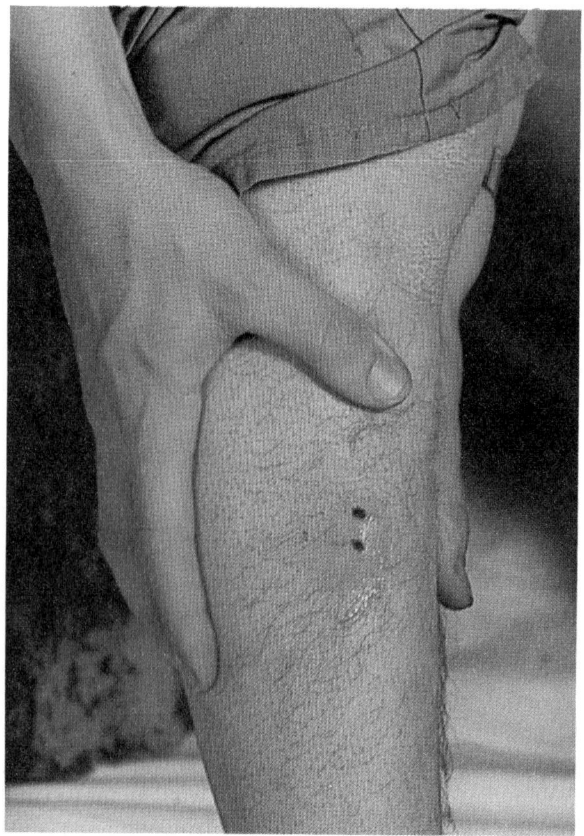

Rattlesnake bite.

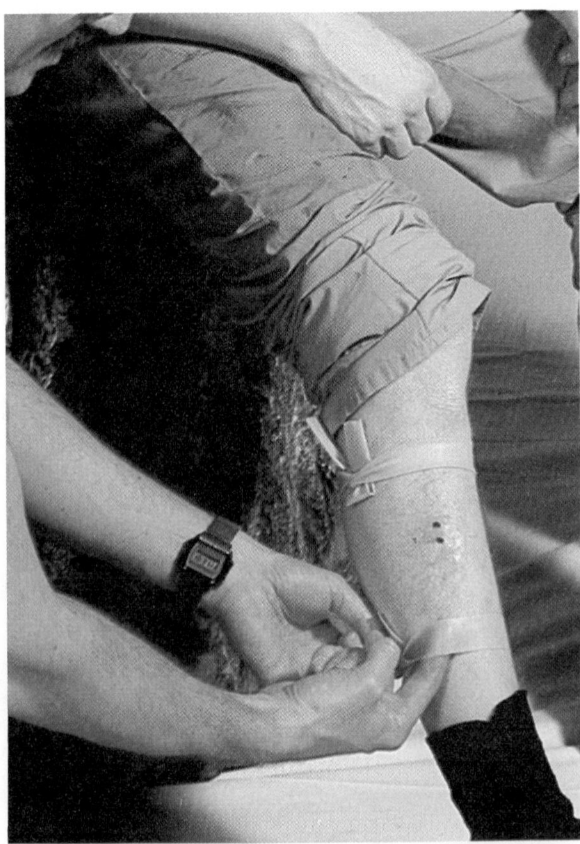

For poisonous snakebite (pit vipers), apply constricting band above and below bite. Bands should be tight enough to slow surface circulation but should not interfere with arterial blood flow. They should be loose enough so that a finger can be inserted under band.

The pit, a heat-sensing organ, makes it possible for the snake to accurately strike a warm-blooded victim, even if the snake cannot see the victim.

4. Appearance of skin. Many venomous snakes have a variety of differently shaped blotches on backgrounds of pink, yellow, olive, tan, gray, or brown skin.

**There is one exception to all of this: the coral snake,** a highly poisonous snake that resembles a number of nonpoisonous snakes, does not have fangs, and has round pupils. Because its mouth is so small and its teeth are short, most coral snakes inflict bites on the toes and fingers. Coral snakes are small and are ringed with red, yellow, and black; the red and yellow touch each other.

Chances for good recovery are great if the victim receives care within two hours of the bite.

## Emergency Care

The care for a snakebite depends on whether the victim was bitten by a pit viper (rattlesnake, copperhead, or cottonmouth) or a coral snake.

To care for a pit viper bite, follow these steps:

1. Have the victim lie down, and keep him/her quiet. Continually reassure the victim. The bitten extremity should be kept slightly lower than the heart.
2. Wipe the wound area with alcohol, soap and water, or hydrogen peroxide.
3. If you do not have a sterile scalpel or razor blade, sterilize a knife in a match flame, in soap and water, in alcohol, or in hydrogen peroxide. Only make an incision if you are thirty minutes or more away from a medical facility.
4. Find the fang marks. Wrap a constricting band around the extremity both above and below the fang marks. It should be tight enough to stop the flow of blood through the veins but not through the arteries.
5. Make longitudinal (vertical) cut marks through each fang mark. Cut marks should be about one-eighth to one-fourth inch in length and should be parallel to each other; they should be made in the direction that the fang entered. The incisions should **not** be cross marks.
6. Apply suction to the wound directly over the incisions. (A suction cup from a snakebite kit is ideal, but you can "milk" the incision with your fingers if necessary.) **Note: There is some controversy about incising and suctioning a snakebite injury, using constricting bands, and when it should be done. Always follow local poison control center instructions.**

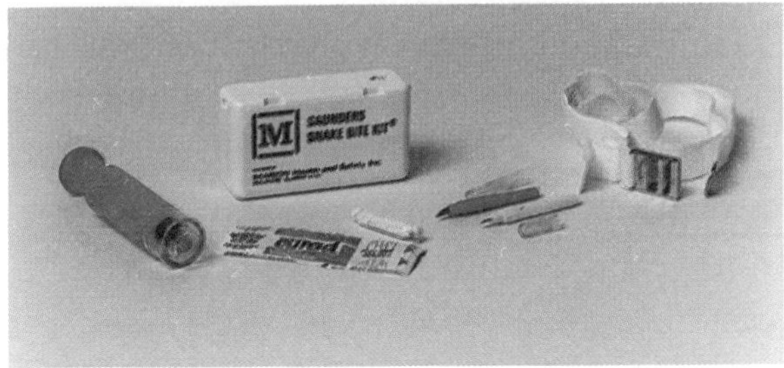

Commercial snakebite kit.

## POISONOUS SNAKEBITES

MOTION OF STRIKE:

Shallow, slanting penetration is typical of snakebite, since snakes tend to hold the head level when striking. Wound depth and venom deposit vary with the species, the length of the fangs, and the snake's excitement. Even if the 1¼ inch fangs of the Eastern diamondback rattlesnake penetrate almost their full length, the slanting wound may be no more than ¼ inch from the skin surface.

Eliptical pupil

Pit

Fang

Poison gland

- Immediate burning pain
- Swelling, discoloration
- Distinct puncture wound
- Blood oozing from wound

Bite pattern:

Pit vipers are characterized by heat-sensitive pits located between the eye and nostril

A pit viper uses fangs to inject its venom. The fang is a tooth that has enlarged and is curved and hollowed out - a kind of hypodermic needle. A fang is attached on each side of the upper jaw to a bone that is movable. Each fang lies against the roof of the mouth and, except for its tip, is sheathed in a casing of flesh. Every few weeks the fangs are replaced by new ones.

The venom to be pumped through the fangs is stored in glands at the side of the snake's head just behind the inner ear. Ducts in these glands extend to the base of the fangs and into openings in the fangs.

As a pit viper strikes and as its jaws open to touch its victim, the fangs come forward. The gland muscles push the venom into the ducts and thus into the fang openings from whence it flows into the puncture wounds in the victim's skin.

New incision technique calls for two parallel slits starting at the punctures and extending downward (along the presumed path of the fangs) at right angles to an imaginary line connecting the punctures. Because of the shallow implantation of venom, the incisions need be only about ⅛ inch deep and about ⅛-¼ inch long. These incisions should reach the main concentration of venom, thought to lie in two parallel oblong pockets. (Some authorities, however, believe the venom spreads rapidly and uniformly in the subcutaneous tissue, so the pockets don't exist for long; they thus include the puncture in the **middle** of the incision.)

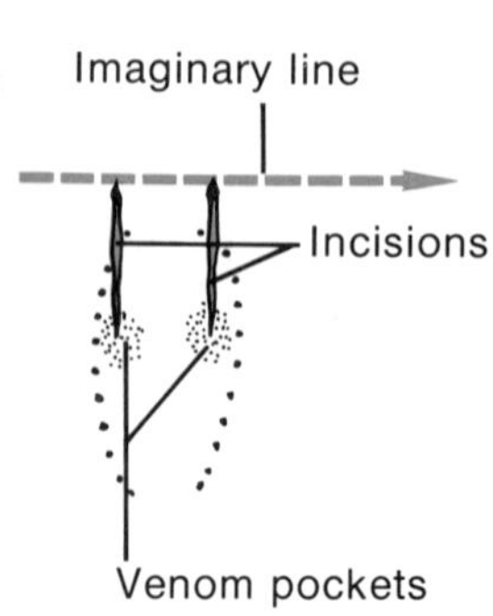

# FIRST AID FOR SNAKEBITE

## POISONOUS OR NONPOISONOUS

Poisonous or nonpoisonous, a snakebite should have medical attention. A snakebite victim should be taken to a hospital *as quickly as possible,* even in cases when snakebite is only suspected.

## FIRST AID

1. As stated above, *get the victim to a hospital fast.* Meanwhile, take the following general first aid measures:
   - Keep the victim from moving around.
   - Keep the victim as calm as possible, preferably lying down.
   - Immobilize the bitten extremity and keep it at or below heart level.

   If a hospital can be reached within 4 to 5 hours and no symptoms develop, this is all that is necessary.

2. *If mild to moderate symptoms develop, apply a constricting band* from 2 to 4 inches above the bite but NOT around a joint (i.e., elbow, knee, wrist, or ankle) and NOT around the head, neck, or trunk. The band should be from ¾ to 1½ inches wide, NOT thin like a rubber band. The band should be snug, but loose enough to slip one finger underneath. Be alert to swelling; loosen the band if it becomes too tight, but do not remove it. To ensure that blood flow has not been stopped, periodically check the pulse in the extremity beyond the bite.

3. *If severe symptoms develop, incisions and suction should be performed immediately.* Apply a constricting band, if not already done, and make a cut in the skin with a sharp sterilized blade through the fang mark(s). Cuts should be no deeper than just through the skin and should be ½ inch long, extending over the suspected venom deposit point (because a snake strikes downward, the deposit point is usually lower than the fang mark). Cuts should be made along the long axis of the limb. DO NOT make cross-cut incisions; DO NOT make cuts on the head, neck, or trunk. Suction should be applied with a suction cup for 30 minutes. If a suction cup is not available, use the mouth. There is little risk to the rescuer who uses his mouth, but it is recommended that the venom not be swallowed and that the mouth be rinsed.

## IF THE HOSPITAL IS NOT CLOSE *(cannot be reached within from 4 to 5 hours)*

1. Continue to try to obtain professional care by transportation of the victim or by communication with a rescue service.
2. *If no symptoms develop,* continue trying to reach the hospital and give the general first aid described above.
3. *If ANY symptoms develop,* apply a constricting band and perform incisions and suction immediately, as described above.

## OTHER CONSIDERATIONS

1. *Shock:* Keep the victim lying down and comfortable and maintain body temperature.
2. *Breathing and heartbeat:* If breathing stops, give mouth-to-mouth resuscitation. If breathing stops and there is no pulse, cardiopulmonary resuscitation (CPR) should be performed by those trained to do so.
3. *Identifying the snake:* If the snake can be killed without risk or delay, it should be brought, *with care,* to the hospital for identification.
4. *Cleansing the bitten area:* The bitten area may be washed with soap and water and blotted dry with sterile gauze. Dressings and bandages can be applied, but only for a short period of time.
5. *Cold therapy:* Cold compresses, ice, dry ice, chemical ice packs, spray refrigerants, and other methods of cold therapy are NOT recommended in the first aid treatment of snakebite.
6. *Medicine to relieve pain:* A medicine *not containing aspirin* can be given to the victim for relief of pain. DO NOT give alcohol, sedatives, aspirin, or other medications.
7. *Snakebite kits:* Keep a kit accessible for all outings in snake-infested or primitive areas.

## SYMPTOMS

1. *Mild to moderate* symptoms include mild swelling or discoloration and mild to moderate pain at the wound site with tingling sensations, rapid pulse, weakness, dimness of vision, nausea, vomiting, and shortness of breath.
2. *Severe* symptoms include rapid swelling and numbness, followed by severe pain at the wound site. Other effects include pinpoint pupils, twitching, slurred speech, shock, convulsions, paralysis, unconsciousness, and no breathing or pulse.

7. The most effective countermeasure is an antivenin shot obtained at a medical facility.
8. Give the victim emergency care for shock. Monitor vital signs; keep the victim warm and lying down.
9. Have the victim transported to a hospital as soon as possible.

## Coral Snake

Emergency care for a coral snake bite is similar to that for a pit viper bite, with a few important additions:

1. Remove the victim's rings and bracelets.
2. Flush off the bite area with water so that any remaining poison is washed away; you will need to use at least several quarts of water.
3. After applying the constricting band (above the bite only), immobilizing the extremity, and giving care for shock, apply a coolant bag or ice bag to the bite site. (**Never** pack the bite area in ice, since you may cause frostbite.)
4. Unlike pit viper bites, coral snake bites should not be cut and suctioned out.

# INSECT BITES

In most cases of insect bite, emergency care consists of:

- Washing the wound thoroughly with soap and water.
- If a victim has an allergic reaction to an insect bite with any of the following symptoms: burning pain and itching at the bite site; itching on the palms of the hands and soles of the feet, neck, and the groin; general body swelling; a nettlelike rash over the entire body; or breathing difficulties, he/she should be seen by a physican.
- Some victims become faint, weak, and nauseated. In cases of severe allergy, victims may develop **anaphylactic shock** (a sudden condition of shock and unconsciousness due to an allergic reaction). These victims should always be transported to the hospital.

In the case of bites involving either the black widow or brown recluse spider, special care must be given. For black widow spider bites:

- Administer care for shock.
- Apply a cold pack (**not** ice) to the bite area.

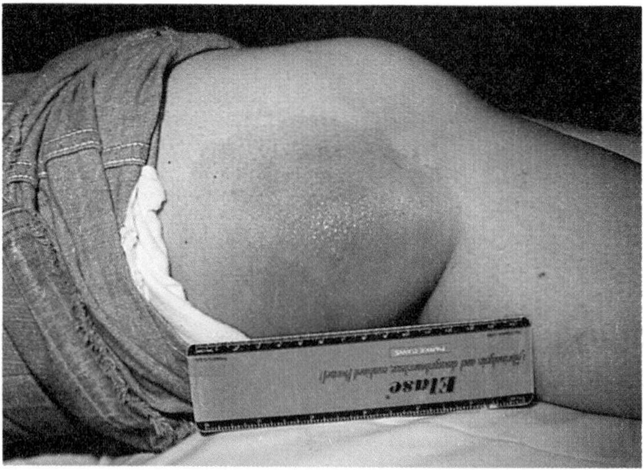

Insect bite.

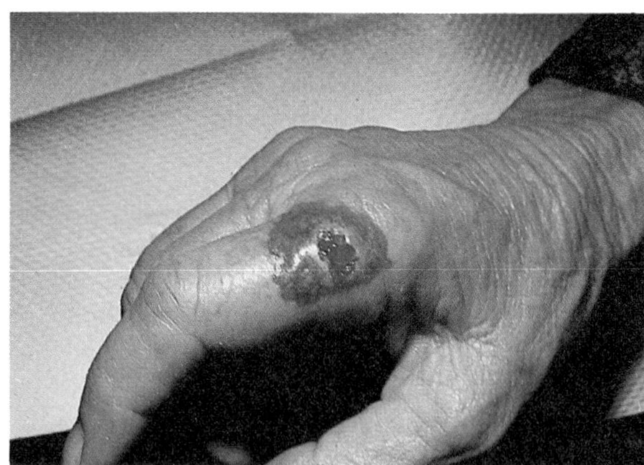

Brown recluse spider bite.

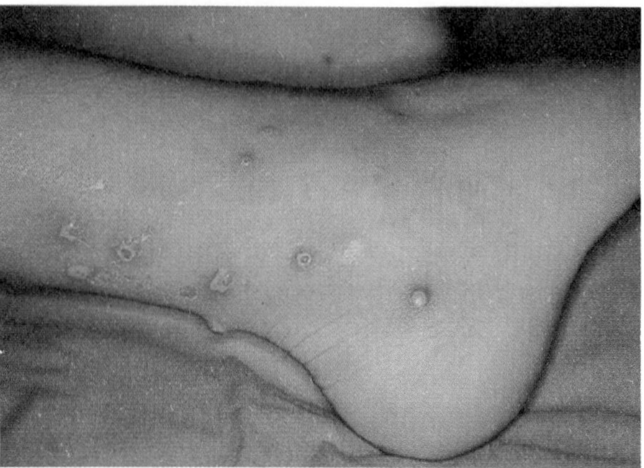

Fire ant bites.

- Have the victim transported to a hospital.
- Since antivenins are available, it is extremely important to get a positive identification of the spider. (If possible — but don't waste time.)

Emergency care for brown recluse spider bites consists of:

- Administering care for shock.
- Administering mouth-to-mouth ventilation, if needed.
- Having the victim transported to a hospital.
- Again, it is important, if possible, that you positively identify the spider so that the correct antivenin can be administered to the victim at the hospital.

Fire ants can also produce serious reactions. The bite causes a stinging pain followed by swelling. There is no specific treatment for the fire ant bite itself. First Aiders should care for systemic and allergic reactions as described for bee stings.

## INSECT STINGS

### Emergency Care

Emergency care for individuals who experience allergic reactions to insect stings consists of the following procedure:

1. Lower the affected part below the heart.
2. Apply a constricting band above the sting site if the sting was inflicted on an extremity. The constricting band should be tight enough to restrict the flow of blood through the veins but not through the arteries. Test for tightness by making sure that you can wedge your finger between the band and the skin. Loosen the band once every three to five minutes to allow the venom to slowly enter the circulatory system. **Do not remove the constricting band until symptoms have been brought under control. Constricting bands are controversial in some areas. Follow local poison control center instructions.**
3. If the sting was inflicted by a honeybee and the stinger is still in the skin, remove the stinger gently by scraping against it with your fingernail or with the edge of a knife or razor blade. Be careful not to *squeeze* the stinger. The venom sac will still be attached, and you will send a new supply of venom into the bloodstream.
4. Apply a cold pack or ice bags to the site to relieve pain and swelling.
5. If the victim develops breathing difficulty, and if an airway cannot be maintained, give mouth-to-mouth ventilation.
6. Keep the victim warm. Have the victim lie down, and elevate the legs and lower the head if he/she shows signs and symptoms of (or danger of lapsing into) shock.
7. Transport the victim to a hospital immediately if more severe signs and symptoms occur.
8. Make sure that the victim will be under strict observation for the first twenty-four hours to eliminate the possibility of later breathing problems or hemorrhage. Tell family members to take the victim to the hospital immediately if any suspicious signs and symptoms develop.
9. If you know that the victim is allergic to stings, do not wait for the signs and symptoms to occur — delay can be fatal. Transport to a hospital immediately.

**See page 204 for discussion regarding allergic reactions to insect venom.**

## POISONOUS PLANTS

**Poison ivy** thrives in sun and in light shade. It usually grows in the form of a trailing vine that sends out numerous kinky brown footlets that are slightly thickened at the tips, but it can also grow in the form of a bush and can attain heights of ten feet or more. **Poison sumac** is a tall shrub or slender tree, usually growing along swamps and ponds in wooded areas. **Poison oak** resembles poison ivy, with one important difference: the poison oak leaves have rounded, lobed leaflets instead of leaflets that are jagged or entire. Poison oak is found mostly in the Southeast and West.

Signs and symptoms of contact with a poisonous plant begin with blisters at the site of contact. It takes two to seven days to develop the rash after initial contact with the plant. In

## Allergic Reactions to Poison Ivy, Oak, Sumac: A Summary of Symptoms and Care

### POISON IVY

**Appearance of plant:** slightly glossy green leaves, growing in groups of three; flowers and berries, when present, are greenish-white; grows as either a trailing vine or erect shrub; most common in eastern and central United States.

**Symptoms of reaction:** initial redness of affected area, followed by development of bumps and blisters; oozing lesions appear and crust over; severe itching accompanies symptoms; symptoms appear anywhere from four to seventy-two hours after exposure and are usually self-limiting.

**Emergency care:** wash skin and clothing with soap and water, making sure all sap is removed; wipe skin with solution of 70 percent alcohol; in self-care use wet compresses of cold water, boric acid, or liquid aluminum acetate to relieve inflammation while lesions are oozing; use calamine location to relieve itching; obtain allergy shots if you are in constant contact with plants or if symptoms are severe.

### POISON OAK

**Appearance of plant:** green leaves, slightly glossy, shaped like oak leaves; plant usually grows in shrublike clusters; found on west coast of the North American continent.

**Symptoms of reaction:** same as for poison ivy.

**Emergency care:** same as for poison ivy.

### POISON SUMAC

**Appearance of plant:** found chiefly in uninhabited areas, such as swamps and damp mountain terrain; leaves grow singly, and are veined; berries are green and drooping (harmless sumac have erect, red berries); grows as a tree, achieving heights of five to six feet.

**Symptoms of reaction:** same as for poison ivy.

**Emergency care:** same as for poison ivy.

cases of more severe exposure, the time is shorter; a rash will usually appear within twelve hours. Itching and swelling accompany the rash; severe reactions may cause pain. The rash usually disappears in one to two weeks in cases of mild exposure and up to three weeks when exposure is more severe.

Toxin on the hands may spread the rash to other parts of the body, but the clear fluid that weeps from the rash will not spread the rash or infect new sites.

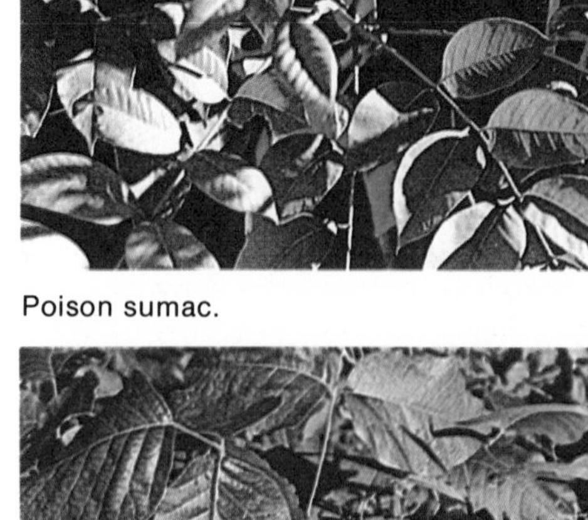

Poison sumac.

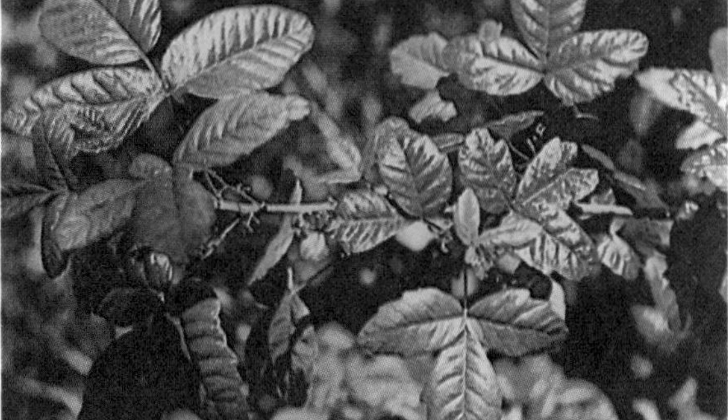

Poison oak.

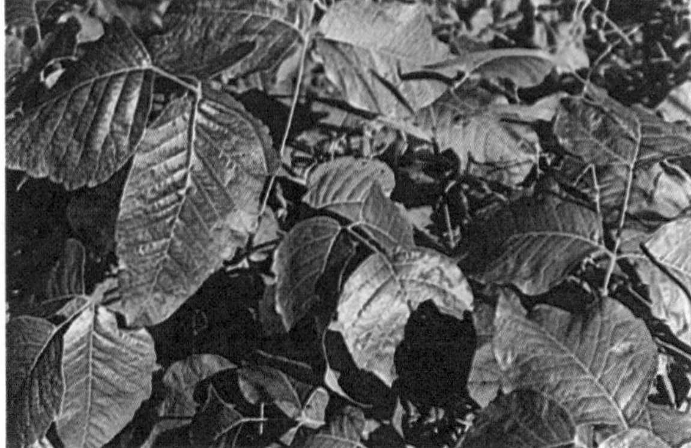

Poison ivy.

The following emergency care is recommended:

1. Wash the exposed bodily parts thoroughly, as soon as possible after contact with the plant.
2. Apply cold compresses to help reduce swelling and irritation.
3. Apply soothing lotions to help reduce swelling and irritation; calamine or calamine/antihistamine are good lotions for this purpose.
4. If severe exposures result in extreme reactions that cannot be controlled comfortably with self-care, a physician should prescribe oral antihistamines and a topical cream.

## FOOD POISONING

Food poisoning occurs when food that contains bacteria or the toxins that bacteria produce is eaten.

The most common food-borne illness, **staphylococcus poisoning,** causes inflammation and irritation of the stomach and intestinal linings. One to five hours after eating the affected food, the patient will experience sudden nausea and vomiting, abdominal cramps, and diarrhea. There is no fever. In severe cases, shock may develop. Recovery is rapid, sometimes within three hours and rarely beyond twenty-four hours.

Emergency care consists of controlling vomiting and diarrhea to prevent dehydration, and giving care for shock. Do not give the victim anything to eat or drink until the vomiting and diarrhea have stopped. Extremely young or old victims may need to be hospitalized to control dehydration.

**Clostridium perfringens** food poisoning results when food is prepared in large quantities and is allowed to sit at room temperature (or in an ineffective steamer). The infection may also result if food is not refrigerated at a low enough temperature (the bacteria thrive in environments anywhere from 40°F. to 140°F.)

Nausea, abdominal cramps, and diarrhea are common symptoms; vomiting is rare. Onset of symptoms occurs usually after six to twenty-four hours; the disease rarely lasts longer than twenty-four hours. To treat, control dehydration.

Symptoms of **salmonella poisoning** usually appear twelve to twenty-four hours following ingestion of a contaminated food. The victim suffers diarrhea, fever, nausea, vomiting, and abdominal cramps with occasional chills. Weakness and dehydration may result.

Emergency care consists of controlling vomiting and diarrhea to prevent dehydration. Antibiotic therapy may be needed for victims under one year of age, elderly victims, persons who have had part of their stomach surgically removed, or persons who suffer from blood disease. All of these victims should be transported to a hospital.

Early recognition of **botulism** and fast care are necessary to save a victim's life. Approximately 60 percent of those infected will die from botulism.

Detection of botulism is difficult because it resembles so many other problems. Suspect botulism in a victim who develops a dry, sore throat and blurred or double vision following a period of fatigue. Other signs and symptoms include weakness or paralysis, limited eye movement, dilated pupils, decreased tendon reflexes, and impaired speech. Any pain that is experienced is generally from a headache in the front part of the head. Breathing difficulty may develop.

A physician must administer antitoxins. Induce vomiting to rid the victim of any remaining spoiled food. Transport the patient to a hospital **immediately.**

## Work Exercises

Poisons are any substances which act to produce harmful effects on the normal body processes. There are numerous ways in which these substances may enter the body.

List four common ways poisons may enter the body.

1.

2.

3.

4.

Complete the following table on ingested poisons by listing the general principles of emergency care.

**INGESTED POISONS**

| Signs/Symptoms | General Principles of Emergency Care |
|---|---|
| Nausea/vomiting<br>Abdominal pain<br>Diarrhea<br>Dilation or constriction of pupils<br>Excessive salivation or sweating<br>Abnormal respiration<br>Unconsciousness<br>Burns, odors, or stains about mouth<br>Convulsions | 1.<br><br>2.<br><br>3.<br><br>Syrup of Ipecac<br>Adults (amount?) ____________ followed by ____________ glasses of water.<br>Children (amount?) ____________ *followed* *by* ____________ glasses of water. |

When should activated charcoal be given?

Match the following poisoning situations with appropriate emergency care procedure.

**WHEN TO INDUCE VOMITING**

| Poisoning Situation | Emergency Care |
|---|---|
| ______ 1. The stuporous or unconscious victim | A. Induce vomiting |
| ______ 2. The pregnant victim | B. Do not induce vomiting |
| ______ 3. The victim with possible acute myocardial infarction | |
| ______ 4. The victim who has ingested corrosives (strong acids or alkalis) | |
| ______ 5. The victim with seizures | |
| ______ 6. The victim who has ingested petroleum products (kerosene, gasoline, lighter fluid, furniture polish) | |
| ______ 7. The victim who has ingested iodides, silver nitrate (styptic pencil), or strychnine | |

## Childhood Poisoning

Approximately 90 percent of all poisoning cases involve children. List five signs/symptoms that may indicate childhood poisoning.

1.

2.

3.

4.

5.

List six emergency care guidelines for inhaled poisons.

1.

2.

3.

4.

5.

6.

Complete the following table by matching the correct characteristic with either poisonous or nonpoisonous snakes.

**DISTINGUISHING BETWEEN POISONOUS AND NONPOISONOUS SNAKES**

| Characteristics | Type of Snake |
|---|---|
| _____ 1. Series of small, shallow puncture wounds. | A. Poisonous |
| _____ 2. Wound begins to swell and discolor. | B. Nonpoisonous |
| _____ 3. Differently shaped blotches on background of pink, yellow, olive, tan, gray or brown skin. | |
| _____ 4. Elliptical pupils (vertical slits, much like those of a cat). | |
| _____ 5. Large fangs that are hollow. | |
| _____ 6. Pain and burning almost immediately. | |
| _____ 7. Pit between the eye and mouth. | |

List the necessary emergency care for a venomous snakebite with severe symptoms (more than 30 minutes away from medical help).

1.

2.

3.

4.

5.

6.

7.

8.

List the emergency care for an allergic insect sting.

1.

2.

3.

4.

5.

6.

7.

## Poisonous Plants

List three emergency care procedures recommended for external (skin) plant poisoning.

1.

2.

3.

## SELF-TEST

### Part I: True and False

If you believe the statement is true, circle the T. If you believe the statement is false, circle F.

T F 1. Do NOT administer activated charcoal at the same time as syrup of ipecac.

T F 2. If vomiting does not occur 10 minutes after the first administration of syrup of ipecac, the dose should be repeated.

T F 3. The vomitus and the poison container should be taken to the hospital along with the victim.

T F 4. Carbon monoxide is probably the most common poisonous gas.

T F 5. When removing a bee stinger, scrape it away rather than squeezing it.

T F 6. Put a cold pack over a spider sting.

T F 7. If a child has burns around his mouth, you can safely assume that the poison is an acid.

T F 8. Household lye should NOT be eliminated by vomiting.

T F 9. Coral snakes are NOT classified as pit vipers.

T F 10. A constricting band applied for a snakebite wound should stop the flow of both arterial and venous blood.

T F 11. Carbon monoxide poisoning is characterized by red skin in early stages.

T F 12. The most common kind of poisoning is inhalation.

T F 13. Induce vomiting in all cases of inhaled poisons.

T F 14. A poisonous snakebite should be treated by placing a constricting band near the wound and elevating the limb above the heart.

T F 15. The most immediate method of first aid treatment for inhaled poisons is to move the victim into fresh air, away from the source of poisoning.

### Part II: Multiple Choice

For each question, circle the one answer that best reflects a true statement.

1. What percent of poisoning cases involve children?

   a. 50 b. 75 c. 30 d. 90

2. Which of the following is *not* a way that poisons may enter the body?

   a. absorption b. emesis c. inhalation d. injection

3. A common sign of ingestion poisoning is:

   a. abdominal cramps
   b. increased respiration
   c. increased circulation
   d. decreased salivation

4. As a general rule, if a victim has ingested a poisonous substance within the past ________ hours, the stomach should be emptied.

   a. 1-3 b. ½-2 c. 4-8 d. 3-6

5. Which of the following poisonous substances should *not* be eliminated by vomiting?

   a. aspirin
   b. household lye
   c. poisonous berries
   d. sleeping pills

6. Syrup of ipecac is an effective means of inducing vomiting. What is the proper dose for eliminating poisons in an adult?
   a. one teaspoon
   b. one tablespoon
   c. two tablespoons
   d. three tablespoons

7. To induce vomiting, syrup of ipecac should be followed by:
   a. rigorous exercise
   b. large doses of activated charcoal
   c. two to three glasses of water
   d. nothing, syrup of ipecac works by itself

8. After vomiting has ceased, give a victim:
   a. activated charcoal
   b. lemon juice in a glass of water
   c. raw egg to coat the stomach
   d. more ipecac and water

9. When should vomiting be induced?
   a. if the poison is a strong acid
   b. if the poison is kerosene
   c. if the poison is an alkali
   d. if the poison is aspirin

10. A late stage symptom often indicating carbon monoxide poisoning results when the skin turns:
    a. cyanotic blue
    b. cyanotic gray
    c. cherry red
    d. pale marble white

11. What is a characteristic symptom of carbon monoxide poisoning?
    a. headache
    b. cool, pale skin
    c. complaints of a strange taste in the mouth
    d. stains around the mouth

12. What is the initial emergency care procedure for inhalation poisonings?
    a. remove the victim to fresh air
    b. begin mouth-to-mouth resuscitation
    c. treat the victim for shock
    d. seek medical care immediately

13. Which of the following is *not* a sign or symptom of a poisonous snakebite?
    a. severe pain and burning
    b. swelling of wound
    c. discoloration of wound
    d. series of small, shallow puncture wounds

14. Most poisonous snakes have:
    a. multicolored rings around the body
    b. elliptical pupils
    c. small teeth
    d. flat heads

15. The constricting band applied for a snakebite wound should:
    a. not stop the flow of either arterial or venous blood
    b. stop the flow of arterial blood, but not venous blood
    c. stop the flow of venous blood, but not arterial blood
    d. stop the flow of both arterial and venous blood

16. If a snakebite wound begins to swell:
    a. remove the constricting band
    b. loosen the band slightly
    c. remove the band for 10 minutes and then reapply
    d. do not loosen or remove the band

17. Of the four types of poisonous snakes found in the United States, which are not classified as pit vipers?
    a. rattlesnakes
    b. coral snakes
    c. moccasins
    d. copperheads

18. Only make incisions in a snakebite wound if:
    a. the wound is from a coral snake
    b. there is numbness and blisters around the wound
    c. you cannot administer an antivenin
    d. you are more than 30 minutes from a medical facility

19. If you need to incise fang marks, the incisions should be:
    a. vertical and parallel
    b. horizontal
    c. cross marks
    d. never incise fang marks

20. Unless contraindicated by local poison control center a First Aider should treat a coral snake bite by:
    a. application of a constricting band and an ice bag
    b. application of a constricting band only
    c. incision and suction of the wound area
    d. application of rubbing alcohol and an ice pack to the wound

21. The emergency care for black widow and brown recluse spider bites always has one of the following in common:
    a. administering mouth-to-mouth resuscitation and/or oxygen.
    b. application of an ice pack
    c. application of a constricting band
    d. try to identify the spider

22. Which of the following should you do as part of the emergency care for a victim of allergic reaction to a sting on the extremity?
    a. apply warm compresses to increase circulation
    b. elevate the extremity to reduce swelling
    c. apply a tourniquet above the sting
    d. apply a constricting band above the sting

23. The proper emergency care for a honeybee sting is:
    a. grasp the sac or stinger with a pair of tweezers and gently pull it out.
    b. apply wet mud to the sting area, let it dry.
    c. apply Arm and Hammer baking soda to the affected area.
    d. remove the stinger by scraping it gently with your fingernail or the edge of a knife.

24. What are the signs and symptoms of poison ivy, poison oak, and poison sumac poisoning?
    a. red rash that doesn't itch
    b. formation of blisters and oozing sores
    c. general body swelling
    d. nausea and vomiting

25. The most common food-borne illness is:
    a. salmonella poisoning
    b. botulism
    c. staphylococcus poisoning
    d. flu

26. After eating a bottle of grandma's canned peaches, a family member develops a dry, sore throat, double vision, and impaired speech. You should suspect:
    a. shigella and get antibiotic treatment
    b. botulism and get medical attention immediately
    c. salmonella and treat for shock
    d. clostridium perfringens and wait it out for 24 hours

Corresponds with:

**American Red Cross**

**Standard First Aid & Personal Safety**

Chapter 8, pages 126-143

and

**Advanced First Aid & Emergency Care**

Chapter 8, pages 118-133

# 12 Drug and Alcohol Emergencies

## GENERAL TERMINOLOGY

**Drug abuse** is defined as the self-administration of drugs (or of a single drug) in a manner that is not in accord with approved medical or social patterns. **Compulsive drug use** refers to the situation in which an individual becomes preoccupied with the use and procurement of the drug. Compulsive drug use usually leads to addiction characterized by physical or psychological dependence.

**Physical dependence** is defined by the appearance of an observable **abstinence syndrome** following the abrupt discontinuation of a drug that has been used regularly. Physical dependence signs and symptoms are different for different drug classes (such as **narcotics, depressants,** or **stimulants**), but physical dependence can always be identified by the presence of an abstinence syndrome.

A physically dependent person will usually have one set of signs and symptoms due to drug use and an opposite set when the drug is withheld. **Opiates,** for example, reduce gastrointestinal activity. When a person who is physically dependent on opiates is denied the drug, he/she suffers the opposite effect of increased gastrointestinal activity.

Physical dependence is not a "normal" physiological condition. It represents adaptation by the bodily systems to the presence of the drug. When a person becomes physically dependent, then, the absence of the drug has a significant physiological impact.

**Psychological dependence** refers to a condition in which a person experiences a strong *need* to experience the drug repeatedly, even in the absence of physical dependence. The state of psychological dependence is sometimes called **habituation.**

While most drug therapy has traditionally centered on treating physical dependence, psychological dependence is often more compelling and critical. Some drugs produce no physical dependence at all but produce intense psychological dependence.

One of the difficulties with psychological dependence is that the victim is "rewarded" for taking the drug. The person becomes motivated, feels good, and thinks that he/she is capable of doing marvelous things. In many cases, the drug is used to escape feelings of depression.

**Tolerance** refers to the situation in which, after repeated exposures to a given drug, achieving the desired effect requires larger doses. The magnitude of tolerance can be measured by comparing the results obtained from the initial dose of the drug with those obtained from subsequent doses.

The extent of tolerance and the rate of its development depend on the individual, the drug, the dose, the frequency of dose, and the method of administration. Most tolerance results from frequent and continuous exposure to the drug. An increase in dosage will again produce the desired results. With some drugs, however, the victim reaches a plateau, and the desired effect cannot be obtained with *any* dosage.

**Addiction** involves physical and psychological dependence, tolerance, and compulsive drug use. It is characterized by overwhelming involvement in the use of a drug.

## SIGNS AND SYMPTOMS OF DRUG ABUSE

Each of the drug classes has unique effects, signs and symptoms of withdrawal and overdose, and patterns of tolerance. See the table, Emergency Consequences of Commonly Abused Drugs for more detailed information.

## ALCOHOL EMERGENCIES

When you encounter an alcohol abuse victim, certain signs indicate that medical attention is needed **immediately:**

1. Signs that the nervous system is depressed — sleepiness, coma, lethargy, decreased response to pain, and so on.
2. Impaired reflexes, coordination, judgment.
3. Tremors (especially if the victim is suffering withdrawal).
4. Withdrawal that has become painful.
5. Inappropriate behavior (especially if it is aggressive).
6. Digestive upsets, including **gastritis,** vomiting, bleeding, and dehydration.
7. Excessively slow or absent breathing.
8. **Grand mal seizures.**
9. Delirium tremens (terrifying mental confusion, constant tremors, fever, dehydration, rapid heartbeat, and fumbling movements of the hands).
10. Disturbances of vision, mental confusion, and muscular incoordination.
11. Disinterested behavior and loss of memory.
12. Injury to bones and joints that is unexplained and that is in various stages of healing.

## GENERAL GUIDELINES FOR MANAGING A DRUG/ALCOHOL CRISIS

Crisis intervention is by definition short term; it involves alleviating the pain and confusion of a specific event or circumstance. The conscious victim with drug- or alcohol-related emergency problems is often experiencing severe emotional stress. In such instances, the most important crisis intervention tools are the verbal and nonverbal communication skills of the attending First Aider.

The following guidelines may be helpful in reducing emotional overreaction by helping the victim make sense out of what is happening:

1. **Provide a reality base.**
   - Identify yourself.
   - Use the victim's name.
   - Anticipate the concerns of the victim, family, and friends.
   - Based on the victim's response, introduce as much familiarity as possible, e.g., persons, objects, newspapers, TV programs.
   - Be calm and self-assured.
2. **Provide appropriate nonverbal support.**
   - Maintain eye contact.
   - Maintain a relaxed body posture. Be quiet, calm, and gentle.
   - Touch the victim if it seems appropriate.
3. **Encourage communication.**
   - Communicate directly with the victim, not through others.
   - Ask clear, simple questions.
   - Ask questions slowly, one at a time.
   - Tolerate repetition; do not become impatient.
4. **Foster confidence.**
   - Be nonjudgmental. Do not accuse the victim.
   - Help the victim gain confidence in you.
   - Listen carefully.
   - Respond to feelings; let the victim know you understand his/her feelings.
   - Identify and reinforce progress.

## MANAGING THE VIOLENT DRUG VICTIM

In managing the violent victim:

1. Do not approach a potentially violent victim alone. Do so only with a sufficient number of people to control an outbreak of violence.

## Emergency Consequences of Commonly Abused Drugs

| DRUG CLUSTER | MOST COMMON DRUG OF ABUSE | CONSEQUENCE OF ABUSE |
|---|---|---|
| **STIMULANTS AND APPETITE SUPPRESSANTS** | AMPHETAMINES<br>Caffeine<br>Cocaine<br>Ephedrine<br>Methylphenidate<br>Nicotine<br>Over-the-Counter Preparations | Moderate dosages cause increased alertness, excitation, euphoria, increased pulse rate and blood pressure, insomnia, loss of appetite. Overdoses can cause agitation, increase in body temperature, hallucinations, convulsions, possible death. Although the degree of physical addiction is not known, sudden withdrawal can cause apathy, long periods of sleep, irritability, depression, disorientation. |
| **CANNABIS PRODUCTS** | Hashish<br>Marijuana<br>THC (Tetrahydrocannabinol) | Moderate dosages cause euphoria, relaxed inhibitions, increased appetite, disoriented behavior. Overdoses can cause fatigue, paranoia, possible psychosis. Although the degree of physical addiction is not known, sudden withdrawal can cause insomnia, hyperactivity, and decreased appetite is occasionally reported. |
| **DEPRESSANTS — NARCOTICS AND OPIATES** | Codeine<br>Heroin<br>Methadone<br>Morphine<br>Opium | Moderate dosages cause euphoria, drowsiness, respiratory depression, constricted pupils, nausea. Overdoses can cause slow and shallow breathing, clammy skin, convulsions, coma, possible death. Sudden withdrawal results in watery eyes, runny nose, yawning, loss of appetite, irritability, tremors, panic, chills and sweating, cramps, nausea. |
| **DEPRESSANTS — SEDATIVES AND TRANQUILIZERS** | Alcohol<br>Antihistamines<br>Barbiturates<br>Chloralhydrate, Other Non-Barbiturate, Nonbenzodiazepine, Sedatives, Over-the-Counter Preparations, Diazepam and Other Benzodiazepines,<br>Other Major Tranquilizers,<br>Other Minor Tranquilizers | Moderate dosages can result in slurred speech, disorientation, drunken behavior without odor of alcohol. Overdose can result in shallow respiration, cold and clammy skin, dilated pupils, weak and rapid pulse, coma, possible death. Sudden withdrawal results in anxiety, insomnia, tremors, delirium, convulsions, possible death. |
| **PSYCHEDELIC DRUGS** | DET (N, N-Diethyltryptamine)<br>DMT (N, N-Dimethytryptamine)<br>LSD (Lysergic Acid Diethylamide)<br>Mescaline<br>MDA (3, 4 Methylenedioxyamphetamine)<br>PCP (PHENCYCLIDINE)<br>STP (DOM-2, 5-Dimethoxy, 4-Methylamphetamine) | Moderate dosages, can result in illusions and hallucinations, poor perception of time and distance. Overdose can result in longer, more intense "trip" episodes, psychosis, and possible death. |
| **INHALANTS** | Medical Anesthetics<br>Gasoline and Kerosene<br>Glues and Organic Cements<br>Lighter Fluid<br>Lacquer and Varnish Thinners<br>Aerosol Propellants | Moderate dosages cause excitement, euphoria, giddiness, loss of inhibitions, aggressiveness, delusions, depression, drowsiness, headache, nausea. Overdoses can cause loss of memory, confusion, unsteady gait, and erratic heart beat and pulse are possible. Sudden withdrawal results in insomnia, decreased appetite, depression, irritability, headache. Death can result from suffocation. |

## ALCOHOL EMERGENCIES

**CAUTION** These signs can mean illnesses or injuries other than alcohol abuse (e.g. epilepsy, diabetes, head injury).

It is therefore especially important that the person with apparent alcohol on his breath (which can smell like the acetone breath of a diabetic) not be immediately dismissed as a drunk.
He should be carefully checked for other illnesses/injuries.

### SIGNS

The signs of alcohol intoxication are familiar to all:

- Odor of alcohol on breath
- Swaying/unsteadiness
- Slurred speech
- Nausea/vomiting
- Flushed face

### EFFECTS

Alcohol affects a person's judgement, vision, reaction time and coordination. In very large quantities, it can cause death by paralyzing the respiratory center of the brain.

### DEPRESSANT

Alcohol is a depressant, not a stimulant. Many people think it is a stimulant since its first effect is to reduce tension and give a mild feeling of euphoria or exhilaration.

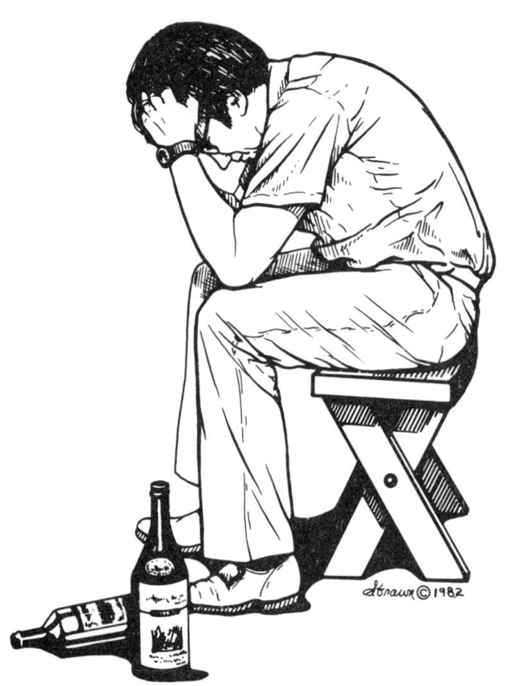


### ALCOHOL COMBINES WITH OTHER DEPRESSANTS

When alcohol is taken in combination with analgesics, tranquilizers, antihistamines, barbiturates, etc., the depressant effects will be added together and, in some instances, the resultant effect will be greater than the expected combined effects of the two drugs.

### MANAGEMENT

The intoxicated victim should be given the same attention given to victims with other illnesses/injuries.

The intoxicated person needs constant watching to be sure that he doesn't aspirate vomitus and that he maintains respirations.

### WITHDRAWAL PROBLEMS

An alcoholic who suddenly stops drinking can suffer from severe withdrawal problems. Sudden withdrawal will often result in DT's (delerium tremens).

**Signs include:**

1. Shaking hands
2. Restlessness
3. Confusion
4. Hallucinations
5. Sometimes maniacal behavior

The victim must be protected from hurting himself.

2. Avoid aggressive actions unless there is the immediate possibility of serious injury. In all other circumstances, only defensive techniques, e.g., holding the arms or legs, or rolling in a blanket, should be permitted.
3. If the First Aider is assaulted, it is possible that he/she ignored the many signals of impending loss of control presented by the victim. These include high degrees of agitation, sweating, and excessive talking while struggling with violent impulses, etc. First Aiders should control their own anxiety, be alert to such signals, and take evasive action (leaving the room or calling in other people) before the victim's impulses are translated into action. There is nothing wrong with running from a room occupied by a physically threatening victim, armed or unarmed.
4. If you can, call for help and have the victim transported to the hospital immediately. If at all possible, keep something familiar with the person — a family member, a friend, a coat, or some other possession.
5. Let the person sit near the door of the room; do not place any obstacle (person or furniture) between the person and the door. In other words, do not block the route of escape. A person who feels trapped will likely become more anxious, which will exaggerate hostility and violence.
6. If the victim is armed, the police must be called. If there are not enough personnel to ensure control of an unarmed but violent victim, the police should also be called.

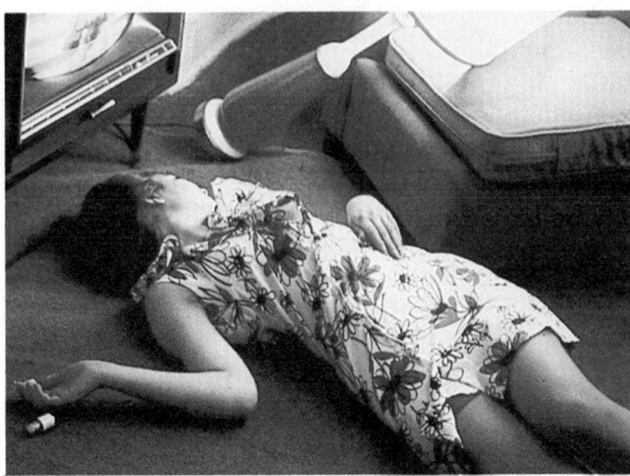

Drug and alcohol emergencies are often serious and life-threatening.

7. The victim must be protected while in the environment of the emergency setting. Needles, sharp instruments, drugs, etc. should not be in the immediate proximity of the victim.

## DEALING WITH HYPERVENTILATING VICTIMS

Hyperventilation is a common emergency situation in drug abusing victims. It can be a manifestation of acute anxiety, but it also may indicate a serious medical problem, severe pain, drug withdrawal, or aspirin poisoning.

Hyperventilation in a drug emergency should be cared for as a medical disorder and **not** as anxiety hyperventilation. **Do not** have the victim breathe into a paper bag.

Often it is difficult to provide a quiet, reassuring environment in an emergency setting. The hyperventilating victim should be removed from the crisis situation as soon as possible. Hyperventilating victims should not be left alone. First Aiders should listen (in a nonjudgmental way) to the problems of the victim and should respond to the victim's questions regarding his/her condition in a calm, professional manner.

## HOW TO DETERMINE IF AN EMERGENCY IS DRUG/ ALCOHOL-RELATED

Because abuse of drugs and alcohol produces signs that mimic a number of diseases, it is often difficult for a First Aider to properly assess a condition as a drug or alcohol emergency. This is especially true if the victim is unconscious.

If you suspect that a victim might be experiencing a drug or alcohol emergency, try the following:

- Inspect the area immediately around the victim for evidence of drug or alcohol use — empty or partially filled pill bottles, syringes, empty liquor bottles, and so on.

## DRUG AND ALCOHOL EMERGENCY INDICATORS

If any of the following six danger signs are present, no matter what caused the crisis, the victim's life may be threatened and there is an immediate need for emergency care and medical assistance.

**1**
**Unconsciousness:**
The victim cannot be awakened from what appears to be a deep sleep or coma. If awakened for a short period of time, he almost immediately relapses into unconsciousness.

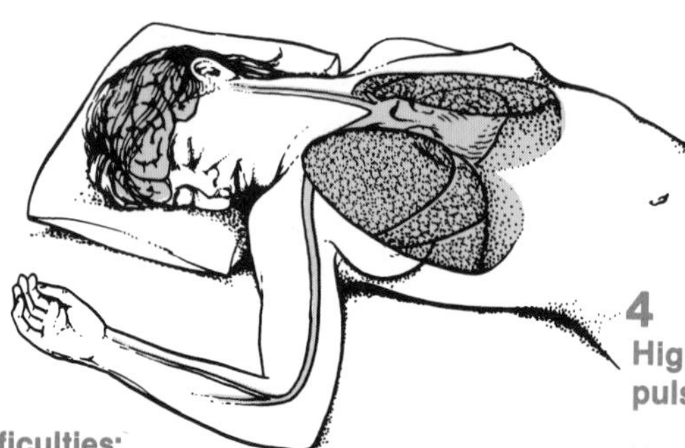

**2**
**Respiratory difficulties:**
The victim's breathing may be very weak, strong and weak in cycles, or may stop altogether. Intake or output may be noisy. If the victim's skin is bluish (cyanotic), he is almost certainly not receiving enough oxygen, but the absence of cyanosis does not necessarily mean that respiratory difficulties are not severe.

**3**
**Raised temperature:**
As a guide it may be stated that any temperature above 100° F. or 38° C. falls into this category.

**4**
**High or low pulse rate, or an irregular pulse:**

Usual range for pulse rate is between 50 and 80 beats per minute for an adult; any pulse that is below or above that acceptable range indicates possible danger, as does a pulse that is irregular (not rhythmical).

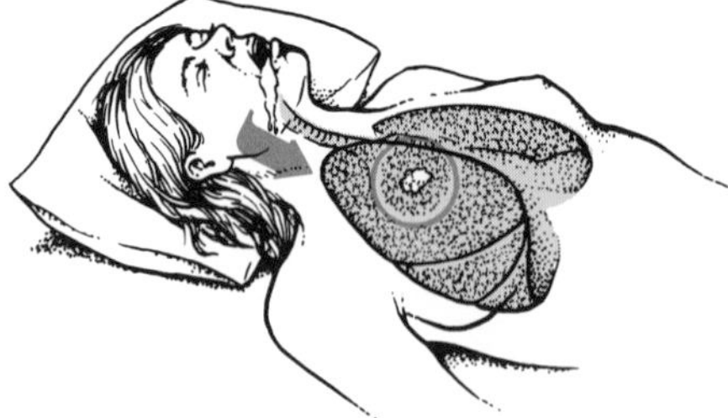

**5**
**Vomiting while semi-conscious or unconscious:**
If the victim vomits while semi-conscious or unconscious the prime danger consists of the possibility that he may breathe vomitus back into his lungs, causing further respiratory difficulties.

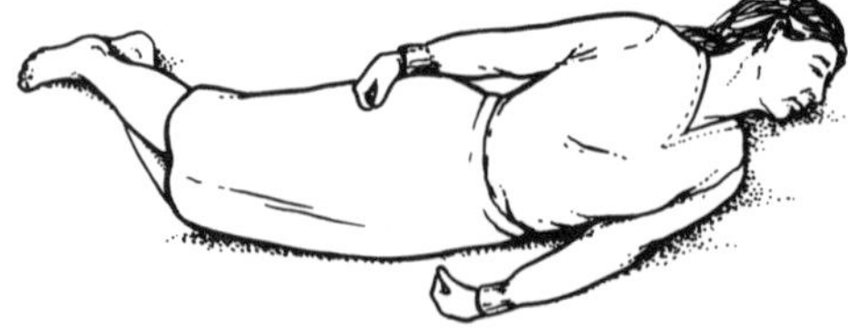

**6**
**Convulsions or seizures:**
Muscle rigidity, spasm, or twitching of face, trunk muscles, or extremities may indicate an impending convulsion with a series of violent muscle spasms and jerking movements.

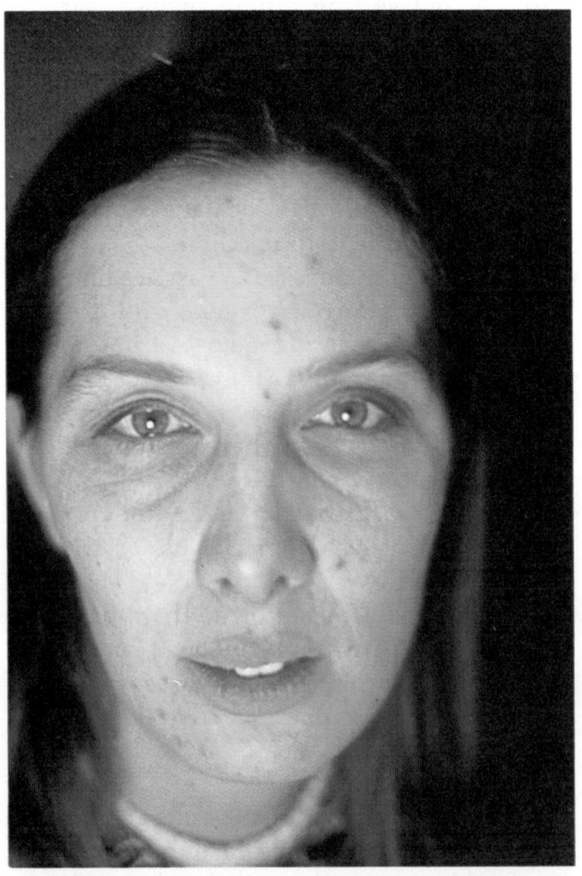

Constricted pupils as seen in narcotic drug use.

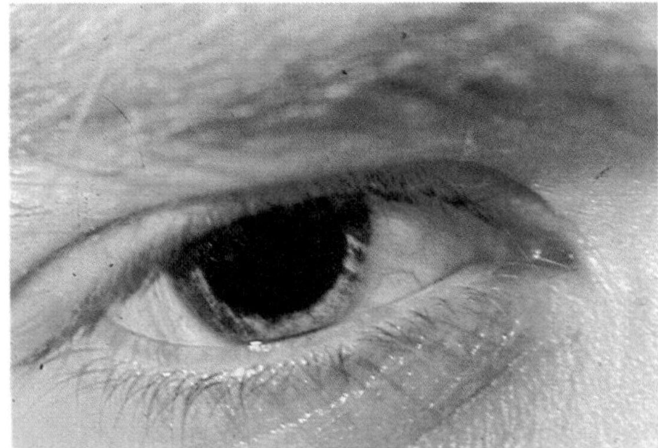

Dilated pupils from use of barbiturate drugs.

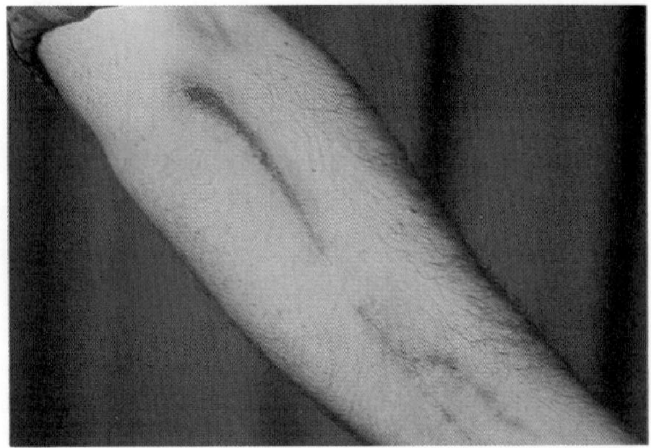

Needle tracks from drug abuse.

- Check the victim's mouth for signs of partially dissolved pills or tablets that may still be in his mouth. (If present, remove.)
- Smell the victim's breath for traces of alcohol. (Be sure that you do not confuse a musky, fruity, or acetone odor for alcohol — all three can be indicative of diabetes.)
- Ask the victim's friends or family members, if they are nearby, what they know about the incident.
- Ask any witnesses who might have seen the victim lose consciousness if they can offer any suggestions about what might have happened.
- Remember — many serious diseases (such as diabetes and epilepsy) resemble drug overdose. Do not make the mistake of assuming that a stuporous, slurry-speeched person has ingested drugs. **Never jump to conclusions.**

## GENERAL PROCEDURES FOR OVERDOSE

An overdose of almost any drug can cause poisoning and should be cared for at once. Emergency care is limited for a person suffering from drug poisoning, but the following procedures can be done. Most of the time, you will be unable to tell exactly which drug a victim has been using. These are guidelines that apply to all alcohol and drug emergencies:

- Do not panic. Treat the victim calmly. Squelch your impulses to throw cold water on the victim or to move him/her around. Of course, you should move a victim if he/she is inhaling a harmful substance or if he/she is in immediate danger (for instance, a victim who has lost consciousness near a burning building).

- Quickly assess the situation. Because symptoms of drug abuse resemble those of other diseases, it is important that you obtain as much information as possible. If the victim is conscious, ask what he/she has taken. If the victim is unconscious, ask friends or family members who may know what has happened. Whatever you do, do not spend a lot of time finding out what has happened at this stage; there may be life-threatening symptoms that need to be handled directly.
- Establish and maintain a clear airway. Remove anything from the mouth or throat that might pose a breathing hazard, including false teeth, blood, mucus, or vomitus.
- Give artificial ventilation if the victim needs ventilation.
- Turn the victim's head to the side and downward toward the ground; in case of vomiting, the victim's mouth and throat will drain more easily in this position.
- Monitor the victim's vital signs frequently. In case of respiratory or cardiac complications, care for the life-threatening situations immediately.
- Watch overdose victims carefully; they can be conscious one minute and lapse into unconsciousness the next.
- Reestablish proper body temperature.
- Take measures to correct or prevent shock.
- If the victim is conscious, induce vomiting, particularly if the drug has been ingested within the last thirty minutes. This course of action depends, however, on where the crisis occurred. If the victim can be taken to a hospital within minutes, inducing vomiting is unnecessary. On the other hand, in an isolated setting where medical care is not promptly available, inducing vomiting is useful. Of course, if the drug has been taken **intravenously** or by inhalation (sniffing), induced vomiting is meaningless. Nor should vomiting be induced in a victim who is not fully conscious. The danger of aspiration of vomitus is too great.
- If the victim is conscious, reassure him/her, and explain thoroughly who you are and that you are trying to help.
- If the victim is convulsing, protect him/her from hurting him/herself by holding the head in your lap so that he/she will not bang it against the ground.
- Speak firmly to the victim. Be understanding and assuring. *Never* ridicule or criticize the victim.
- Obtain brief information so that you know what kind of drug or alcohol was consumed. Perform a brief physical assessment to eliminate possibilities of complications or other injuries.
- Call for assistance.
- If there is time before the emergency team arrives, search the area around the victim for tablets, capsules, pill bottles or boxes (especially empty ones), syringes, prescriptions, hospital attendance cards, or physician's notes that might help identify what drug the victim has taken. Give any such evidence to the emergency team.
- If the victim is agitated, move him/her to a quiet place where he/she can be observed and where there will be little interaction with others. It is critical that you calm the victim who seems to be agitated or paranoid.
- If the victim becomes increasingly excited and approaches or reaches a delirious phase, be firm but friendly. Some victims will be in an excited phase when the emergency team arrives. This excitement period, often a prelude to coma, may last for several hours.
- DO NOT jump to conclusions — do not make decisions based solely on the victim's personal appearance, the fact that you detect an alcoholic odor, or the victim's companions.
- DO NOT accuse or criticize the victim.
- DO NOT leave intoxicated victims alone; make sure that they are attended and observed at all times.

### Directions for Making the Victim Vomit

- Give two tablespoonfuls (30 ml) Syrup of Ipecac (one tablespoon for a child). Follow this with two to three cups of water. If no vomiting occurs after twenty minutes, this dose may be repeated one time only.

### Administration of activated charcoal

- Activated charcoal (two to four tablespoonfuls in a glass of water) may be given after vomiting has occurred or if ipecac has failed to cause vomiting within an hour. Do not give activated charcoal before ipecac has had an opportunity to cause vomiting.

## The Talk-Down Technique

The dangers associated with the **hallucinogens** and with **marijuana** are primarily psychological in nature. These may be evident as intense anxiety or panic states (**"bad trips"**), depressive or paranoid reactions, mood changes, disorientation, and an inability to distinguish between reality and fantasy. Some prolonged psychotic reactions to psychedelic drugs have been reported, particularly with persons already psychologically disturbed.

The "talk-down" technique has been established as the preferred method for handling bad trips. This technique involves nonmoralizing, comforting, personal support from an experienced individual. It is aided by limiting external stimulation, such as intense light or loud sounds, and having the person lie down and relax.

The goal of talking-down is to reduce the victim's anxiety, panic, depression, or confusion. Follow these steps:

1. Make the victim feel welcome. Remain relaxed and sympathetic. Because a victim can become suddenly hostile, have a companion with you.
2. Reassure the victim that this strange mental condition is a result of ingestion of the drug and that he/she *will* return to normal. Help the person realize that he/she is not mentally ill.
3. Help the victim verbalize what is happening. Ask him questions. Outline the probable time schedule of events.
4. Reiterate simple and concrete statements. Be absolutely clear in letting the victim know where he/she is, what is happening, and who you are.
5. Listen for clues that will let you know whether the victim is anxious, and, if he/she is, discuss those anxieties. Help the victim work through them. Help the person conquer guilt feelings.
6. Forewarn the victim about what will happen as the drug begins to wear off. He/she will probably be confused one minute, and will experience mental clarity the next. Again, help the person understand that this is due to the drug, not to mental illness.
7. Always call for emergency assistance in a drug and/or alcohol emergency.

### Summary Comments Regarding Care For Drug/Alcohol Emergencies

- Vomiting should be induced if the overdose was taken in the preceding thirty minutes.
- Hyperactive victims should be protected from hurting themselves and others. They should be reassured and treated calmly.
- Level of consciousness should be maintained.
- Respirations should be carefully monitored since overdoses of depressants can cause respiratory depression and death.
- The First Aider should instill confidence. The victim should be assured that he will be all right.
- The First Aider should be alert for possible allergic reactions and shock.
- Evidence should be preserved.
- Prompt transportation to a hospital is required.

## Work Exercises

Complete the following table by matching the terms with the correct definition.

### General Drug Terminology

| Terms | Definitions |
|---|---|
| ______ 1. Drug Abuse | A. Condition in which the victim experiences a strong need to experience the drug repeatedly. |
| ______ 2. Compulsive drug use | B. Leads to addiction characterized by physical or psychological dependence. |
| ______ 3. Physical dependence | C. Refers to the situation in which, after repeated exposures to a given drug, achieving the desired effect requires larger doses. |
| ______ 4. Psychological dependence | D. Involves physical and psychological dependence, tolerance, and compulsive drug use. |
| ______ 5. Habituation | E. The self-administration of drugs (or of a single drug) in a manner that is not in accord with approved medical or social patterns. |
| ______ 6. Tolerance | F. Sometimes called psychological dependence. |
| ______ 7. Addiction | G. Appearance of an observable abstinence syndrome following the abrupt discontinuation of a drug that has been used regularly. |

List five signs that indicate that medical attention should be sought immediately for an alcohol abuse victim.

1.

2.

3.

4.

5.

### Managing Drug/Alcohol Crises

The goal of crisis intervention is to establish and maintain rapport, create trust, and build a short-term working relationship that will lower anxiety, produce a clearer understanding of the problem at hand, and identify the resources to cope with it. Specifically, a First Aider should provide a ______________________ for the victim. Maintain ____________ contact with the victim. Encourage ______________________. Foster ____________________.

List five important considerations when dealing with a victim who has taken drugs and/or alcohol and is aggressive, hostile, violent, or psychotic.

1.

2.

3.

4.

5.

If you suspect drug/alcohol ingestion at a dangerous level, you should observe the victim for six signs and symptoms that indicate the victim's life is in danger. List them.

1.

2.

3.

4.

5.

6.

## General Procedures for Managing Overdose Emergencies

An overdose of almost any drug should be cared for at once. List eight emergency care guidelines for alcohol/drug overdose.

1.

2.

3.

4.

5.

6.

7.

8.

## SELF-TEST

### Part I: True and False

If you believe the statement is true, circle the T. If you believe the statement is false, circle F.

T F 1. Almost every drug — including aspirin and alcohol — can be misused or abused.

T F 2. It is easy to tell what drug a person has taken by simply observing the symptoms and signs.

T F 3. The use of some drugs — such as alcohol — is legal and widely accepted, but prolonged use or misuse can become extremely detrimental.

T F 4. Hallucinogen abuse is difficult to treat because its effects are highly variable and unpredictable.

T F 5. Physical effects of marijuana use are related in intensity to dose, and first aid for marijuana use is rarely required.

T F 6. Narcotic withdrawal is often intense, and there is little an amateur First Aider can do.

T F 7. While normal and controlled use of amphetamines produces alertness and a feeling of well-being, an overdose can result in unpleasant effects such as confusion, disorientation, and antisocial behavior.

### Part II: Multiple Choice

For each question, circle the answer that best reflects an accurate statement.

1. A victim of alcohol intoxication does not require immediate first aid unless:
   a. he/she is unresponsive
   b. he/she shows signs of shock
   c. he/she is breathing abnormally
   d. any of the above

2. ________________ refers to a condition in which a victim experiences a strong need to experience a drug repeatedly.
   a. physical dependence
   b. withdrawal
   c. intoxication
   d. psychological dependence

3. Drug tolerance refers to:
   a. the body's ability to normally function when a drug has been administered
   b. the amount of a certain drug that would be considered lethal
   c. the body requiring progressively larger doses of a drug to achieve the same desired effect
   d. a strong need to experience the drug repeatedly

4. Drug addiction involves:
   a. a physical dependence on a drug
   b. physical and psychological dependence, tolerance, and compulsive drug use
   c. chronic tolerance, habituation, and frequency
   d. psychological dependence on a drug

5. Delirium tremens occur as a result of:
   a. alcohol overdose
   b. alcohol taken with tranquilizers
   c. high alcohol concentrations ingested very quickly
   d. alcohol withdrawal

6. The signs of acute intoxication may be mimicked by a ________________ victim.
   a. comatose
   b. diabetic (coma)
   c. convulsive
   d. violent

7. When you encounter an alcohol abuse victim, which of the following signs indicates that medical attention is needed immediately?
   a. grand mal seizures
   b. high blood pressure
   c. hypoglycemia
   d. increased breathing rate

8. Which of the following is *not* a guideline for managing a drug/alcohol crisis?
   a. encourage the victim to communicate
   b. provide appropriate nonverbal support for the victim
   c. provide a reality base for the victim
   d. let the victim make decisions on what he/she needs to do

9. Which of the following is *not* a guideline for managing a violent victim?
   a. let the person sit near.the door
   b. approach a violent victim alone so as not to cause him/her undue alarm
   c. protect the victim while in the environment of the emergency setting
   d. avoid aggressive action toward the violent patient if possible

10. The most important information to be gathered from an emergency drug/alcohol victim concerns:
    a. the type of drug taken
    b. whether a lethal dose of the drug has been taken
    c. level of consciousness and vital signs
    d. whether a victim is armed

11. A common emergency among drug abusing victims is:
    a. hyperventilation
    b. cardiac arrhythmias
    c. convulsions
    d. tremors

12. Which of the following may indicate an alcohol/drug emergency is life-threatening?
    a. pancreatitis
    b. impaired coordination
    c. vomiting while not fully conscious
    d. disturbance of vision

13. A pulse rate should be considered as indicating a life-threatening emergency if it is:
    a. below 80 and above 100
    b. below 60 and above 100
    c. below 60 and above 120
    d. below 50 and above 130

14. Which of the following is *not* a guideline for dealing with an overdose victim?
    a. if the victim is conscious, induce vomiting
    b. throw a little cold water on a victim who appears semi-conscious
    c. be alert for allergic reactions
    d. be firm but friendly in dealing with the victim

15. What is the preferred method for handling an individual experiencing a "bad trip?"
    a. throw cold water on the victim
    b. the "talk down" technique
    c. get the victim to walk around
    d. put the victim in an isolated room where he/she cannot hurt him/herself

16. Which of the following is part of the "talk down" technique for communicating with a drug/alcohol emergency victim?
    a. forewarn the victim about what will happen when the drug starts to wear off
    b. restrain a violent victim if necessary
    c. allow the victim some time alone
    d. encourage the victim to rest and sleep

17. Serious potential danger from inhalants includes:
    a. altered heart rhythm
    b. allergic reaction that produces hay fever symptoms
    c. hallucinations and delusions
    d. psychic dependence

18. The greatest medical danger associated with inhalant use is:
    a. severe irritation of the respiratory passages
    b. loss of consciousness
    c. alteration of the heart rhythm
    d. pathological changes in the liver

19. A first priority in treating barbiturate withdrawal is to:
    a. increase circulation
    b. maintain an open airway
    c. keep convulsions under control
    d. ease nausea and vomiting

Corresponds with:
**American Red Cross**
**Standard First Aid & Personal Safety**
Chapter 12, pages 170-176
and
**Advanced First Aid & Emergency Care**
Chapter 15, pages 225-246

# 13 Common Emergencies and Sudden Illnesses

## CARDIAC EMERGENCIES

When something goes wrong with the circulatory system, the result is often heart disease — a major medical problem that affects about twenty-nine million Americans. Of those people, almost four million have suffered at least one heart attack or have had chronic chest pain related to malfunction of the heart muscle (**angina pectoris**).

### Myocardial Infarction (Heart Attack)

When the oxygen supply to the heart muscle is cut off for a long period of time — usually by a blood clot (**coronary thrombosis**) in the artery of the heart or by a severe narrowing of the artery — part of the heart muscle actually dies, a condition known as **myocardial infarction** (heart attack).

Because the left side of the heart pumps harder and sustains the systolic blood pressure, it requires more oxygen than the right side. Therefore, most myocardial infarction affects the left side of the heart. Three serious consequences result from myocardial infarction:

1. **Cardiogenic shock.** The heart muscle is damaged so much that it can no longer sustain the systolic blood presure, and the patient lapses into shock within twenty-four hours.
2. **Sudden death.** Almost 50 percent of those who suffer a myocardial infarction die within the first hour, and many suffer

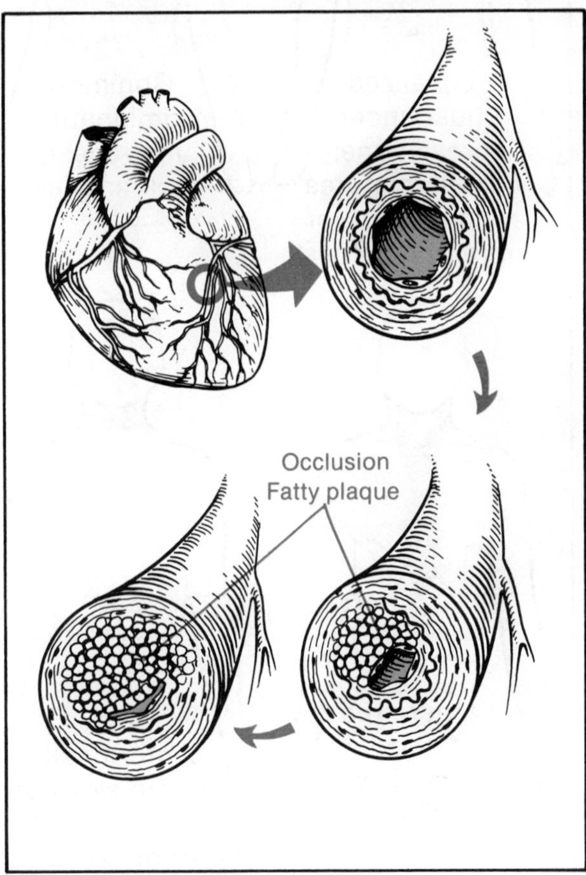


Fatty deposit buildup in arteries. The deterioration of a normal artery is seen as atherosclerosis develops and begins depositing fatty substances and roughening the channel lining until a clot forms and plugs the artery to deprive the heart muscle of vital blood, which results in heart attack.

## EARLY SIGNALS OF A HEART ATTACK

PAIN, in one form or another, almost always accompanies a heart attack and ranges from a mild ache to unbearable severity. When severe, pain is often felt as constricting, like a vise on the chest. Pain also often includes the burning and bloating sensations that usually accompany indigestion. Pain may be continuous and then might subside, but don't ignore it if it does. Pain could occur in any one or combination of locations shown below.

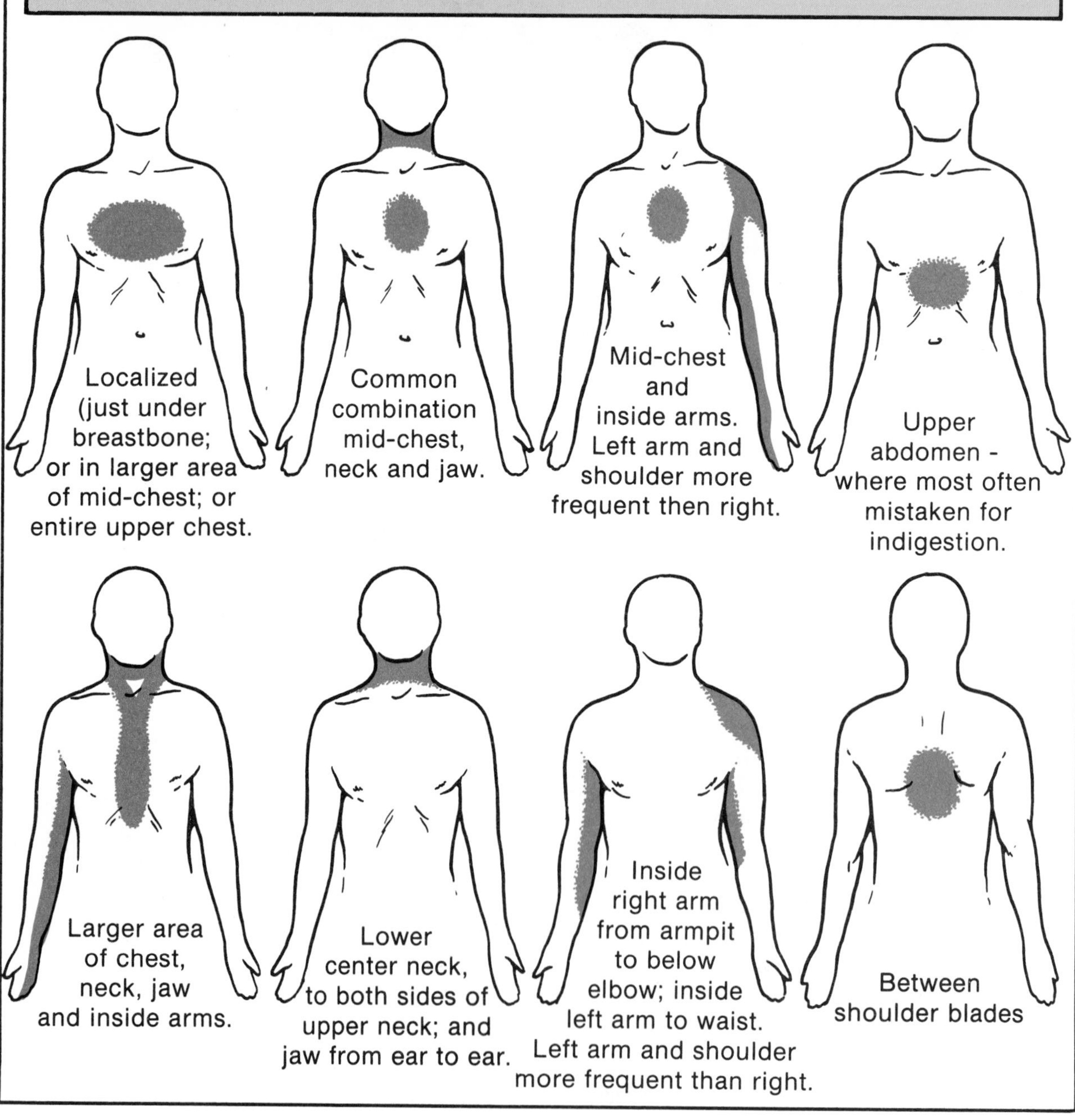

RISK FACTORS IN CORONARY HEART DISEASE
• Lack of physical exercise
• Heavy cigarette smoking
• Excessive caffeine intake
• Dietary indescretion, overindulgence
• Obesity (extreme)
• Coronary sclerosis due to hypercholesterolemia
• Hypertension (above 140/90)
• Family history of premature coronary heart disease (usually under age 60), oral contraceptives use in women over 40.
• Heart pain may be caused by extreme physical or psychic stress.
©SMS
• Age (increasing incidence over 30 years of age)
• Aging and hypertension, which aggravate aterioscIerosis, are extremely important; the latter is amenable to control.
• Happiness appears to be a most important prerequisite for a long, healthful life; chronic dissatisfaction and disappointment seem to contribute to coronary disease.
• Tension, frustration, and hostilities may predispose to myocardial infarction.

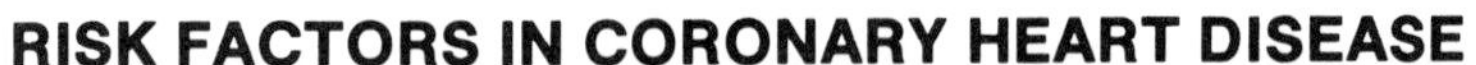

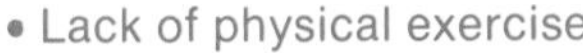

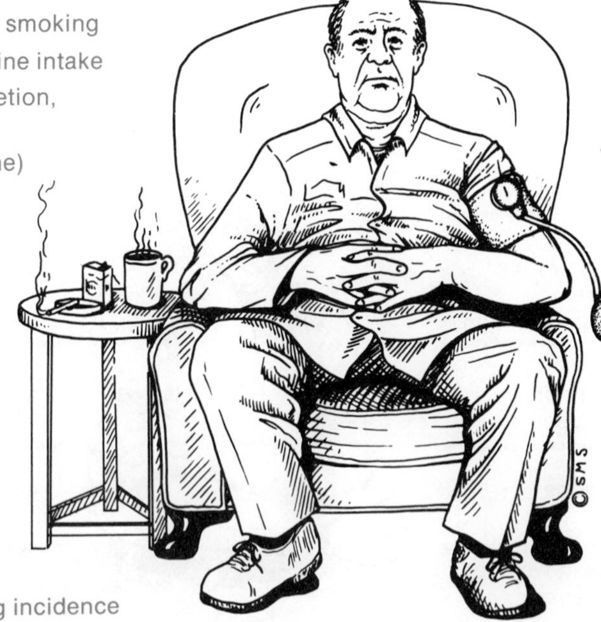

Each additional risk factor increases the likelihood of premature myocardial infarction. The risk of myocardial infarction in a patient with high cholesterol levels, high blood pressure, and heavy smoking is ten times that in a victim without them.

recurrences of the attack within three to five hours. Death results because the heart cannot effectively pump blood due to an upset in its normal beating pattern.

3. **Congestive heart failure (CHF)**. This occurs usually between three and seven days following a myocardial infarction if the heart loses its capability to pump effectively.

## Angina Pectoris

The heart circulates blood to the lungs, where it is freshly supplied with oxygen. The freshly oxygenated blood is then circulated to the tissues and organs of the body, including the heart. When the heart needs more oxygen than it is getting, and the lack of oxygen lasts for more than a few seconds, the result is a sharp chest pain called angina pectoris.

Angina pectoris can result from:

1. Strenuous exercise, causing the heart to pump so quickly that the oxygenated blood is not returned as soon as needed.
2. **Atherosclerosis** (fatty deposits in the arteries) of the arteries that take oxygenated blood to the heart.
3. Emotional stress.
4. Extremes in weather — including extremely hot, cold, humid, or windy weather.

### DISTINGUISHING ANGINA PECTORIS FROM MYOCARDIAL INFARCTION

| | ANGINA PECTORIS | MYOCARDIAL INFARCTION |
|---|---|---|
| Location of Pain | Substernal or across chest | Same |
| Radiation of Pain | Neck, jaw or arms | Same |
| Nature of Pain | Dull or heavy discomfort with a pressure or squeezing sensation | Same, but more intense |
| Duration | Usually lasts 3 to 8 minutes rarely longer | Usually lasts longer than 30 minutes |
| Other Symptoms | Usually none | Perspiration, weakness, nausea, pale gray color |
| Precipitating Factors | Extremes in weather, exertion, stress, meals | Often none |
| Factors Giving Relief | Stopping physical activity, reducing stress, nitroglycerin | Nitroglycerin may give incomplete, or no relief |

If in doubt as to which condition the victim has, always treat as if it is an acute myocardial infarction.

## Emergency Care for Cardiac Emergencies

A victim with heart difficulty can be given the following general care:

1. Have the victim cease all movement.
2. Place the victim in a semireclining or sitting position.
3. If the problem is a suspected angina attack, ask the victim if he/she has medication. If so, place it underneath the tongue.
4. Make sure that the airway is open and assist ventilations as needed.
5. Loosen constricting clothing.
6. Maintain body temperature as close to normal as possible.
7. Comfort and reassure.
8. Administer CPR if cardiac arrest occurs.
9. Call for emergency medical aid immediately.

# STROKE

## Emergency Care for Stroke

The following steps should be initiated:

1. Handle the victim calmly and carefully; be particularly gentle with paralyzed parts.
2. Position the victim on his/her back with head and shoulders slightly raised to relieve the pressure in the skull.
3. Assess the victim's airway and respiration. If the victim manifests breathing difficulty, assist respirations. If you believe that the victim may choke on vomitus or mucous, turn his/her head to the side to aid drainage.

4. If the victim develops further difficulty in breathing, turn him/her on the side (preferably with the paralyzed side down). If the unconscious victim begins to vomit, turn him/her on the side, clear the airway, and assist ventilations as needed.
5. Call for emergency medical aid immediately.
6. Remove all dentures and dental bridges or false teeth.
7. Keep the victim warm, but do not overheat. Excessive heat speeds brain damage.
8. Keep the victim absolutely quiet. Shield him/her from curious onlookers.
9. **Never give the victim anything to drink;** paralysis of the throat is common. Never use any kind of stimulant (such as smelling salts).
10. If you move the victim, carefully support the paralyzed limbs.
11. Even though a victim may be unconscious or in a coma, he/she may be able to hear and understand what goes on. It is critical that you avoid saying anything that will increase the victim's anxiety, because it can aggravate and worsen the stroke considerably.

## CAUSES OF STROKE

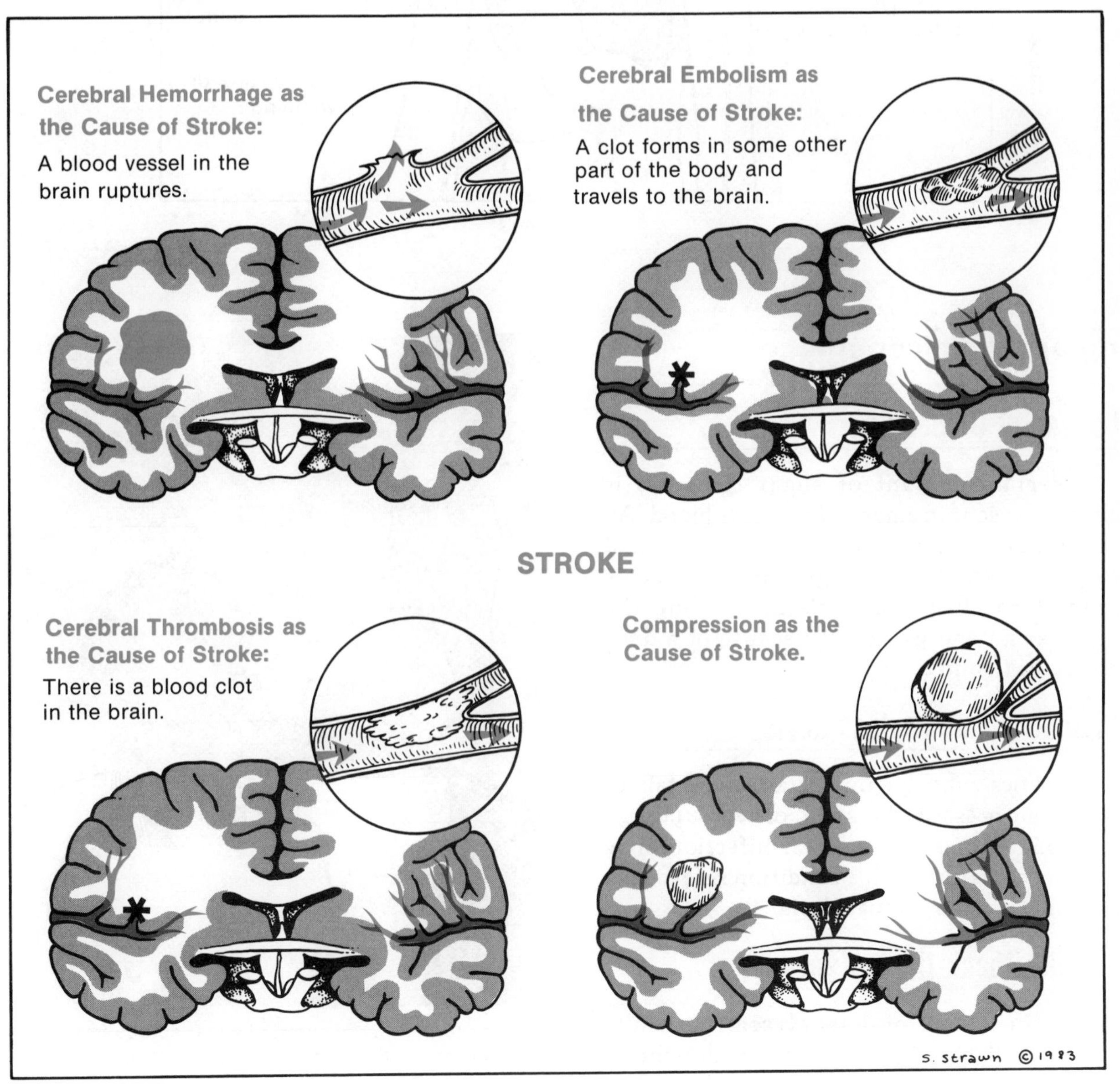

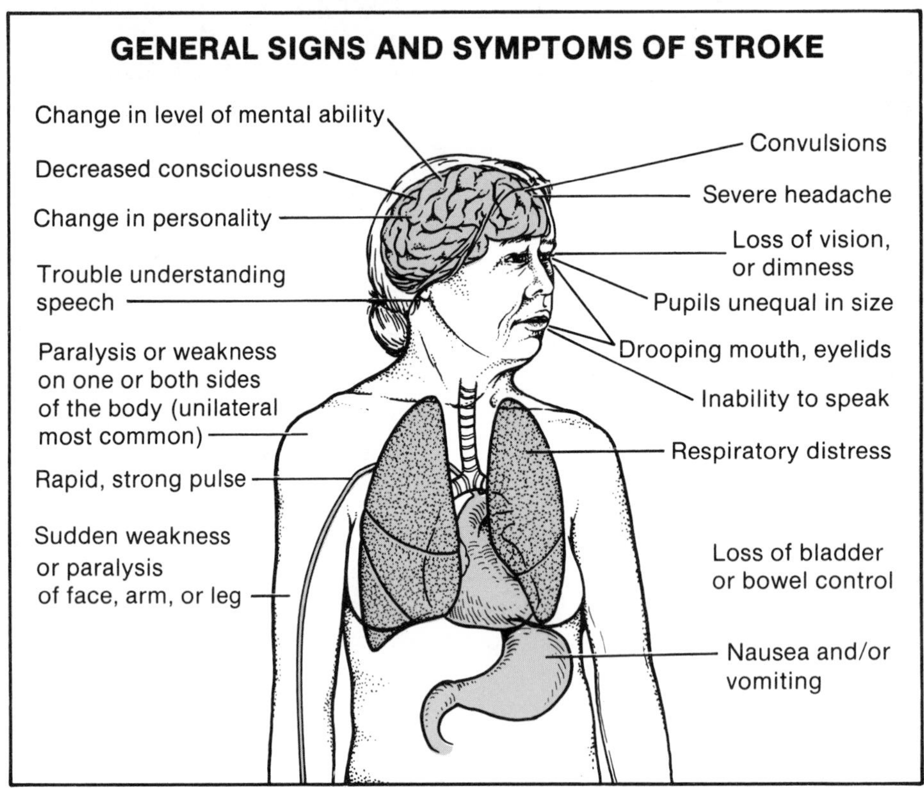


# DIABETIC EMERGENCIES

## Causes of Diabetes

A certain amount of sugar (glucose) is always present in a normal person's blood. All cells require sugar for normal functioning and for conversion as an energy source. Diabetes renders the body incapable of utilizing the sugar as an energy source because of a deficiency in **insulin**.

## Diabetic Coma (Ketoacidosis)

Diabetics who go untreated, who fail to take their prescribed insulin, or who undergo some kind of a stress (such as infection) may become comatose with a condition referred to as diabetic coma (**ketoacidosis**).

## Insulin Shock (Hypoglycemia)

**Insulin shock**, or **hypoglycemia**, results when the diabetic has too much insulin. Sugar

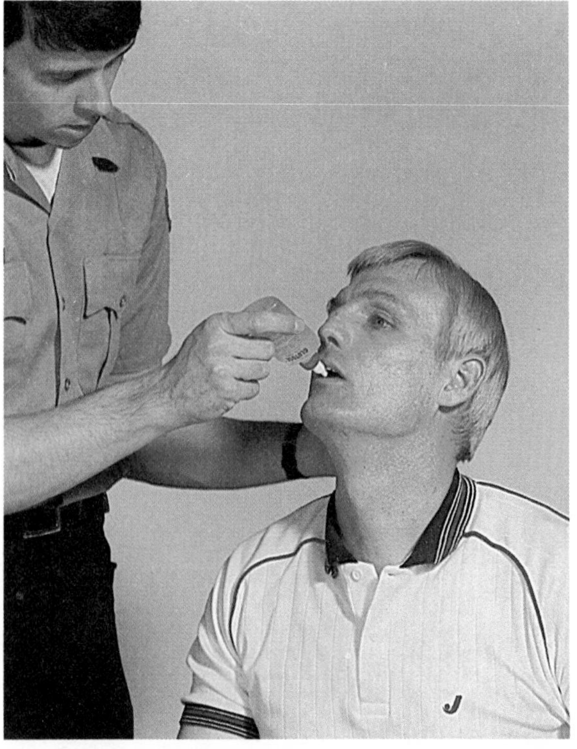

Administering a concentrated sugar source to a conscious insulin shock (hypoglycemic) victim.

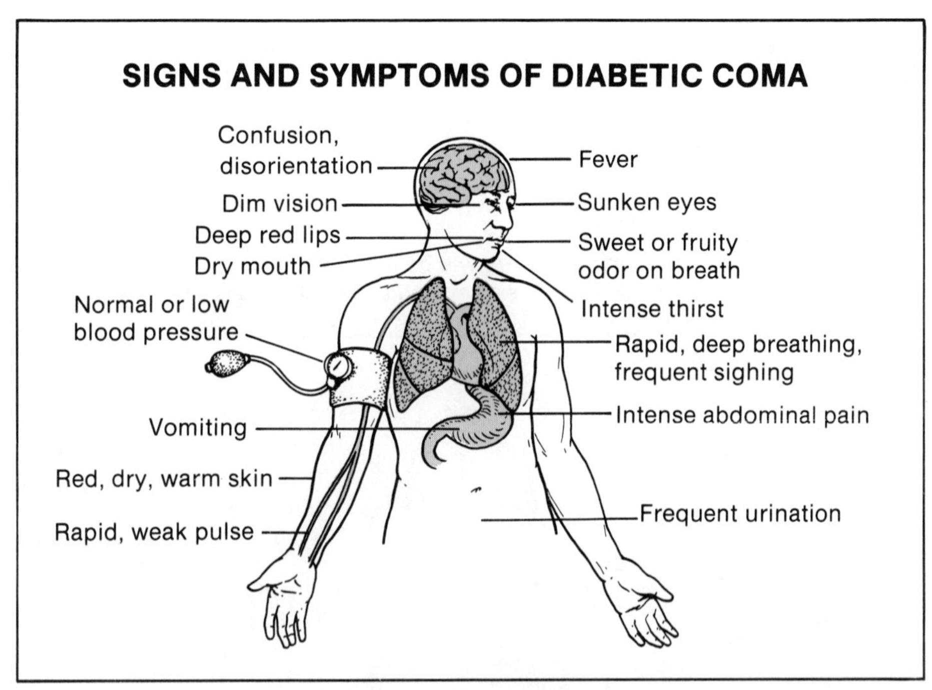


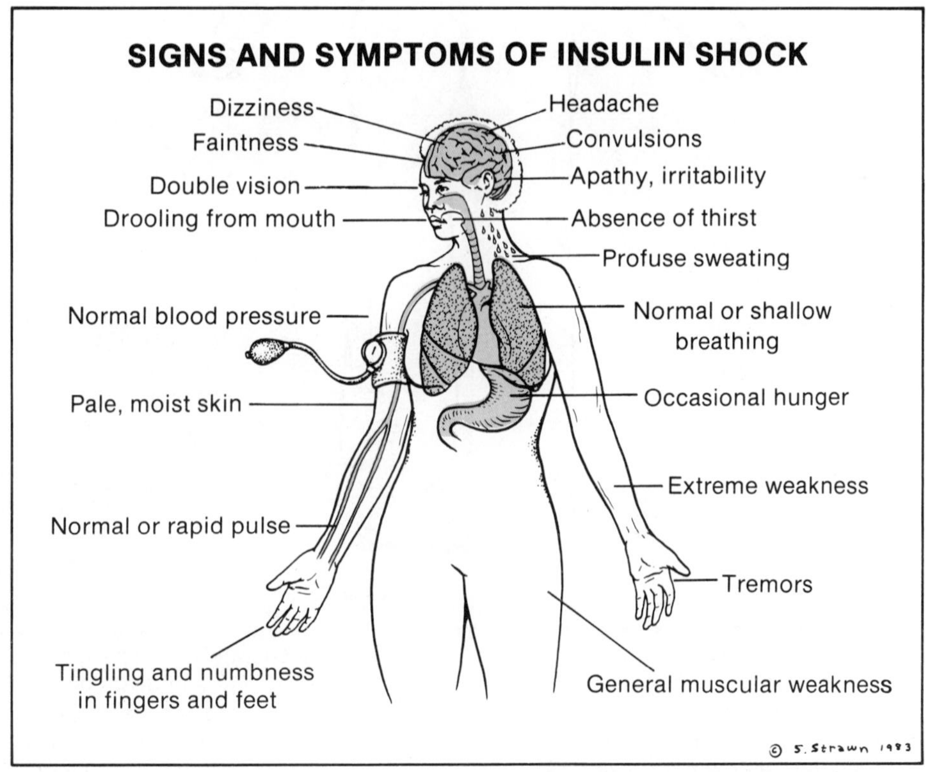


moves rapidly out of the blood and into the cells, resulting in an insufficient blood sugar level to maintain normal brain function. Because the brain is as dependent on glucose as it is on oxygen, permanent brain damage or death can result from insulin shock if emergency care is not given immediately.

Diabetes is a condition in which the body is unable to use sugar normally.
Body cells need sugar to survive.
Insulin in the body permits sugar to pass from the blood stream to body cells.
If there is not enough insulin, sugar will be unable to get to body cells and they will starve.
If there is too much insulin, there will be insufficient sugar in the blood stream and brain cells will be damaged since they need a constant supply of sugar.

## DIABETIC COMA

Note: The onset of diabetic coma is gradual over a period of days.

There is insufficient insulin and therefore too much sugar in the blood and not enough in the body cells. The diabetic:

has eaten too much that contains or produces sugar, or
has not taken his insulin.

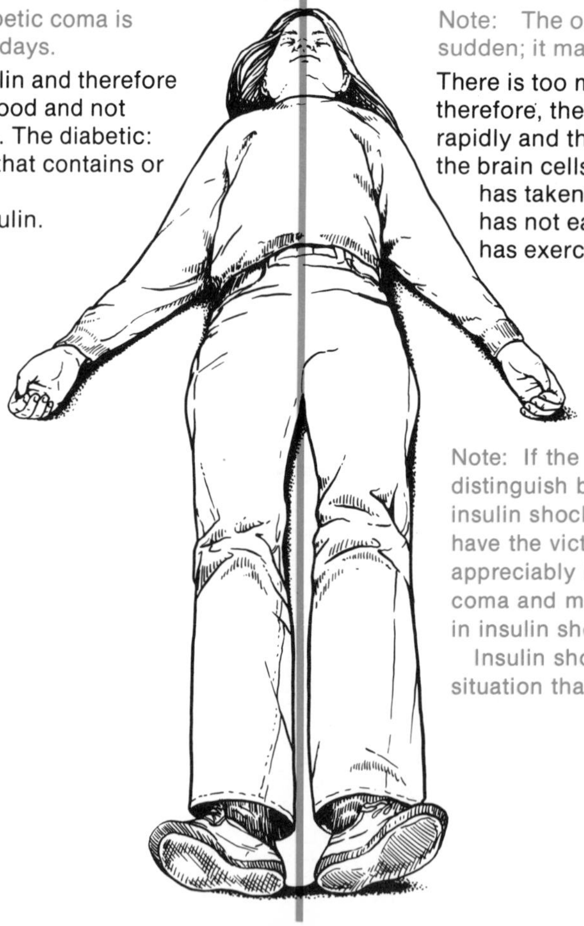

## INSULIN SHOCK

Note: The onset of insulin shock is sudden; it may occur within minutes.

There is too much insulin in the body; therefore, the sugar leaves the blood rapidly and there is insufficient sugar for the brain cells. The diabetic:

has taken too much insulin, or
has not eaten enough food, or
has exercised excessively.

Note: If the First Aider cannot distinguish between diabetic coma and insulin shock and sugar is available, have the victim take it. It can't appreciably hurt the victim in diabetic coma and may save the life of a victim in insulin shock.

Insulin shock is a much more critical situation than diabetic coma.

## EMERGENCY CARE

**Diabetic coma:**

This victim needs immediate transportation to a medical facility.
Monitor vital signs.
Follow procedures for any unconscious victim regarding airway maintenance.
Keep victim lying flat with head and shoulders slightly elevated.
If vomiting occurs put in coma position with head turned to aid draining and prevent aspiration.

**Insulin shock:**

This victim desperately needs sugar before brain damage and death occur. Rubbing sugar on the tongue of an unconscious victim should arouse him (use only what the tongue can absorb). Sugar in any form can be given to a conscious victim. He needs immediate transportation to a medical facility.

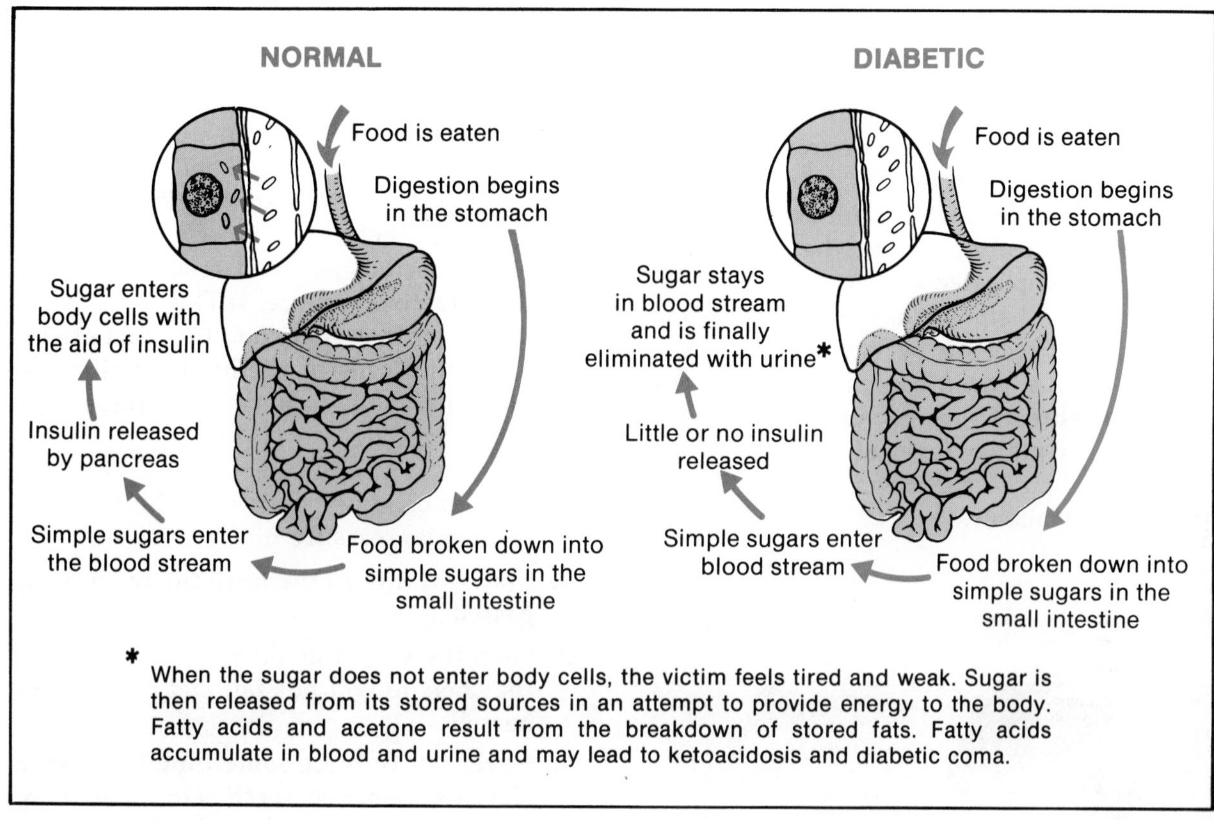


Normal versus diabetic use of sugars.

## HYPERVENTILATION

Hyperventilation means that the victim "overbreathes" or breathes too rapidly. The causes of this phenomenon are varied but usually involve psychological stress. In isolated instances, blood clots that have migrated to the lung and formed a pulmonary embolism may cause hyperventilation. Also, if a medical situation such as diabetes causes the pH level of the blood to become acidic, the body will try to compensate by varying the respiratory rate. The speeding up of respirations is an attempt to blow off carbon dioxide.

### Signs and Symptoms of Hyperventilation

Whatever the cause of hyperventilation, the overbreathing lowers the arterial carbon dioxide to an abnormal level. The body experiences aklalosis, which results in some of the signs and symptoms of hyperventilation.

A victim who possesses three or more of the following symptoms may be suffering a hyperventilation attack:

- A feeling in the top of the head that is hard to describe.
- Dizziness or lightheadedness.
- Blurring vision.
- Dryness or bitterness of the mouth.
- Tingling of the hands and feet or around the mouth.
- Tightness or a "lump" in the throat.
- Shortness of breath.
- Pounding of the heart.
- A feeling of great tiredness or weakness.
- A feeling of being in a dream.
- A feeling of impending doom.
- Drawing-up of the hands at the wrist and knuckles, but with straight fingers in severe attacks only.
- Fainting.
- Rapid breathing; and heart rate.

## Emergency Care For Hyperventilation

Your initial care while you are assessing the victim is kindness and reassurance. Listen carefully, show understanding consideration, and try to help the victim calm down. Try to talk the victim into slowing the respiration rate. In uncomplicated anxiety hyperventilation you can help build the blood carbon dioxide level back up by having the victim breathe into a paper bag. This causes the victim to rebreathe his/her own exhaled air, which has a higher level of carbon dioxide than normal air. A sufficient amount of oxygen is also available.

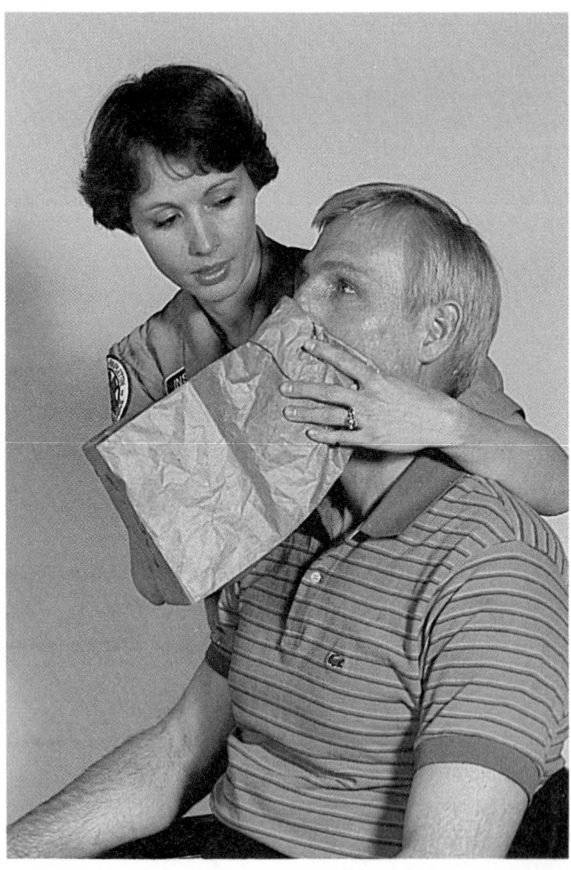

For anxiety hyperventilation, have victim breathe into a paper bag to increase carbon dioxide intake. **Do not use this method if there is a medical cause for the hyperventilation. Call for emergency medical aid.**

**Never have a victim breathe into a paper bag if you suspect anything other than anxiety as the cause of hyperventilation.**

# SEIZURES AND EPILEPSY

Among the most common — and puzzling — of central nervous system disorders is **epilepsy**. Seizures represent sudden changes in sensation, behavior, muscle activity, or level of consciousness and result from irritated, overactive brain cells. They are beyond voluntary control. Any condition that affects the structural cells of the brain or alters its chemical metabolic balance may trigger epileptic seizures.

1. Stay as calm as possible. If the victim is conscious, reassure him/her.
2. **Stay with the victim until the seizure has passed.**
3. Help the victim lie down on the floor so that he/she will not fall and injure him/herself.
4. **Never try to force something between a victim's clenched teeth.** Doing so may result in injury to both you and the victim.
5. Remove or loosen any tight clothing.
6. Turn the patient on his/her side with head extended and face turned slightly downward so that secretions and vomit can drain quickly out of the mouth.
7. Maintain an airway.
8. Place a padding (pillow, folded jacket, or other object) underneath the victim's head.
9. Do not move the victim unless he/she is near something dangerous that cannot be moved, such as a radiator.
10. Do not attempt to restrain the victim unless he/she is in immediate danger.
11. If possible, keep the victim from becoming a spectacle.
12. Reassure and reorient the victim following the seizure. Allow him/her to rest, and make him/her as comfortable as possible.
13. If the victim lapses into a second seizure without regaining consciousness from the first one (status epilepticus), transport him immediately, and consider him a medical emergency.

## EPILEPSY — GRAND MAL SEIZURES

A Grand Mal Seizure is a sign of an abnormal release of impulses in the brain. It is a physical, not a psychological, disorder.

**1**

The victim may have an "aura" or premonition before the seizure occurs. An aura is often described as an odd or unpleasant sensation that rises from the stomach toward the chest and throat.

For some victims the aura is always the same, such as numbness or motor activity (like turning of head and eyes, spasm of a limb) or it may consist of a peculiar sound or taste.

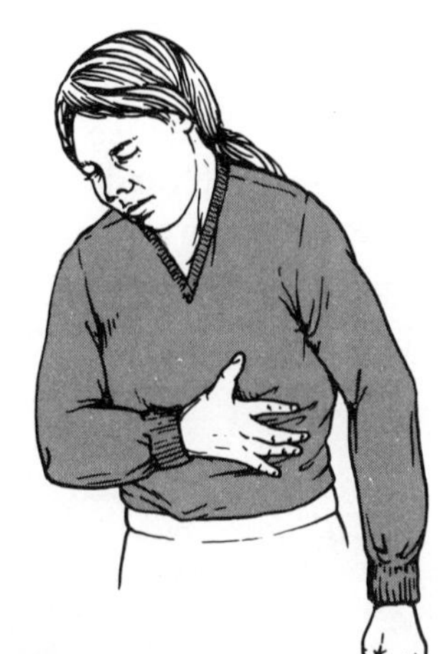

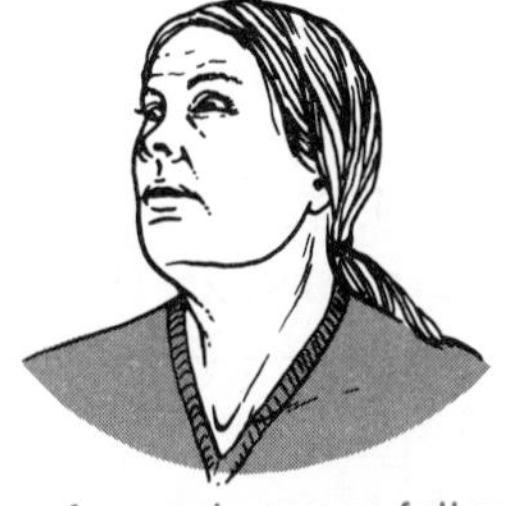

**2**

Loss of consciousness follows the aura. The forced expulsion of air caused by contraction of the skeletal muscles may cause a high pitched cry sound. The victim may be pale at this point with possible spasms of the muscles, causing the tongue to be bitten.

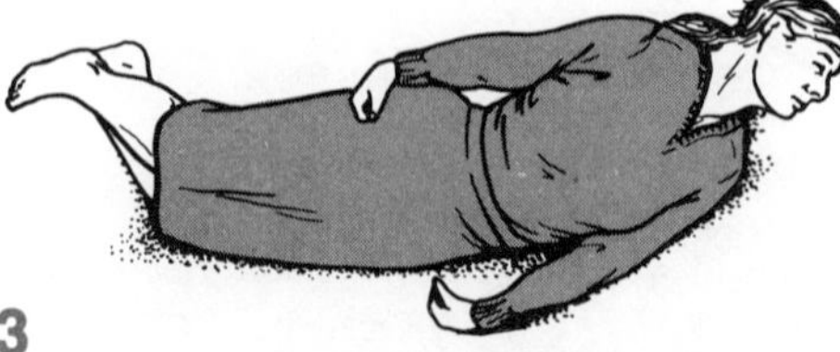

**3**

The victim will usually fall with convulsions and loss of consciousness. Cyanosis may accompany the seizure because breathing stops during the phase of prolonged muscle contraction. Within seconds the victim will manifest an arched back and alternating contraction and relaxation of movements in all extremities (clonic convulsive movements). Frothing at the mouth occurs, which may be bloody as the result of cheek or tongue biting. The attack usually lasts from about 30 seconds to five minutes. The patient may lose bladder and bowel control.

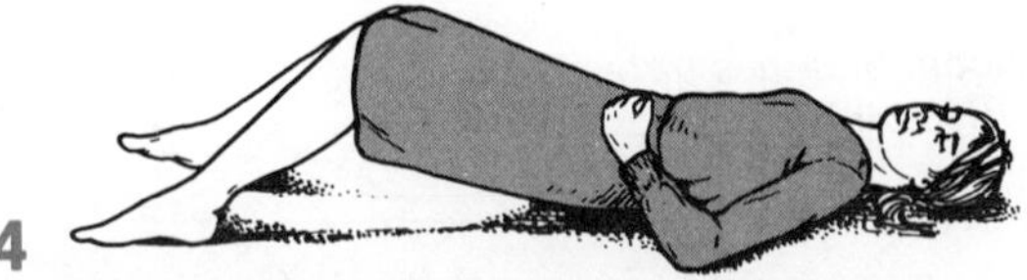

**4**

Gradually the clonic phase (convulsions) subsides. It is followed by a **postictal state**, characterized by a deep sleep with gradual recovery to a state of transient confusion, fatigue, muscular soreness, and headache. The victim should be encouraged to rest since activity could precipitate another attack.

### EMERGENCY CARE

- If the victim seems to stop breathing, do not be concerned. Do be concerned if the victim passes from seizure to seizure without regaining consciousness (status epilepticus). This situation requires immediate medical attention.
- The major requirements of the First Aider is to protect the victim from hurting himself during a seizure.
- The victim should not be physically restrained in any way unless he is endangering his own welfare.
- Move objects, not the victim.
- Position the victim to allow for drainage.
- Loosen tight clothing.
- Do not use a bite stick or other object between teeth.
- If status epilepticus (a continuation of seizure) occurs or breathing ceases assist breathing, check vital signs, and call for emergency medical aid immediately.
- Keep victim from being a spectacle.
- Reassure and reorient victim following the seizure.
- Allow him to rest.
- An ambulance is often called for a grand mal seizure, but if the victim responds normally he may not need transport. If in doubt always call for emergency aid.

## STATUS ASTHMATICUS

**Status asthmaticus** is a severe, prolonged asthmatic attack. It is a dire medical emergency. Upon examination, the victim's chest is greatly distended. The victim fights desperately to move air through the obstructed airways and prominently uses accessory muscles of respiration.

When dealing with any asthmatic patient, maintain a calm, reassuring attitude.

A note of caution: **all that wheezes is not asthma**. Among the many other causes of diffuse wheezing are acute left heart failure ("**cardiac asthma**"), smoke inhalation, chronic bronchitis, and acute pulmonary embolism.

### STATUS ASTHMATICUS

**Status asthmaticus** is a severe, prolonged asthmatic attack. The acute asthmatic attack involves airway obstruction due to bronchospasm, swelling of mucous membranes in the bronchial walls, and plugging of bronchi by thick mucous secretions. Allergic reactions, respiratory infection, or emotional stress may bring on an attack.

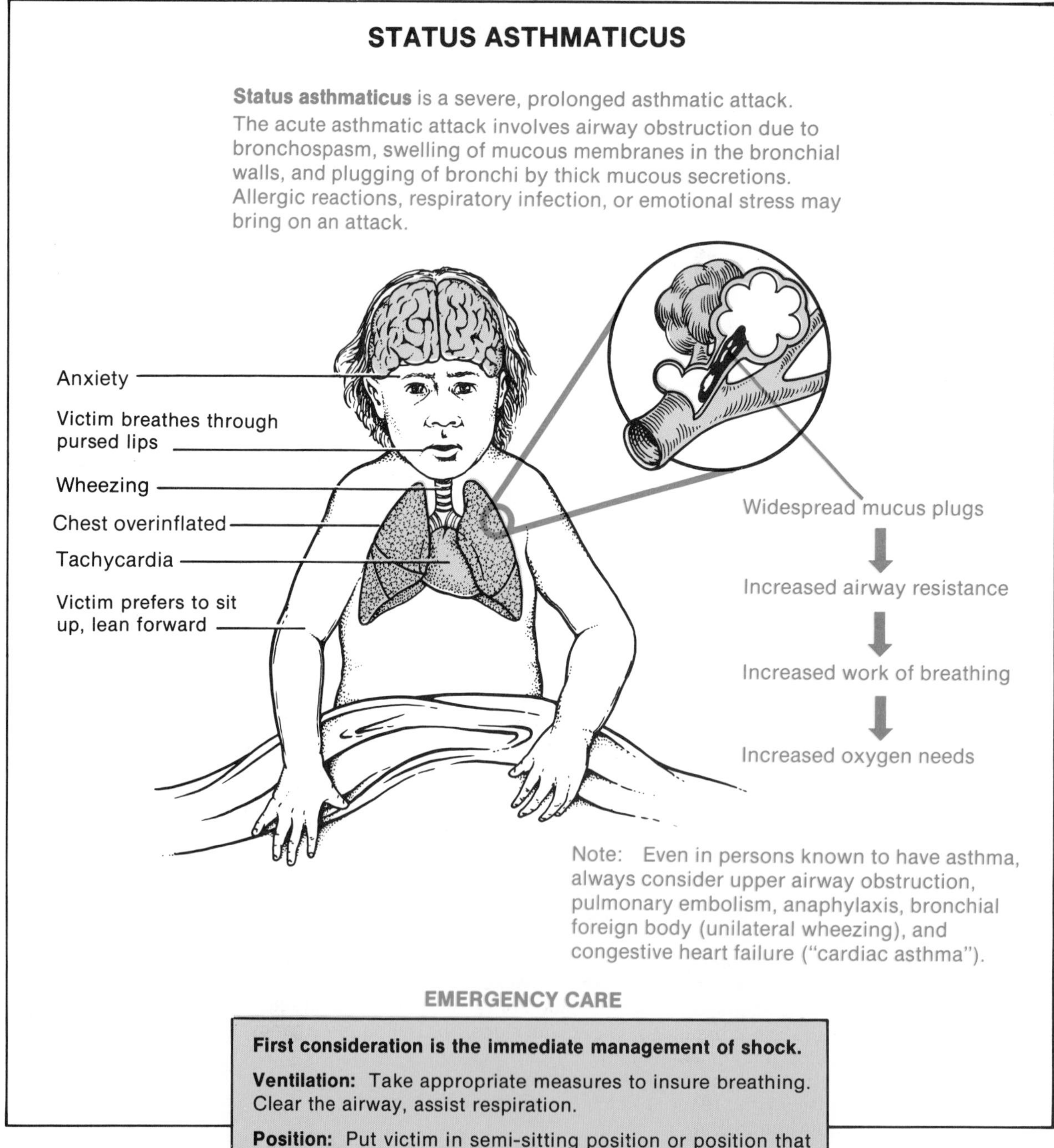


Note: Even in persons known to have asthma, always consider upper airway obstruction, pulmonary embolism, anaphylaxis, bronchial foreign body (unilateral wheezing), and congestive heart failure ("cardiac asthma").

#### EMERGENCY CARE

**First consideration is the immediate management of shock.**

**Ventilation:** Take appropriate measures to insure breathing. Clear the airway, assist respiration.

**Position:** Put victim in semi-sitting position or position that helps victim breathe easiest.

**Transport:** Call for emergency medical aid immediately and monitor vital signs.

# Work Exercises

## Heart Attack

1. The degree of pain is not necessarily indicative of heart attack, but the location of the pain is. Circle any pain location listed below that may be a sign of heart attack.

| | | |
|---|---|---|
| upper abdomen | right arm | left shoulder |
| lower abdomen | left arm | back, between shoulders |
| chest | jaw | lower back |
| neck | right shoulder | |

2. List seven emergency care procedures for cardiac victims.

    1.

    2.

    3.

    4.

    5.

    6.

    7.

## Stroke

Label the figures in the following illustration by indicating the three general causes of blood supply interference in the brain:

### CAUSES OF STROKE

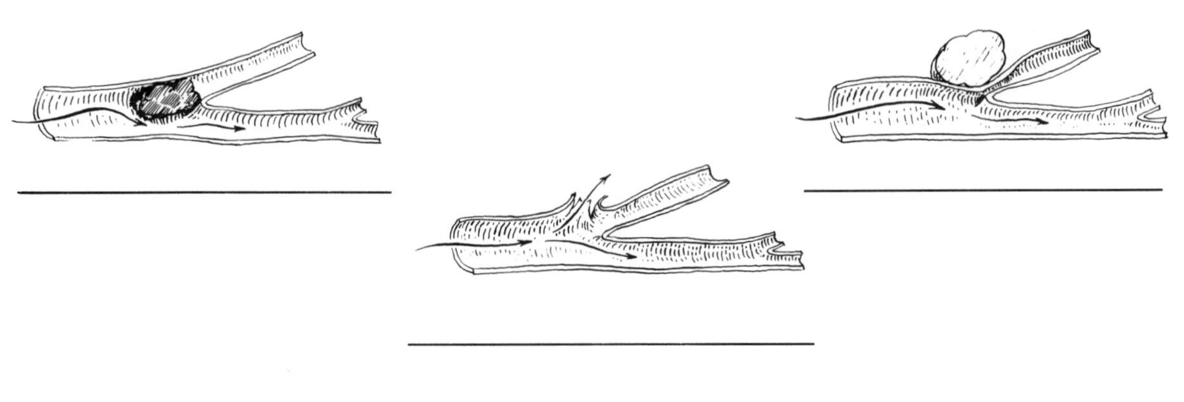

List the six most important emergency care procedures when caring for a stroke victim.

1.

2.

3.

4.

5.

6.

## Insulin Shock and Diabetic Coma

List the necessary emergency care procedures when caring for a victim of diabetic coma and insulin shock.

### Diabetic Coma

1.

2.

3.

4.

### Insulin Shock

1.

2.

3.

4.

5.

## Epilepsy

List eight emergency care procedures for grand mal seizures.

1.

2.

3.

4.

5.

6.

7.

8.

## SELF-TEST

### Part I: True and False

If you believe the statement is true, circle the T. If you believe the statement is false, circle F.

T F 1. A stroke victim should be positioned on the back with legs elevated.

T F 2. The First Aider should place an object between the teeth of a victim of convulsions in order to prevent the tongue from being bitten.

T F 3. It is important that the jerking and rigidity of muscle groups that occurs during some seizures be prevented and restrained.

T F 4. Shortness of breath is one of the primary symptoms of heart attack.

T F 5. Unequal pupil size may indicate that the victim has suffered a stroke.

T F 6. Because a victim of diabetic coma has too much sugar in his/her blood, it would be fatal to give him/her sugar.

T F 7. Insulin shock is not serious because as the insulin disperses into the system, the reaction will correct itself.

T F 8. A person suffering from diabetic coma usually has deep and rapid breathing with a peculiar fruity breath odor.

T F 9. Insulin shock may be caused by eating too much.

T F 10. First aid for insulin shock is to raise the victim's blood sugar level concentration as quickly as possible.

T F 11. A conscious person experiencing insulin shock can be given candy, soft drinks, sugar or fruit juice.

T F 12. Pale, moist skin are common symptoms of diabetic coma.

T F 13. A person suffering from insulin shock may appear to be intoxicated with alcohol.

T F 14. Stroke may be indicated by paralysis of one side of the body, unequal pupils, and paralysis of some facial muscles.

### Part II: Multiple Choice

For each question, circle the one answer that best reflects a true statement.

1. In most cases, the pain from myocardial infarction is:
   a. located beneath the breastbone and feels like someone is squeezing the chest
   b. very sharp, especially during inhalation
   c. in the upper abdomen and feels like indigestion
   d. between the shoulder blades in the back

2. A myocardial infarction victim will manifest which of the following?
   a. hypoxia, increased pulse rate, falling blood pressure
   b. decreased pulse rate, shortness of breath
   c. slowed respirations, decreased pulse rate, increased blood pressure
   d. bright blushed skin, hypoxia, increased blood pressure

3. Which of the following is *not* a symptom of stroke?
   a. chest pain
   b. difficulty in breathing
   c. inability to talk (or slurred speech)
   d. loss of bladder and bowel control

4. A person having a grand mal seizure should be:
   a. placed in a tub of water
   b. gently restrained
   c. placed in a sitting position to secure an adequate airway
   d. kept from hurting him/herself

5. Diabetic coma is characterized by:
   a. rapid onset
   b. gnawing hunger
   c. acetone breath
   d. recent insulin shot

6. In acute heart attack, the pain usually is over the heart and:
   a. in the lower abdomen
   b. down the right arm
   c. down the left arm
   d. in the legs

7. A sudden blocking of the coronary arteries that normally supply the heart muscles with blood causes a condition known as:
   a. chronic heart failure
   b. heart attack
   c. stroke
   d. angina

8. An insufficiency of insulin, which usually results when a diabetic patient has not taken insulin or has overeaten, is called:
   a. diabetic coma
   b. diabetic shock
   c. insulin coma
   d. insulin shock

9. An excess of insulin, which may result when a diabetic patient has taken too much insulin, has not eaten, or has overexercised, is called:
   a. diabetic coma
   b. diabetic shock
   c. insulin coma
   d. insulin shock

10. Which symptom is the characteristic clue indicating diabetic coma?
   a. cherry red lips
   b. moist, clammy skin
   c. involuntary muscular twitching
   d. a sickly sweet breath odor

11. A heart condition, often mistaken for indigestion, is brought on by emotional stress, strenuous exercise or agitation and is characterized by pain in the chest or arm. This condition is known as:
   a. chronic heart failure
   b. heart attack
   c. stroke
   d. angina pectoris

12. Which of the following is *not* an emergency care measure for a cardiac victim?
   a. loosen constrictive clothing
   b. place the victim in a semireclining position
   c. have the victim cease all movement
   d. do not help victim administer his/her medication until a physician has seen the victim

13. When the blood supply to part of the brain is cut off impairing the function of cells in that part of the brain, the victim is said to have suffered a(n):
   a. stroke
   b. epileptic seizure
   c. angina pectoris attack
   d. coma

14. Which of the following is *not* a cause of blood supply interference in the brain?
   a. compression
   b. clotting
   c. convulsions
   d. hemorrhage

15. What are the signs and symptoms of stroke?
   a. total paralysis, constricted pupils
   b. weak, rapid pulse and paralysis on one side of the body
   c. slurred speech, unequal pupils
   d. labored breathing, no paralysis

16. Before the actual stroke, a person may suffer:
   a. convulsions
   b. speech loss
   c. aneurysm
   d. loss of bladder control

17. The most critical stroke victim is the:
    a. one who loses consciousness completely and becomes weak on the involved side
    b. one who becomes rigid and completely paralyzed on the involved side
    c. one who has severe headache and unequal pupils
    d. one who has loss of vision and inability to speak

18. What is the emergency care for a stroke victim?
    a. give the victim sips of water
    b. keep the victim lying down and elevate the feet
    c. begin CPR
    d. keep the victim quiet and reassure him/her

19. The initial care for a hyperventilating person is to:
    a. establish an airway
    b. begin CPR
    c. loosen restrictive clothing
    d. show kindness and reassurance

20. The onset of diabetic coma generally occurs:
    a. in 5-20 minutes
    b. in 10-12 hours
    c. in 24 hours
    d. in 48 hours

21. The major emergency care procedure for a victim in diabetic coma is:
    a. to administer insulin
    b. to treat for shock
    c. to give a glass or orange juice
    d. to try to keep him/her awake

22. Insulin shock onset generally occurs within:
    a. 5-20 minutes after injection of insulin
    b. 10-12 hours after injection of insulin
    c. 24 hours after injection of insulin
    d. 48 hours after injection of insulin

23. A diabetic is exhibiting the following signs: rapid, weak pulse; cold, clammy skin; and convulsions. What do these signs indicate?
    a. insulin shock
    b. diabetic coma
    c. insulin coma
    d. diabetic shock

24. If the First Aider can't distinguish between diabetic coma and insulin shock, what should he do?
    a. nothing, the wrong treatment can be deadly
    b. treat for shock and transport
    c. give a shot of insulin or put an insulin tablet in the mouth
    d. assist victim in taking some type of sugar

25. What is the emergency care for insulin shock if the victim is unconscious?
    a. administer a glass of orange juice
    b. do nothing; activate EMS system
    c. put an insulin tablet in his/her mouth or give an insulin shot
    d. rub a sugar cube on the tongue

26. Which of the following emergency care measures is used when dealing with an epileptic victim.
    a. rush the victim to the hospital; this is a true emergency
    b. move objects around the victim which may harm him/her
    c. forcibly restrain the victim until the convulsions pass
    d. force a padded object in between the victim's teeth

27. The most serious threat in status epilepticus is:
    a. lack of oxygen due to impaired breathing
    b. fractures
    c. swallowing the tongue
    d. dehydration

| Corresponds with: |
|---|
| **American Red Cross** |
| **Advanced First Aid & Emergency Care** |
| Chapter 16, pages 246-253 |

# 14

# Emergency Childbirth

The delivery of a baby is a natural function. At times, complications arise that lead to emergency situations outside the hospital setting. The role of the First Aider in a normal delivery is merely to assist the mother and baby.

## STRUCTURE

The accompanying illustration shows the normal structures involved with a full-term pregnancy.

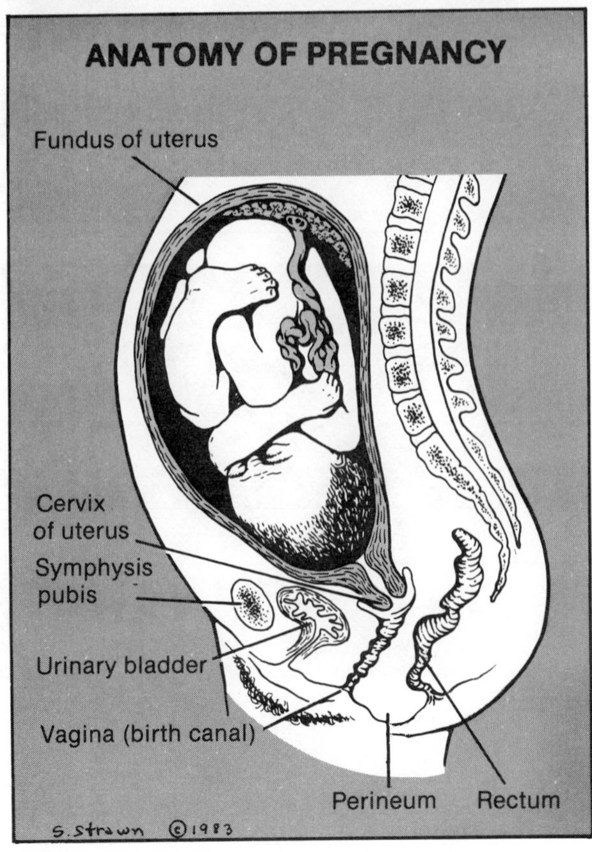


- The baby usually lies head down in the uterus or womb.
- The umbilical cord, attaching the baby to the placenta, supplies the baby's nutritional and oxygen needs.
- The amniotic sac surrounding the baby contains amniotic fluid, which acts as a "shock absorber," among other functions.
- The placenta is the organ of exchange between the mother's blood and the baby's blood.
- The birth canal is made up of the cervix and vagina.

## EVALUATING THE MOTHER

Childbirth is a natural, normal process. If you are called to the scene of an imminent childbirth, there are two important first aid actions:

1. Give the mother calming reassurance. Let her know you are there to help and that she is going to be okay.
2. Evaluate the mother to decide if she should be transported to the nearest medical facility, or if she should have the baby at her present location.

The First Aider can decide whether to transport the mother or to prepare for a delivery by asking the mother a few questions and conducting a simple evaluation. Mom is usually nervous and apprehensive, so be gentle and kind, showing confidence and support.

## CHILDBIRTH

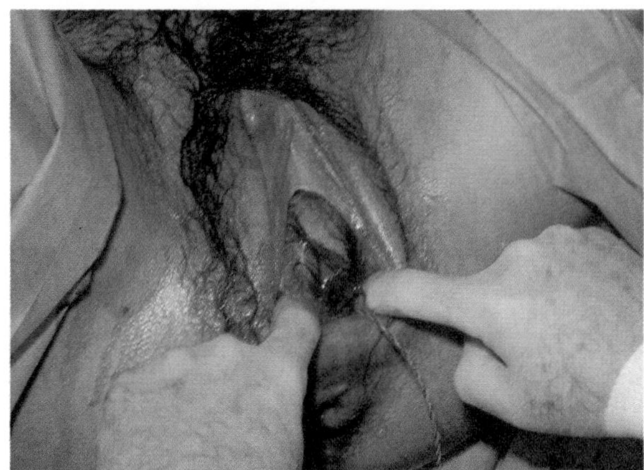

**1**
Early crowning.

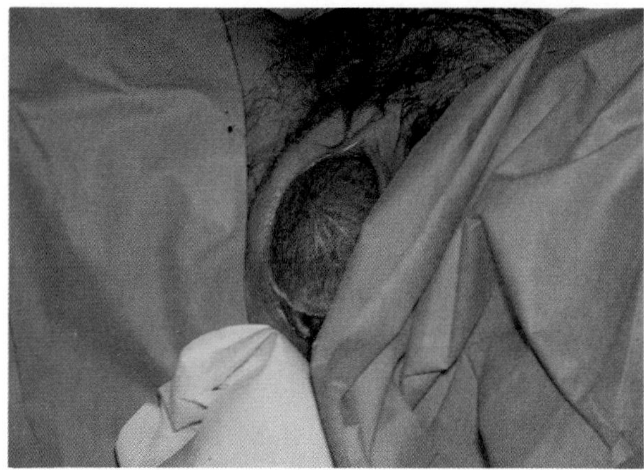

**2**
Late crowning.

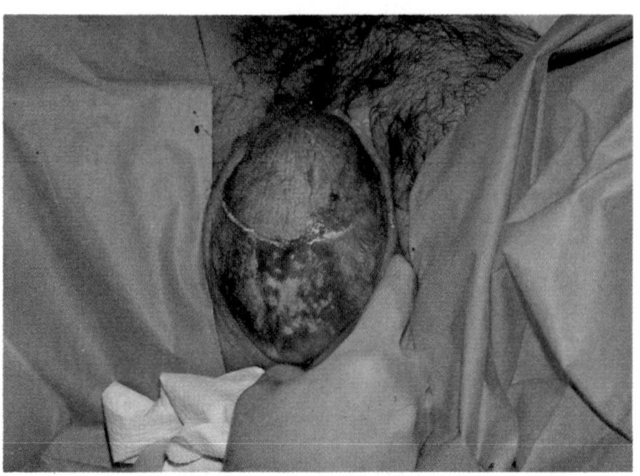

**3**
Head delivering.

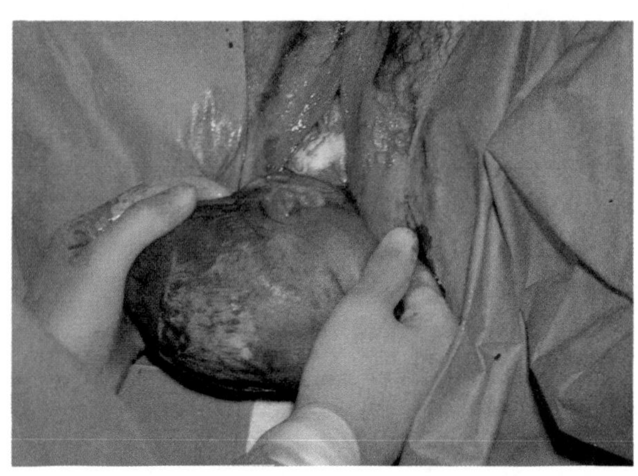

**4**
Head delivers and turns.

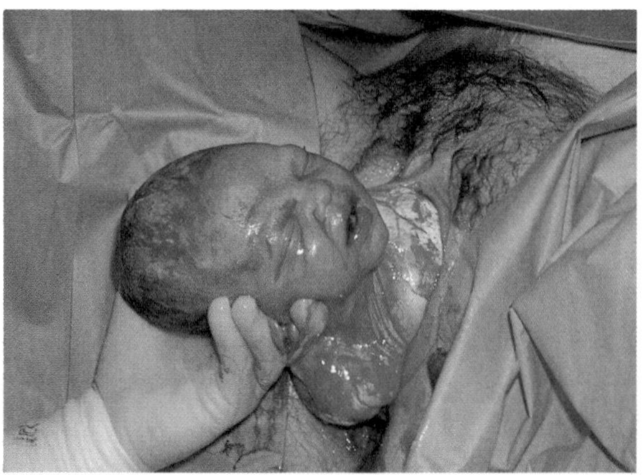

**5**
Shoulders deliver.

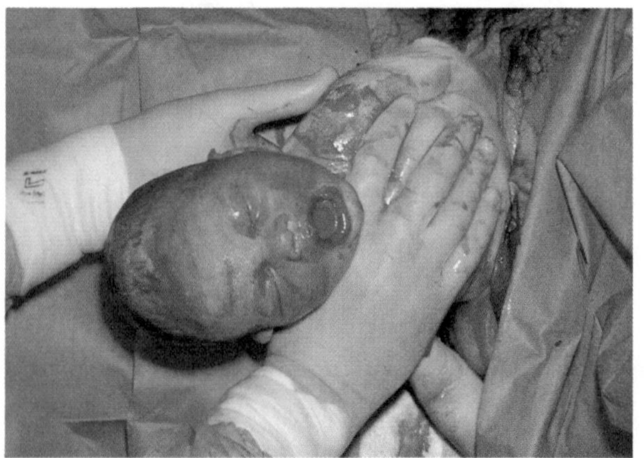

**6**
Chest delivers.

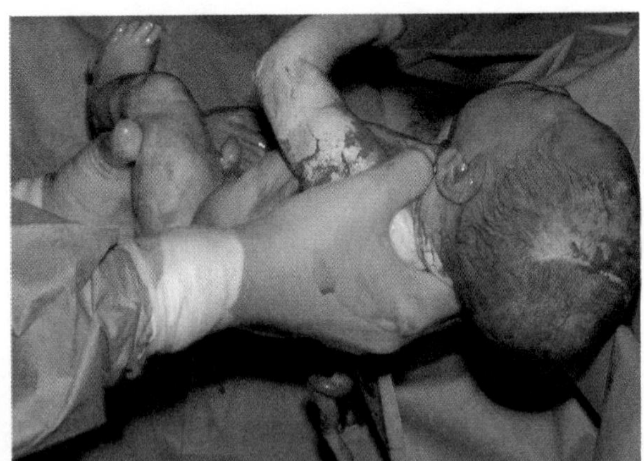

**7**
Infant delivered.

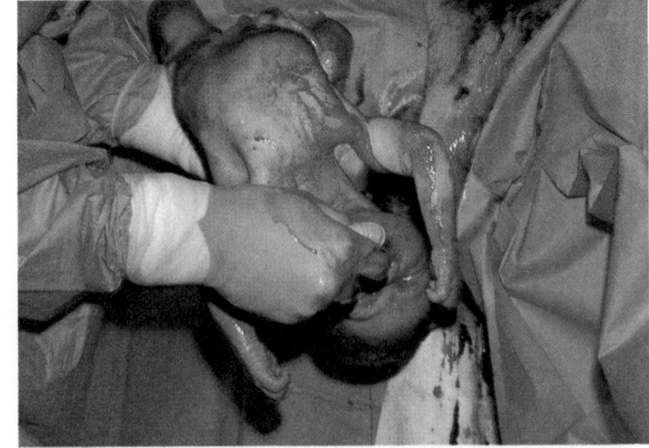

**8**
Clearing the airway.

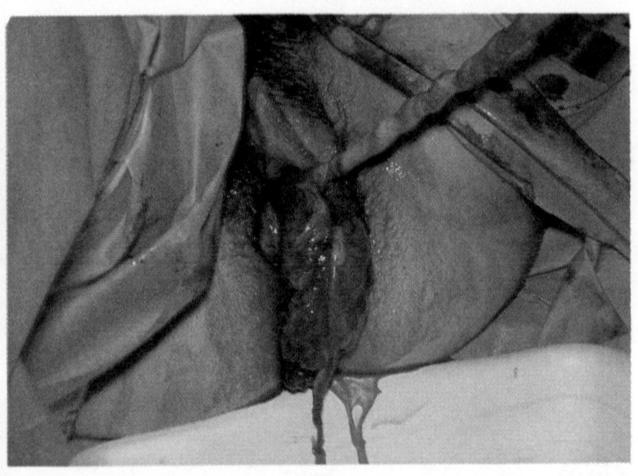

**9**
Placenta begins delivery.

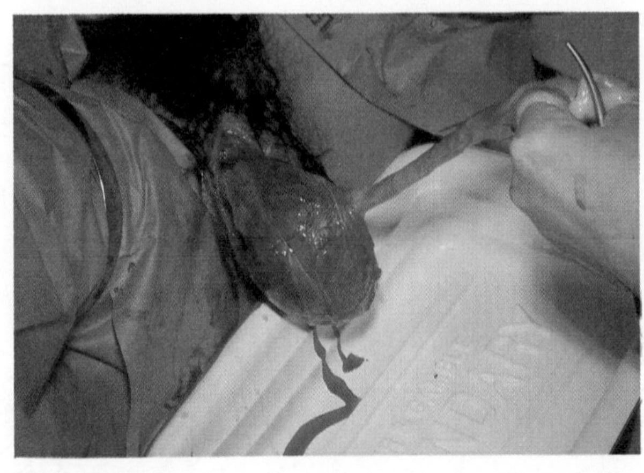

**10**
Placenta delivers.

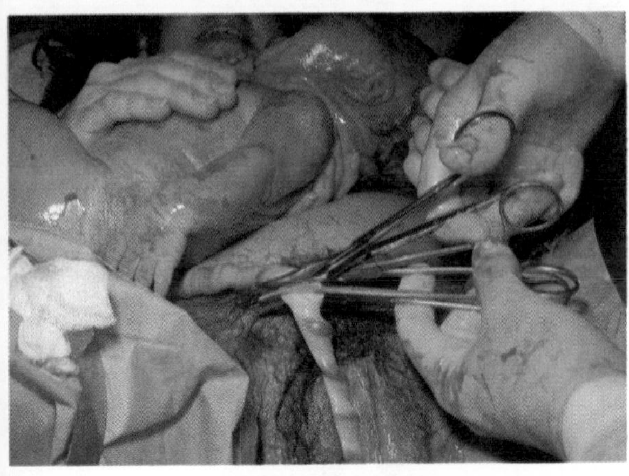

**11**
Cutting of cord.

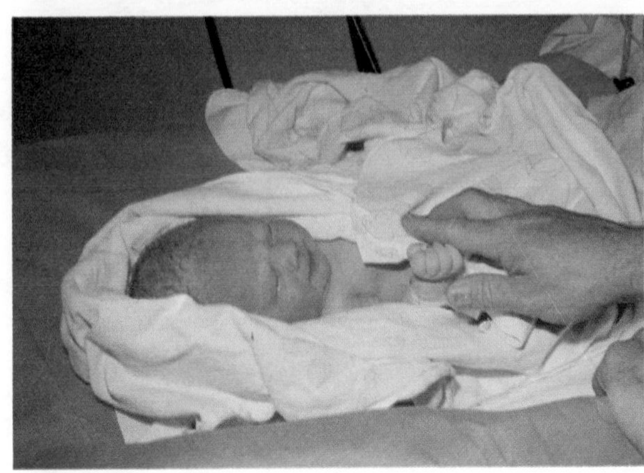

**12**
Wrap the baby.

Ask these questions:

- Have you had a baby before? The birth process will take longer with a first pregnancy, allowing for more transportation time.
- Are you having labor pains or contractions? How far apart are they? Contractions thin out and dilate the cervix so the baby can come through the birth canal. If contractions are five minutes or more apart, TRANSPORT; two minutes or more apart, DO NOT transport.
- Has the amniotic sac (bag of waters) ruptured? If so, when? This usually signifies the end of the first stage of labor, with the birth of the baby not far behind.
- Do you feel the sensation of a bowel movement? These are bearing-down sensations which bring the baby through the birth canal. The baby will shortly be born. DO NOT let Mom sit on the toilet.
- Do you feel like the baby is ready to be born?
- Place the mother on her back with her legs spread and examine the vaginal area. DO NOT touch the vagina. Look to see if the crown of the baby's head, or other presenting part, is pushing out of the vagina. If there is a bulging in the vaginal area, or a part of the head is visible, prepare to deliver the baby where you are.

During the interview and examination process make sure that you have sent a *specific* person to phone an ambulance and the mother's doctor if possible.

## STEPS OF NORMAL DELIVERY

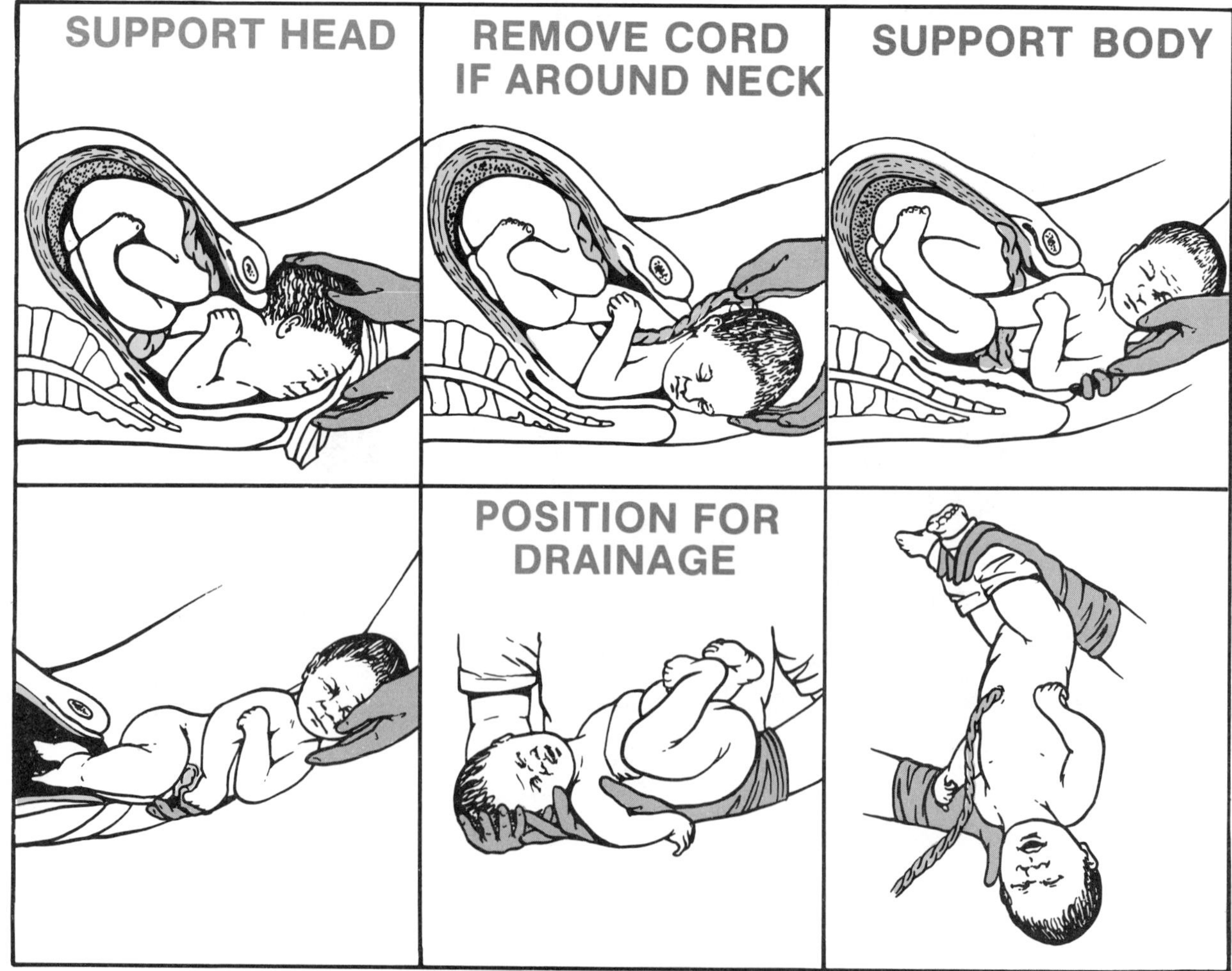

## DELIVERING THE BABY

The birth process has three major stages, known as the first, second, and third stages of labor. Understanding what goes on in each stage will help you to be of greater benefit to the mother and baby.

First Stage of Labor (opening of the cervix).

- This is also known as the early stage of labor.
- Contractions are 5-10 minutes apart and last 45-60 seconds.
- How long this stage lasts depends on the number of pregnancies the mother has had. (From 10-12 hours in a first pregnancy, to 5-6 hours in a succeeding pregnancy.)
- The purpose of the rhythmic contractions is to force the cervix (neck of the uterus) to open to allow the infant to pass from the uterus into the birth canal.
- The mother experiences bearing-down sensations to push the baby along the birth canal.
- The breaking of the bag of waters (amniotic fluid) typically signifies the end of this stage.

Second Stage of Labor (birth of the baby).

- In this stage the infant descends and is delivered.
- As the baby proceeds through the birth canal, bulging in the vaginal area, or crowning will appear.
- Crowning is when the baby's head is visible between the vaginal lips, between contractions.
- The head usually comes out face down.
- The baby's face then rotates itself toward the mother's thighs.
- One shoulder is born, then the rest of the baby will slide out.

Third Stage of Labor (delivery of the placenta).

- The placenta will "be born" just like the baby, and will usually take 5-15 minutes to deliver.

## WARMING THE BABY

An infant moving from a temperature of 98° to 99° F. to the current environmental temperature may experience hypothermia quickly if not protected. Cover the baby with a soft blanket or infant swaddle.

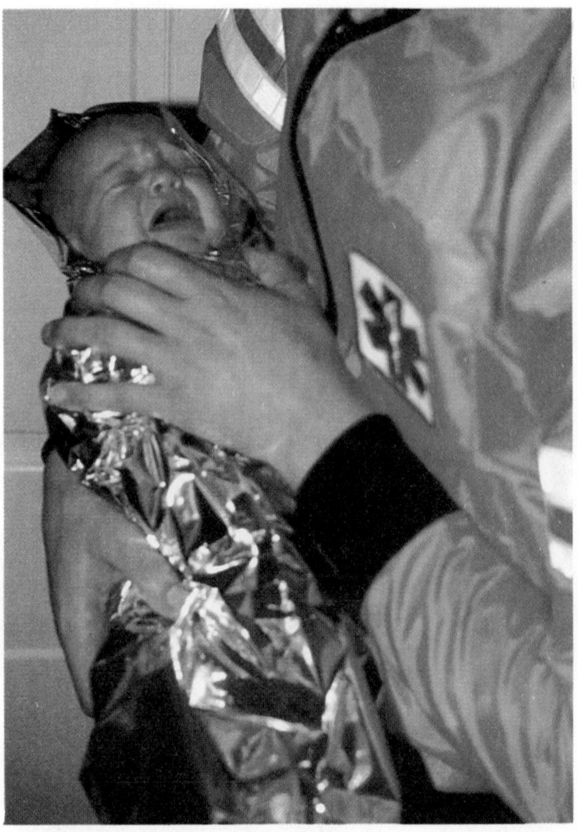

An infant swaddle to warm the baby.

## EMERGENCY CARE

- Stay calm and remember that childbirth is a natural process.
- Give the mother calming reassurance and support.
- Decide whether there is time to get to the hospital.
- If there is not time, have someone contact the ambulance and hospital, then prepare the delivery area.
- Have the mother lie on her back with her knees bent and separated.
- Remove any clothing that is in the way and place clean material under her buttocks.

- Wash your hands well.
- Do not place your hands inside the vagina.
- Inspect the opening of the birth canal (vagina) to determine if the baby's head is visible during contractions. If the exposed area of the baby's head is the size of a 50-cent piece or larger, the delivery will probably occur in minutes.)
- Encourage the mother not to bear down or strain during each contraction. Have her breathe in and out rapidly with short, panting breaths.
- NEVER try to hold back the baby's head or tell the mother to hold her legs together to prevent childbirth.
- As the baby's head begins to emerge, make sure that the amniotic membrane is torn. If not, tear it with your fingernails *before* the baby is born.
- As the head emerges, gently place one hand over the head and apply gentle pressure to keep the head from suddenly emerging.
- Feel the baby's neck for a possible loop of umbilical cord. If present, slip it over the baby's head.
- Now wipe out the baby's mouth and nose with facial tissues, gauze, or a clean cloth.
- DO NOT try to push, pull, or turn the baby in any direction.
- Support the baby's head and neck with your hands, and lift SLIGHTLY upward to help the shoulder emerge.
- Support the body as it emerges, remembering to get a firm hold on the baby.
- Dry the baby immediately and keep it warm.
- Keep the baby's head slightly lower than the rest of its body to facilitate drainage of the throat and mouth.
- Rub the baby's back and flick the soles of its feet to stimulate the baby's breathing. If there is a mucous obstruction problem, firmly grasp the ankles with your hand, hold the baby upside down, and stroke the baby's neck towards the mouth, then wipe out the mouth.
- If the baby does not breathe within one minute after birth, begin CPR.
- Keep the umbilical cord slack, and place the baby with its head extended back and a pad under its shoulders to keep an open airway. The mother can do this by holding the baby on her abdomen if need be.
- Try to keep the baby at the same level as the vaginal opening (i.e. between the mother's legs), but be careful that the baby does not fall from this position.
- Allow the placenta to be born like the baby was (20-30 minutes). Do NOT pull on the cord. To help the mother deliver the placenta, tell her to push or bear down as if she were having a bowel movement.
- If the area between the mother's vagina and anus is torn and bleeding, treat it like an open wound. (Direct pressure with gauze or sanitary pads.)
- The umbilical cord does not have to be cut; in fact it can stay intact for up to two days if necessary without undue concern. After the placenta is born, place it in a plastic bag along with three-quarters of the umbilical cord. Loosely bind the top of the plastic bag.
- Massage the mother's uterus until it is firm.
- Jot down any important information that the physician at the hospital should know about, i.e., time of delivery, appearance and color of amniotic fluid, cord around neck, etc.
- Tag the mother and baby with tape around their wrists and write the mother's name on both, with the sex of the baby and the time of delivery.
- Make sure that the mother and baby along with the placenta in a plastic bag are properly transported to the hospital.

## COMPLICATIONS

If complications occur, do the following:

- If the cord is wrapped tightly around the baby's neck, immediately clamp it in two places and cut it.
- If an arm, leg or shoulder emerges first, do NOT pull. Transport the mother to the hospital immediately.
- If the buttocks emerge first (breech birth) support the emerging body. DO NOT pull. Use two fingers into the vagina to locate and pull down slightly on the baby's mouth. If the baby does not emerge, transport immediately.

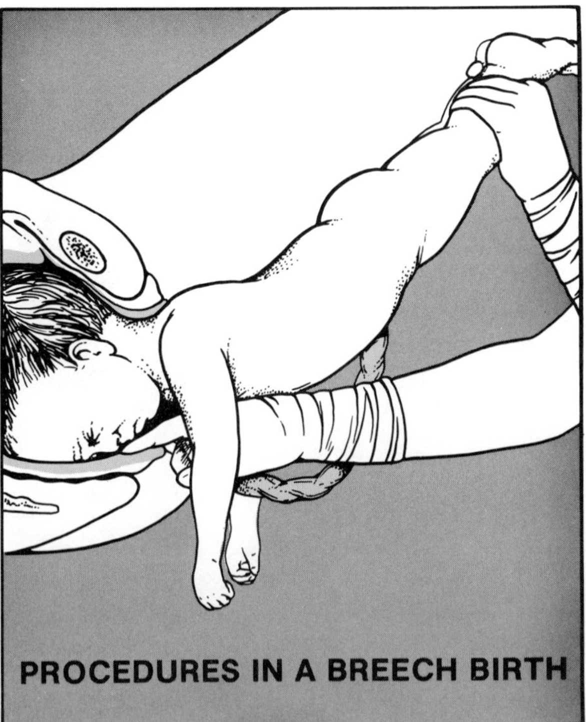


A breech delivery. Support the baby's chest and abdomen with your hand. Do not pull the baby.

- If a cord emerges before the baby (prolapsed cord), put your hand into the vagina and gently push the baby's head back until a pulse is felt in the umbilical cord. Stay in this position and transport immediately.

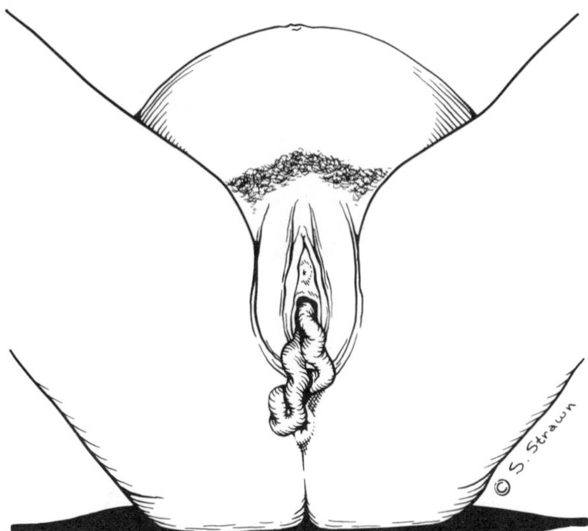


Prolapsed cord. Elevate the mother's hips with a pillow and keep her warm. With a surgical-gloved hand, gently push the baby up the vagina several inches to relieve the pressure on the cord. Keep the mother in this position while she is transported to the nearest medical facility.

## ABORTION

In cases of spontaneous abortion:

1. Provide basic life support for the woman.
2. Give her care for shock.
3. Call an ambulance as soon as possible.
4. Have any passed tissue or evidences of blood loss (bloody sheets, towels, underwear) taken to the hospital.

### SIGNS AND SYMPTOMS OF SPONTANEOUS ABORTION

- Passage of tissue
- Heavy vaginal bleeding
- Inability to feel the uterus
- Cramplike pains in lower abdomen
- Uterus located below woman's navel
- Mother's knowledge of pregnancy

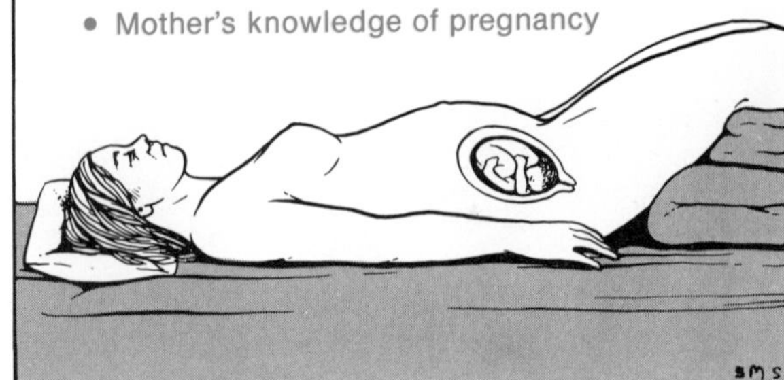

## Work Exercises

### Physiology of Childbirth

Label the diagram with each of the terms italicized in the following discussion.

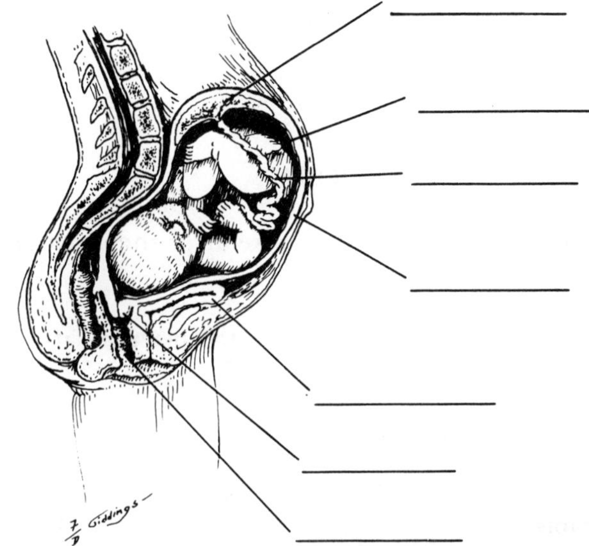

The developing baby, called a *fetus*, grows in the mother's *uterus*. Attached to the wall of this muscular organ is a special organ called the *placenta*. Its major purpose is to provide oxygen and nourishment to the fetus from the mother. The placenta is expelled from the uterus shortly after the birth of the baby.

The fetus is joined to the placenta by a rope-like structure called the *umbilical cord*. This cord carries the blood — and consequent oxygen and nourishment — that circulates between the placenta and the fetus. The umbilical cord is also expelled from the uterus after the birth of the baby.

While the baby is developing in the uterus, it is enclosed in a "bag of waters" called *amniotic fluid*. This fluid acts as a "shock absorber" for the baby and has other important purposes. The thin, membranous sac which holds the fluid is called the *amniotic sac*. When the baby is being born the amniotic sac breaks and the fluid gushes from the *birth canal*.

The lower part of the uterus is called the *cervix*. It is the "neck" of the uterus. During childbirth the cervix dilates to approximately ten times it's normal size to allow the baby to pass through. The baby passes from the cervix into the *vagina* or birth canal.

### Assisting With The Delivery

In the space provided, give a description of the assistance necessary for each area.

**Delivery position and preparation of the mother.**

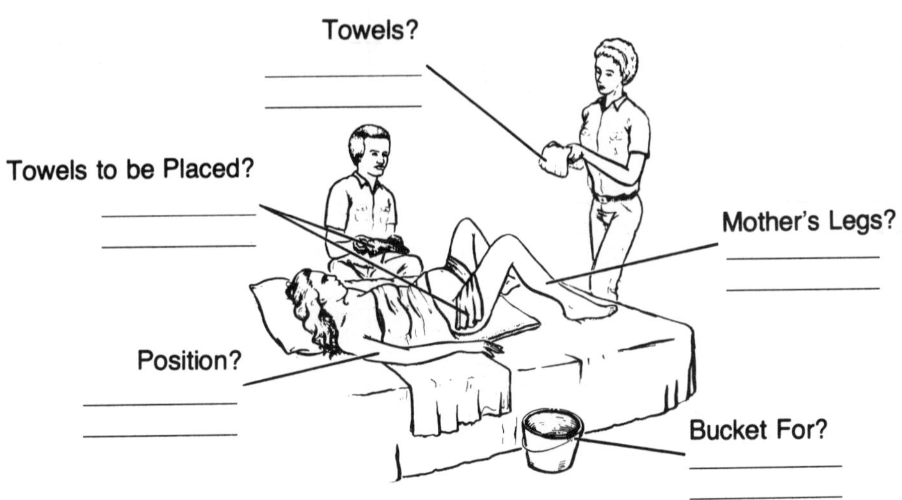

What is the most important first aid procedure in emergency childbirth?

## Delivery of the Placenta

1. How long does it take after the birth of the baby?

2. What do you do with the placenta after it is expelled?

## Care of the Mother

What are the important points to remember in caring for the mother after the birth is complete?

1.

2.

3.

4.

5.

## Labor and Birth Complications

Complete the "Emergency Care" column in the following table.

| Complication | Description | Emergency Care |
|---|---|---|
| Cord around neck | Umbilical cord wrapped once or more times around the baby's neck. | |
| Breech birth | Delivery in which the baby's buttocks appear first instead of the head. | |
| Prolapsed Cord | The umbilical cord protrudes from the vagina ahead of the baby. | |
| Abortion | Fetus is born before it is old enough to sustain life. | |

## SELF-TEST

### Part I: True and False

If you believe the statement is true, circle the T. If you believe the statement is false, circle F.

T F 1. Emergency childbirth is just that — measures that should be taken under an emergency when it is impossible for the mother to reach a hospital or physician.

T F 2. The birth will probably occur within a few minutes when the visible part of the baby's head is the size of a dime.

T F 3. If the woman is having her first child and the visible part of the baby's head is smaller than a fifty-cent piece, the birth is probably about twenty minutes away, and you should try to transport her if a hospital is close enough.

T F 4. If you are close to a medical facility and the birth begins, instruct the woman to clamp her legs tightly together and try to keep the baby's head inside the birth canal.

T F 5. If the umbilical cord is wrapped around the baby's neck as it emerges from the birth canal and you are unable to slip it over the baby's head, you should cut it immediately.

T F 6. Cutting the umbilical cord is critical, since an infant left attached to the placenta is in danger of bleeding to death.

T F 7. The cervix is a muscular organ that surrounds and holds the fetus.

T F 8. The umbilical cord carries blood between the fetus and the placenta.

T F 9. In breech delivery, the buttocks are presented first.

T F 10. It is acceptable to hold the mother's legs together during crowning if you are rushing to the hospital.

T F 11. A gentle pull on the baby as it is being born will give a more efficient delivery.

T F 12. An umbilical cord that is wrapped around the baby's neck must be quickly, but gently, removed.

T F 13. If there is difficulty in delivering the baby's shoulders, the First Aider can gently guide the baby's head downward.

T F 14. If the baby doesn't breathe immediately after birth, the First Aider should give mouth-to-mouth and nose resuscitation.

T F 15. It is important to take the placenta to the hospital with the mother and baby.

T F 16. It is NOT essential for the First Aider to cut the umbilical cord.

T F 17. After delivery, gentle massage of the uterus helps to control the mother's bleeding.

T F 18. The mother and baby should always be taken to the hospital after the birth.

T F 19. If the umbilical cord protrudes into the birth canal when the bag of waters ruptures, take the mother to the hospital *immediately.*

T F 20. A baby is usually born with its face up.

T F 21. It is vital that the umbilical cord be cut as soon after birth as possible.

T F 22. The baby needs to have its white, greasy coating on its skin washed off as soon as possible.

T F 23. A First Aider should gently pull on the umbilical cord to help expel the afterbirth.

T F 24. If the baby is still encased in the bag of waters when the head is delivered, you should tear it with your fingers.

T F 25. If medical assistance is not available, you can gently push on the baby's head to delay delivery.

T F 26. The cord should be cut as close to the baby's body as possible.

**Part II: Multiple Choice**

For each question, circle the answer that best reflects an accurate statement.

1. The umbilical cord should be cut no closer than how many inches from the infant's body?
   a. one
   b. two
   c. three
   d. four

2. If the baby's head emerges from the birth canal and the amniotic sac is still unbroken, you should:
   a. wait for the baby to emerge completely
   b. tear the bag with your fingers so the fluid can drain
   c. carefully puncture the bag, taking care not to injure the baby

3. A woman should be given immediate help instead of transport when her labor contractions are regularly spaced:
   a. five minutes apart
   b. three minutes apart
   c. two minutes apart
   d. one minute apart

4. During labor, the baby's head should be visible at the opening of the birth canal:
   a. during the actual contraction
   b. between contractions
   c. all the time
   d. none of the time

5. A baby should be breathing within how much time after birth?
   a. ten seconds
   b. one to two minutes
   c. five minutes
   d. thirty to forty-five seconds

6. In order to decide whether to transport the mother prior to delivery, the First Aider should:
   a. ask the mother if she is having her first baby
   b. examine the mother for signs of crowning
   c. ask the mother if she feels as if she has to move her bowels
   d. all of the above

7. If the cord is presented first, you should:
   a. not worry — proceed with the delivery
   b. get medical assistance immediately
   c. push the cord back in
   d. pull gently on the cord to expedite delivery

8. As the baby's head emerges, you should:
   a. push gently on top of the head
   b. pull gently on top of the head
   c. apply downward pressure
   d. guide and support the head

9. If the baby does not begin to breathe by itself, you should:
   a. start mouth-to-mouth and nose resuscitation
   b. hyperextend its neck
   c. use the Holgar-Nielson method of resuscitation
   d. turn the baby upside down and gently shake it

10. To make a final decision about delivery at the scene:
    a. ask the woman how far apart her pains are
    b. examine the vaginal opening for signs of crowning
    c. feel the woman's abdomen for signs of movement
    d. check the perineum for signs of bulging

11. If a First Aider starts for the hospital with the mother and the delivery starts during the trip, the First Aider should:
    a. stop and prepare for the delivery
    b. have the woman hold her legs together tightly
    c. pack the vaginal opening with sanitary napkins
    d. place the hand firmly against the vaginal opening

12. When the umbilical cord comes out of the vagina before the baby comes, there is a danger that:
    a. the cord may tear during the delivery
    b. the baby may suffocate due to lack of oxygen
    c. the cord may strangle the baby
    d. the cord may pull the afterbirth free when the baby is delivered

Corresponds with:
**American Red Cross**
**Standard First Aid & Personal Safety**
Chapter 9, pages 144-159
and
**Advanced First Aid & Emergency Care**
Chapter 9, pages 134-144

# 15 Burn Emergencies

Over two million burn accidents occur each year in the United States. Of those who are burned (in fires, by chemicals, by the sun, in automobile accidents, or in other kinds of accidents), more than 70,000 require hospitalization; almost 10,000 of them die as a result of their burns. Burns are a leading cause of accidental death in the United States.

| Signs/Symptoms and Common Causes of Burns | | | | |
|---|---|---|---|---|
| **First-Degree** | Redness or discoloration<br>Mild swelling<br>Pain<br>Rapid healing | May be fatal if 2/3 surface involved<br>Outer layer of skin only | Least serious — only outer layer of skin<br>Rarely requires medical attention | Overexposure to sun<br>Slight contact with hot objects<br>Scalding by hot water or steam |
| **Second-Degree** | Red or mottled skin<br>Blister formations<br>Much swelling over several days<br>Wet skin surface<br>Very painful<br>New skin grows back | Outer layer of skin as well as dermis | Plasma loss through burned skin layers<br>Undestroyed nerve endings increase pain<br>Infection prevents new skin growth | Deep sunburn<br>Contact with hot liquids<br>Flash burns from gasoline, kerosene |
| **Third-Degree** | Charred epidermis, dermis, fat, muscle<br>Skin coagulation, destruction of red blood cells<br>Loss of skin, healing only at margins, scar tissue replaces rest of area<br>No pain | Hair follicles, dermis, epidermis, and some vessels | Nerve endings destroyed<br>Often resembles second-degree at first<br>Usually combination of all degrees of burns | Flame<br>Ignited clothing<br>Immersion in hot water<br>Contact with hot objects<br>Electricity |
| **Deep Third-Degree** | Charred sub-cutaneous tissue, underlying bone and muscle<br>Skin coagulation<br>Destruction of red blood cells<br>Complete skin loss<br>No pain | Hair follicles, epidermis, dermis, sebaceious glands, sweat glands, vessels, subcutaneous tissue, and bone | Very serious; regeneration of these tissues impossible<br>Grafting necessary | Caught in burning house<br>Exposure to flame — in steel mill or from torch<br>Serious electrical burns |

## BURN CLASSIFICATION

Burns strike every age group and with varying degrees of severity. They are classified by degree of damage to the skin and underlying tissues.

## DETERMINING EXTENT: THE RULE OF NINES

The **"Rule of Nines"** can be used to quickly calculate the amount of skin surface that has received burns. Most areas of the adult body can be divided into portions of 9 percent or multiples of nine.

The hand can be used as a good reference, as it represents about 1 percent of the body. For determining the severity of burns in children and infants, the same percentages as used in adults may be used, with the exception of the head and legs.

The Rule of Nines utilizes a method of dividing the body into regions, each of which represents 9 percent of the total body surface (or a multiple of 9 percent). Head and neck composes 9 percent; anterior (front) trunk, 18 percent; posterior (back) trunk, 18 percent; each upper extremity, 9 percent; the genital area, 1 percent; and each lower extremity, 18 percent. Using the Rule of Nines, you can determine the extent of burns suffered by a victim who you find at the accident site.

## LOCATION OF THE BURN

Certain areas of the body are more critically damaged by burns than others, and it is essential that you recognize which areas represent the greatest hazard to a burn victim.

Burns on the face or neck should be examined immediately because of possible burns to the eye area or respiratory complications. Check the eyes to make sure that no injury has occurred. Then assess whether respiratory damage is present.

Other locations of burns that are particularly critical include the hands, feet, and external genitalia. Any burn to the upper body is more serious than a burn of similar extent

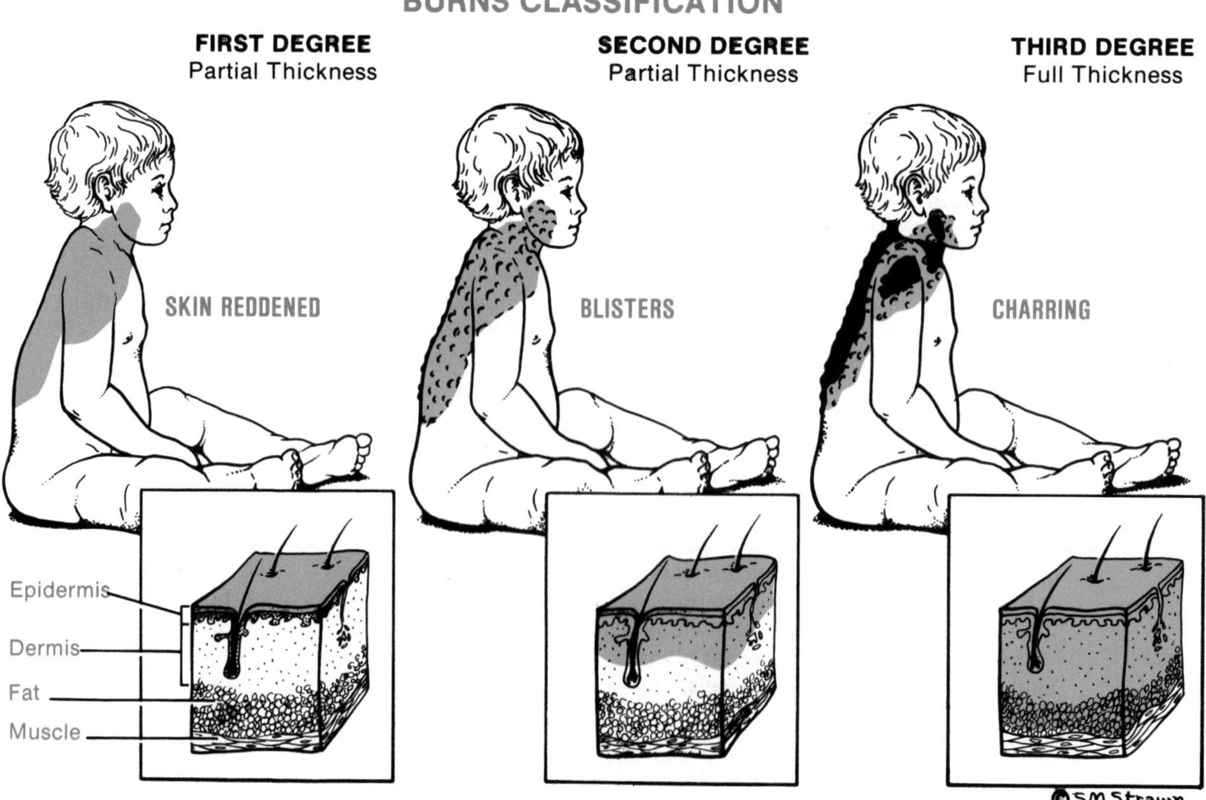

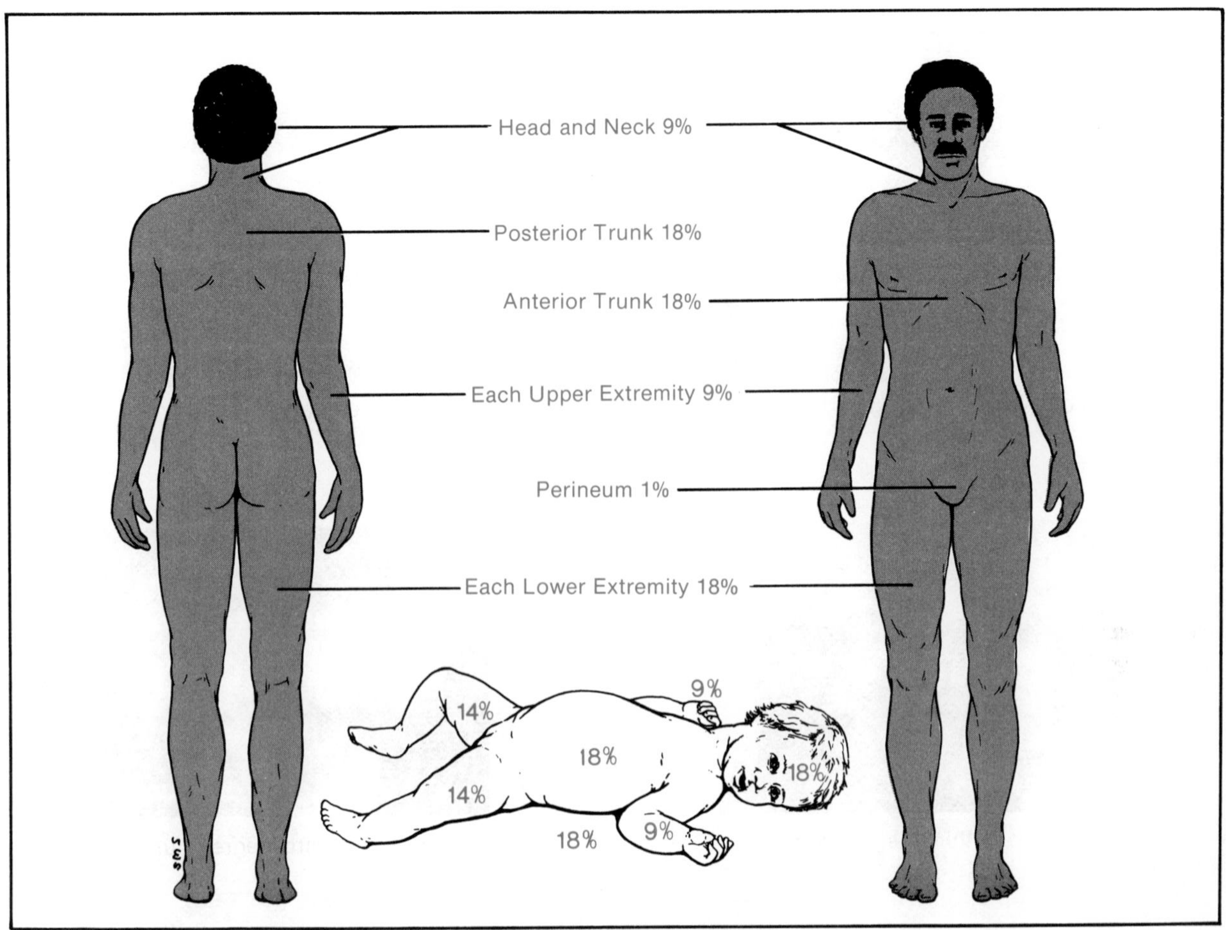


The rule of nine: A method for estimating percentage of body surface involved with burns. The body surface is divided into regions, each of which represents 9% or a multiple of 9% of the total surface.

and degree on the lower body. Victims with burns in any of these areas need to be transported to a hospital or burn center immediately.

## AGE OF THE VICTIM

Children under the age of five and adults over the age of sixty tolerate burns very poorly. In an elderly patient, a burn covering only 20 percent of the body can often be fatal.

Because the elderly and the very young have extremely thin skin, they will sustain much deeper burns from a much less severe source. An additional problem is disease immunity — it is incomplete in the young child and is usually compromised in the elderly.

## PROBLEMS ASSOCIATED WITH BURNS

The problems most often associated with burns are:

- Airway or respiratory difficulties.
- Related musculoskeletal injuries.
- Loss of body fluids, contributing to shock.
- Pain contributing to shock.
- Anxiety contributing to shock.
- Swelling.
- Infection due to destruction of skin tissue.

### Emergency Care

1. **Remove the victim from the source of the burn.** If the victim was burned by a fire, take him/her as far away as possible without inflicting further injury.

## TYPES OF BURNS

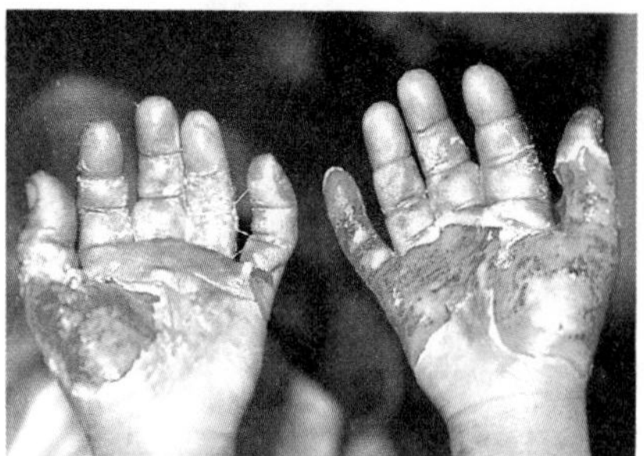

Second- and third-degree burns.

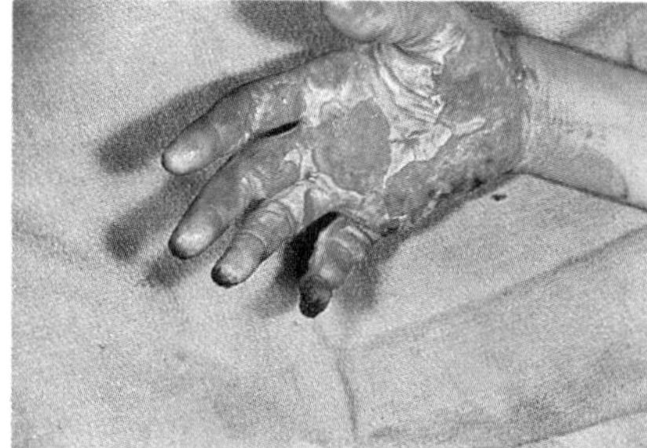

Third-degree flare burns.

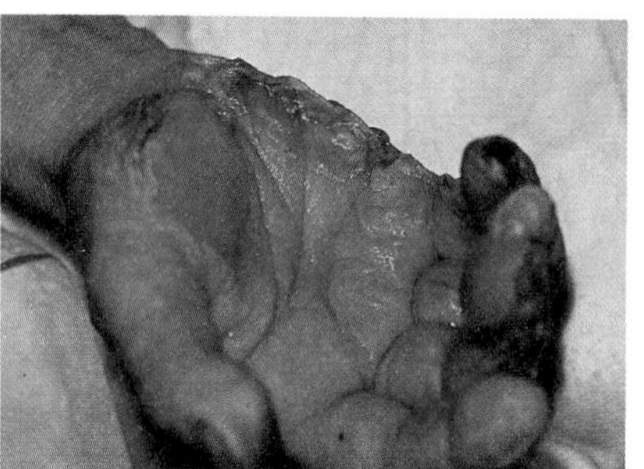

Second- and third-degree burns.

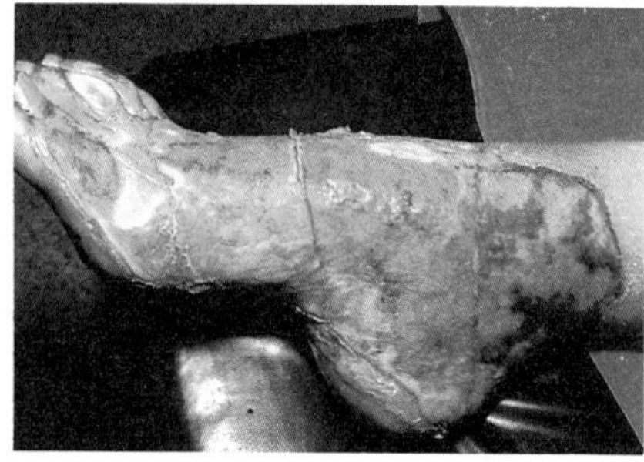

Second- and third-degree burns.

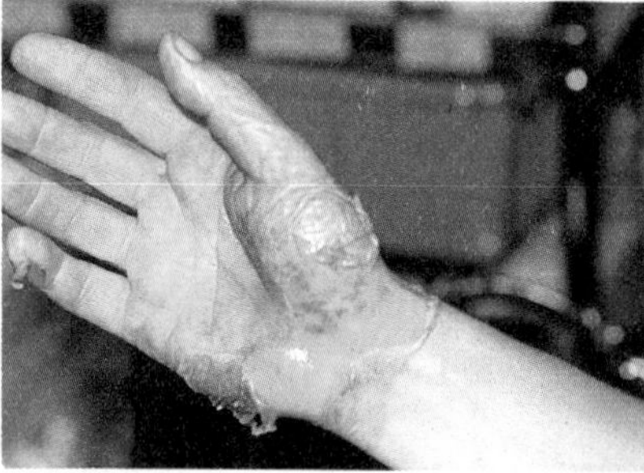

Second-degree burn.

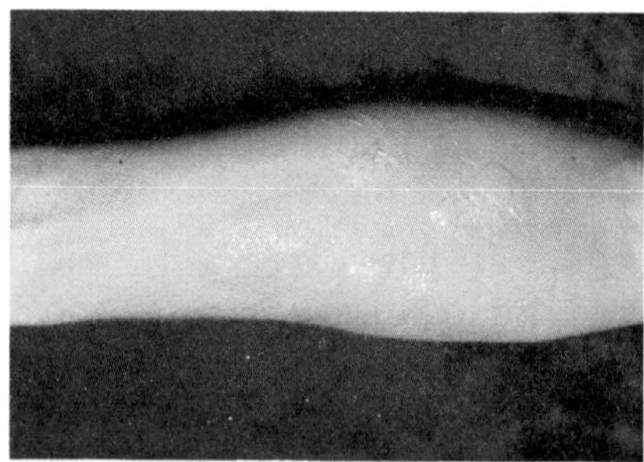

Second-degree burn.

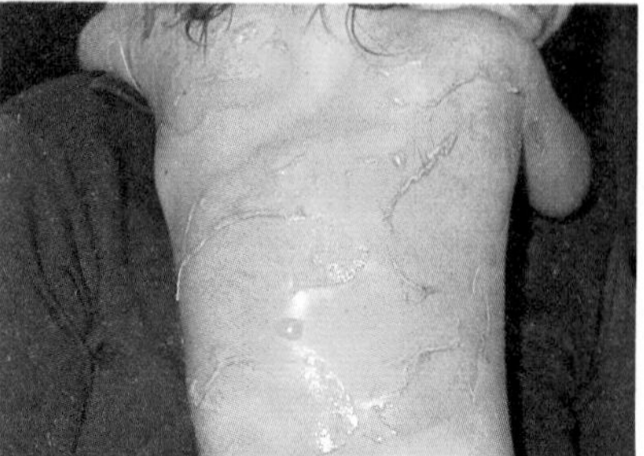

Second-degree burn.

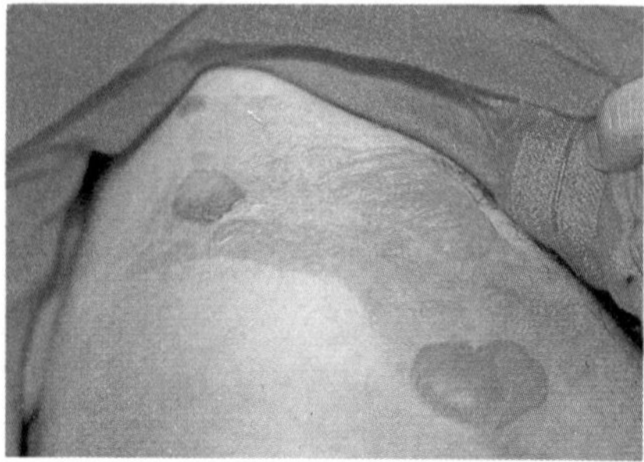

Second-degree burn.

## CRITICAL BURNS

**Note: The general condition of the victim must also be considered. For example, a moderate burn in an aged or critically ill person might be serious.**

**CRITICAL BURNS** are burns complicated by respiratory tract injury and other major injuries or fractures.

**THIRD-DEGREE** burns involving the critical areas of the face, hands and feet

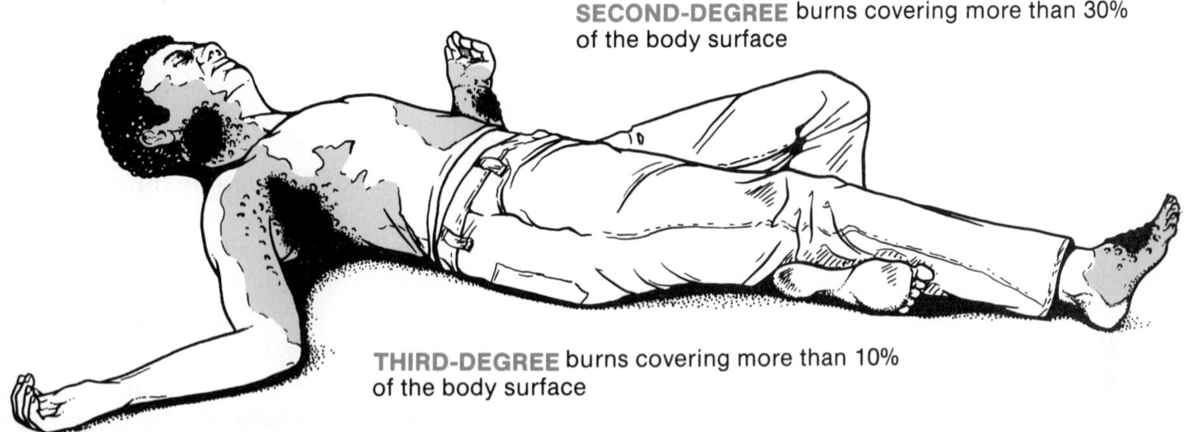


### GENERAL EMERGENCY CARE

- For first- and second-degree burns, the burned part should be immersed in cold water for 2 to 5 minutes if possible.
- The burned area should be covered with a clean dressing.
- If possible, cold wet applications should be used to relieve pain unless burn is extensive.
- If smoke inhalation is suspected, assist ventilation if necessary.
- **Note:** Never use grease (e.g. butter, lard, vaseline) on a burn.

2. **Eliminate the cause of the burn.** Put out the fire. Wash away the chemicals. Disconnect live electric wires.
3. **Determine the severity of the burn.** Decide immediately how critical the burn is and how extensive the injury has become. Take into account the factors previously discussed: the extent of total body surface involved, the depth of the burn, the age of the victim, the location of the burn, and the possibility of preexistent disease or additional injury.
4. **Assess for respiratory/cardiac complications.** Check the victim thoroughly to determine whether breathing or heartbeat have stopped. If the victim is still breathing, look for signs of possible injury to the respiratory system. Be especially alert for wheezing or coughing as the victim breathes, for a sooty or smoky smell on the breath, for particles of soot in the saliva, and for burns of the mucous membranes in the mouth and nostrils. If any of these signs are present, immediately begin to aid breathing.
5. **Do not put anything on the burn.** Under no circumstance should grease, oil, ointment, butter, or any other substance be applied to the burn.
6. **Remove all clothing and jewelry from the burned area.** Do not pull off any item that is sticking to the skin, but remove any clothing or jewelry that might be dangerous if swelling should occur.
7. **Immediately immerse the burned area in cool water.** In addition to providing pain relief, cool water can stop the spread of the heat damage to surrounding tissues. Make sure that the victim does not get immersed in ice water — the rapid temperature extreme can cause severe complications. Di-

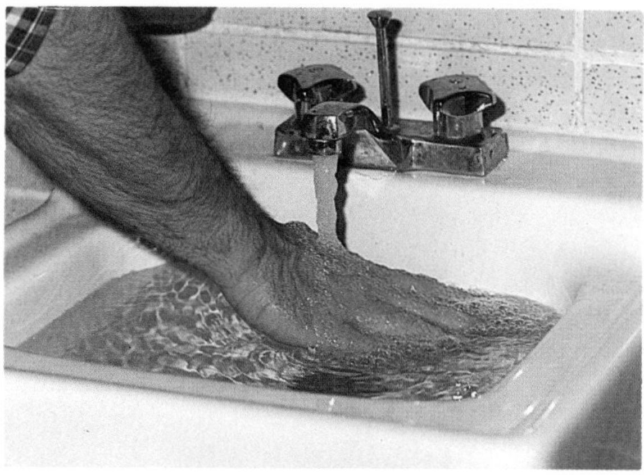
Cooling a burn by submerging in cold running water.

rect application of ice to the burn can cause frostbite and complicate the severity of the burn.

Halt the application of cool water after thirty minutes. Further treatment by immersion is ineffective and may actually lead to complications, such as causing a chill that may induce shock.

8. **If possible, leave first-degree burns uncovered.** The burn will heal more rapidly and more completely if it is not covered. If a dressing *is* necessary, apply only a clean (sterile if possible) cloth and leave it as loose as possible. Applying constricting bandages will further damage the burned area and may even tear burned skin loose from the body.
9. **Give the victim emergency care for shock.** Even if the victim manifests no signs and symptoms of shock, have him/her lie down, drink fluids, and stay warm.

## INHALATION INJURIES

Three causes of inhalation injury accompany burns: (1) heat inhalation; (2) inhalation of noxious chemicals or smoke; and (3) inhalation of carbon monoxide gas.

Most of the damage done to the upper airway is a result of heat inhalation — mucous membranes and linings get scorched, and **edema** (swelling) partially blocks the airway. Specific signs and symptoms of upper airway injuries are respiratory distress accompanied by restlessness, difficulty in swallowing, hoarseness, coughing, and a bluish skin color.

The usual direct cause of death in inhalation injury cases is pneumonia. At first the

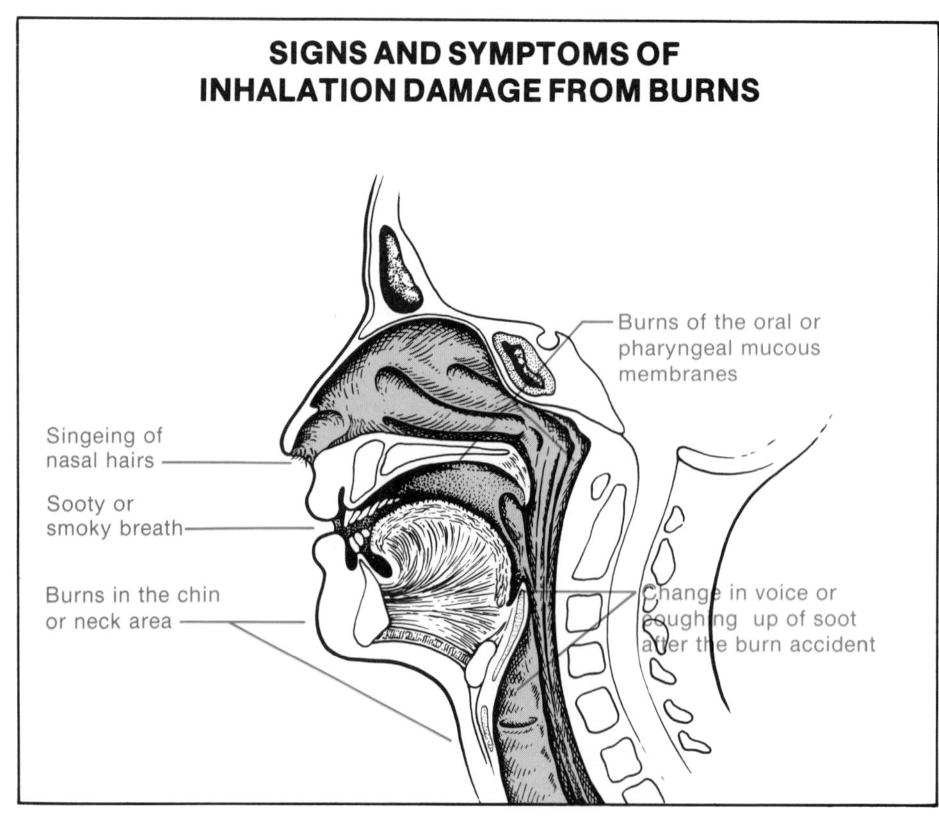

victim will wheeze; later, he/she will manifest increased difficulty in breathing and will cough up mucous and fluid.

The following signs and symptoms indicate **respiratory injury:**

1. Wheezing.
2. Carbon particles in the victim's saliva.
3. A sooty or smoky smell on the breath.
4. Burned or singed nasal hairs.
5. Hoarseness.
6. Restricted movement of the chest.
7. Burns of the oral mucous membranes.
8. A victim who was trapped in a confined or extremely smoky area during a fire.

Victims who have sustained severe pulmonary or respiratory injury may experience no change in skin color and no unusual signs of injury in the chest area. If any of the signs and symptoms listed above are present, take measures to prevent further damage:

1. Maintain open airway and assist ventilations if necessary.
2. Remove the victim as far as possible from the source of the burn — especially if it is a fire. Mouth-to-mouth ventilation may be required to help the victim breathe.
3. Remove any clothing that may restrict chest movement or breathing. Remove neckties if they have not burned and if they are not sticking to the skin.
4. Call for emergency medical aid as soon as possible.

## CHEMICAL BURNS

Speed is essential in caring for chemical burns. The more quickly you are able to remove the cause of the burn and initiate care, the less severe the burn will be.

1. Flush the burned area with water immediately. If the victim is at home, the shower or garden hose is ideal. Flush the area for at least five minutes under a steady stream of water — make sure that no traces of the chemical remain on or around the burned area.
2. Immediately remove the victim's clothing, shoes, and stockings and any other jewelry or apparel that might have become contaminated with the chemical. Take care not to contaminate your own skin, eyes, or clothing.
3. After you remove the victim's clothing, continue flushing the entire body for about thirty minutes. Do not waste time trying to find an antidote — flushing with water is more effective and most available.
4. Make sure to flush the eyes if any chemicals splash into them. Have the victim remove contact lenses. **Never use chemical antidotes in the eyes.**

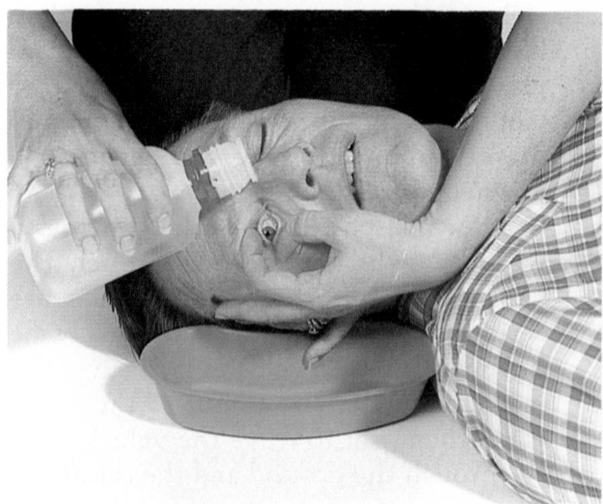

Flushing a chemical burn to the eye.

5. Have someone call for emergency medical aid while flushing burned area.
6. Do not neutralize a burned area with alkali or acid solutions. You may guess wrong about the content of the chemical agent and may worsen the burn by attempting to neutralize it. You may also miscalculate the quantity needed to neutralize it. Worst of all, neutralization reactions generate heat that can extend the depth of tissue damage and intensify the injury.

## ELECTRICAL BURNS

Follow these guidelines when approaching an accident that involves downed power lines or other electrical hazards:

1. Look for downed wires that you may not notice whenever an accident has involved a vehicle that has struck a power pole. How can you tell if a line might be downed

and hidden in the grass or brush? Carefully look at the next pole down the line, and count how many power lines are at the top crossarm of the undamaged pole. There should be the same number of lines at the top crossarm of the damaged pole. If there aren't, watch out! If it is dark, use a flashlight or spotlight to inspect the poles and surrounding area.

2. **NEVER** attempt to move downed wires! Only authorized repairmen from the power company should be allowed to touch a high-voltage wire; they have the skill and the proper equipment (including high-voltage rubber gloves and fiberglass prods).
3. Get help from the power company **immediately** upon entering the scene of a downed power line.
4. If a downed power line is lying across a wrecked vehicle, **DO NOT** touch the vehicle, even if the victims inside are seriously injured. You will most likely die if you touch the vehicle. If the victims inside are conscious, shout to them and warn them not to leave the vehicle — if they touch the ground and the car at the same time, the current will kill them.
5. If the car begins to burn and the victims inside are at risk of dying in the fire, instruct them to open the car door and jump as far as they can away from the car. In any case, they should not touch the car and the ground at the same time.
6. If a downed power line is in the area but is **not** near or touching the vehicle, you can proceed as needed.
7. If a downed power line is sparking and flipping around, use extreme caution and roll a spare tire over to the line slowly so that it falls on the wire. Do **not** touch the tire as it rolls.
8. If the downed wires are household current wires (they are the ones at the eighteen- to twenty-two-foot level, or second down the pole), you can safely handle them in **dry** weather if you use gloved hands, a folded dry sheet, or a wooden stick. If the weather is humid, don't attempt to move even a household current line. Truly dangerous wiring is always placed at the top of the pole.
9. If the downed lines are television cable or telephone lines, you can safely handle them with gloved hands, even if they are slightly moist.
10. When in doubt, **don't touch a downed line.** NEVER assume that a downed line is dead unless power company officials confirm it.
11. Call for emergency aid.
12. Master electrician, Clyde Tomboulian, reminds us of several other important concepts:

    - Relatively low voltages such as household 120 volts can cause burns to tender tissue such as the mouth (when a child chews on an electrical cord, for example). However, many victims of **electrocution** (such as swimmers when a poolside radio falls into the water) will show no visible signs of injury.

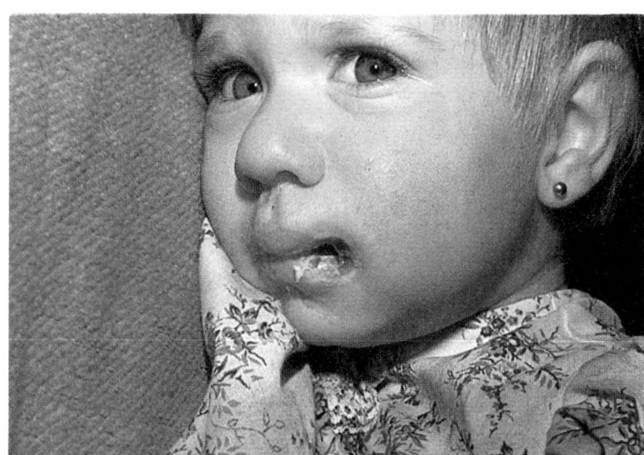

Electrical burn caused by chewing on an electrical cord.

    - The best clue for scene evaluation is to make a visual sweep for power cords that may be routed to the tool the victim is still holding. (Remember, a power tool does not have to be "on" to present a shock hazard!) If you have a possible pool drowning victim, check quickly in the water for any electrical cord or hazard. Before entering the water to remove the victim, brush the ends of the fingers of one hand very lightly against the water. If you feel a tingle, get all the power turned off at the main switch before putting even a toe in the water.

| Emergency Care For Electrical Injuries | |
|---|---|
| **Signs and Symptoms — Physical and Behavioral** | Breathing stops with high-frequency electrical current or lightning. Two burns — where power enters and leaves. Entry point wound small, but burn area large below surface. Electric shock: Unconsciousness or dazed and confused condition, weak and irregular pulse or no pulse. |
| **Factors Affecting Severity** | • Frequency of current; voltage and amperage.<br>• Amount of moisture on patient.<br>• Amount of insulation (clothing, rubber shoes) worn by patient.<br>• Area of body through which the current passes. |
| **Emergency Care** | • Separate the victim from electrical source carefully.<br>• Check for breathing and pulse immediately.<br>• Start CPR if necessary.<br>• Treat for shock.<br>• Treat burns as for heat burns.<br>• Check for entrance and exit burns — cover with dressing.<br>• Call for emergency medical aid immediately.<br>• Maintain body temperature; keep victim quiet and lying down.<br>• Provide emotional support to victim.<br>• Assess for other injuries such as head trauma or fractures — stabilize as appropriate. |

- If you find a victim in a bathtub with a radio, portable heater, or other appliance, be sure that you **pull the plug** before you touch the victim. A victim may be found leaning across a kitchen counter with one hand in the sink (which is grounded) and the other on some appliance (toaster, mixer, etc.). The shock did not come from the sink; the sink only completed the circuit. The shock came from the appliance, when an accidental connection occurred, causing the metal parts to become energized with respect to ground. The cure is simply to **pull the plug** to remove the shock hazard before starting victim care.

## Types of Electrical Burns

There are three kinds of electrical burns: (1) **contact burns** (when the current is most intense at the entrance and exit sites); (2) **flash burns** (when an extremity is close to an electrical flash or is struck by a flash of lightning); and (3) **arcing injuries** (when a current jumps from one surface to another).

## Signs and Symptoms of Electrocution

If you are unsure whether or not a person has been shocked, examine the victim for signs and symptoms of electrocution:

1. Dazed and confused condition.
2. Obvious and severe burns on the skin surface.
3. Unconsciousness.
4. Weak, irregular, or missing pulse.
5. Shallow, irregular, or missing breathing.

## Emergency Care

1. Your first and immediate responsibility is to get the victim away from the source of electrocution.
2. Start CPR immediately **if** indicated (no carotid pulse), even if you are unsure about the extent of injury.
3. A victim sustaining electrical shock may become hysterical and start to run around in circles and behave erratically. Force the victim to lie down and keep quiet. Make sure to maintain the body temperature. Cover the victim with several heavy blankets to help offset shock.
4. Get emergency medical aid immediately.

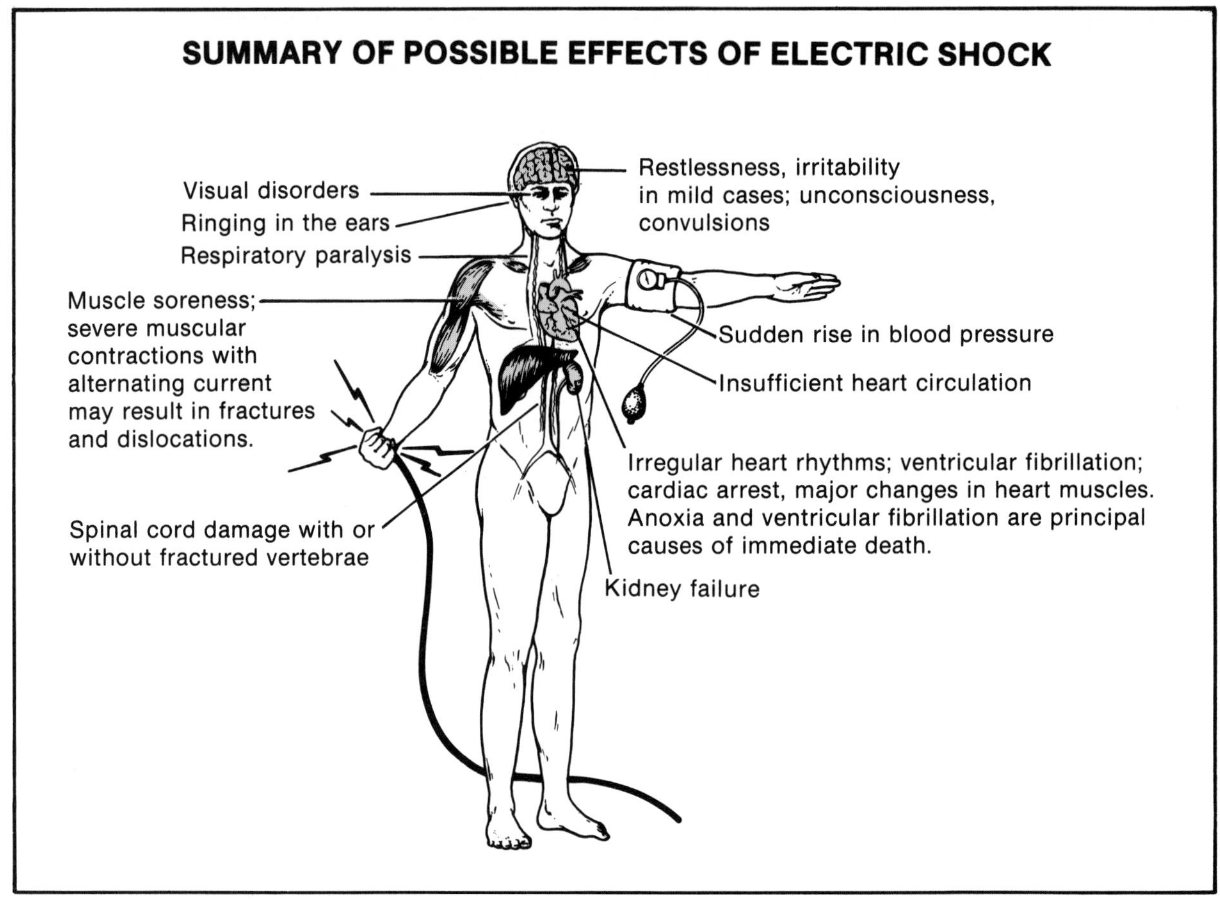


## Lightning Injuries — Emergency Care

1. Survey the entire scene. Assess what happened, and make sure that the victim is free from further damage. For example, remove any debris that has fallen on him/her, move him/her away from sources of conduction, and so on. Persons who are struck by lightning do not contain a current and are safe to handle — it is impossible to become electrocuted by touching them.
2. Assess breathing and circulation status. Begin measures to maintain breathing and heartbeat.
3. Check skin color.
4. If the victim is conscious, check movement in all the extremities.
5. Determine the victim's reaction to pain.

In administering artificial ventilation to lightning strike victims, do not tilt the head backward because of the probability of spinal injuries. Hold the head in a neutral position, and bring the jaw gently forward. Care for shock immediately, and examine the victim to ascertain whether he/she has any obvious open wounds that need care or fractures that need to be immobilized. Assume the worst if it is necessary to move the victim — take care not to jostle the victim in such a way as to further injure him.

Remember — respiratory or cardiopulmonary arrest is the most immediate life-threatening complication. CPR should be administered to all lightning victims and should continue until vital functions are restored or until you are relieved by medical personnel. Call for emergency medical aid immediately.

## Emergency Burn Care

### GENERAL PRINCIPLES

**The emergency care rendered to a burn victim largely depends on the cause of the burn and the degree of severity. Regardless of the severity of the burn, however, infection can be a serious problem. Certain principles need to be kept in mind when dealing with any burn victim.**

- Remove the victim from the burn source.
- Maintain the airway and monitor respiration.
- Control any bleeding.
- Treat for shock and maintain body heat.
- When a burn and soft tissue wound are in the same area, treat as if a burn only — except to control bleeding.
- Remove clothing, jewelry, and loose debris, unless they are sticking to the burned surface.
- Do NOT try to clean the burn.
- Separate burned surfaces from contact with one another.
- Never use ointments, lotions, or sprays unless recommended by a physician.
- Never use industrial grease or oil, butter, or similar cooking fats on burns.
- Do not break blisters.
- Splint fractures.
- Do not administer fluids — may cause vomiting.
- Assess for related injuries.

### EMERGENCY CARE FOR MINOR BURNS

- Smother and remove smoldering material.
- Remove restrictive clothing and jewelry.
- Assess extent of burn.
- To relieve pain, cold water applications can be applied, or the burned area can be submerged in cold water. Cool running water is best.
- Unclean areas should be cleaned with soap and water and left open to air or covered with a clean, dry dressing.
- If sunburned areas are clean, they should not be washed.
- Do not break blisters.
- Do not try to remove pieces of clothing that adhere to a wound.
- Elevate burned arms or legs.

### EMERGENCY CARE FOR MODERATE TO CRITICAL BURNS

- First Aiders should protect self against flames, noxious gases, smoke, explosions, falling debris, etc.
- If victims clothes are smoldering, wet them using any available water or smother with coat, blanket, etc. Don't waste time trying to remove clothing first.
- If clothing still retains heat as in a scald, cool by pouring water over area and then remove clothing.
- Maintain airway — breathing difficulties are common with burns around face, neck and mouth.
- Do not try to clean burn.
- Never use ointments, lotions, sprays, industrial grease, or oil, butter, or similar products on burns.
- Do not break blisters.
- Cool smaller thermal burns with water, flush chemicals from the surface, and/or remove victim from electrical source.
- Do not use cold applications on extensive burns; cold could result in chilling and hypothermia.
- Check for signs of smoke inhalation — if suspected, assist ventilations.
- Assess for other injuries — about half of burn patients have associated injuries — skeletal are most common.
- Control bleeding by direct pressure despite burn.
- Immobilize fractures despite burn.
- Remove restrictive clothing and jewelry.
- Remove clothing not adherent to burn.
- Estimate extent of burn.
- Cover burn with a clean, dry, sterile burn dressing or sheet.
- Treat for shock and maintain body heat.
- Elevate burned legs or feet and elevate burned hands higher than the patient's heart unless elevation increases pain.
- Check vital signs.
- Monitor need for airway care.
- Reassure victim.
- Call for emergency medical aid.

*(continued)*

## Emergency Burn Care — Continued

### SPECIAL CONSIDERATIONS

**Chemical:**

- Remove all clothing containing the chemical agent. The First Aider should not remove clothing first. The clothing should be removed while area is being flushed with water.
- Do not use neutralizing solutions; this may increase heat — dilution is always the best treatment in the field.
- Dilute with copious amounts of water.
- If the victim is stable and has no other serious injuries, irrigate with water (in shower or under hose) for fifteen to twenty minutes. For lye, irrigate for one hour.
- If you have time, protect yourself by using a pair of rubber gloves.
- If the chemical gets on the victim's face and/or in eyes, flush face and eyes with a cool, gentle flow of water for up to thirty minutes. Remove victim's contact lenses.
- For dry alkali burns like lime, always brush alkali from skin first before flushing with copious amounts of water. Adding water first can create a corrosive substance.
- Never flush a phosphorus burn with water or other solution. It can cause serious tissue damage and sloughing. Instead, soak the affected area in water.
- If possible, determine type of chemical and/or send container if small enough to hospital personnel.
- Call for emergency medical aid so victim can be transported to hospital.
- Reassure victim.

**Electrical:**

Electrical burns can be more serious than they appear, since they can penetrate the skin deeply; the burn may even enter in one place and leave the body in another so that there are two wounds.

The severity of electrical burns often is difficult to determine because the deeper layers of the skin, muscles, and internal organs may be involved. Also, the burns may be followed by paralysis of the respiratory center and an irregularity of the beat of the heart. Unconsciousness or instant death may occur.

General care for electrical burns is as follows:

- Remove the victim from contact with the electrical source without coming into contact with the current yourself. The best approach is to unplug or disconnect the current or, where safe, use a dry insulation. See information on downed power lines.
- Conduct a primary survey, as cardiac and respiratory arrest can occur in cases of electrical burns.
- Check for points of entry and exit of current.
- Cover the burned surface with a clean dressing.
- Cool minor burns with cool, running water or cool compresses.
- Splint all fractures. (Violent muscle contractions caused by the electricity may result in fractures and/or head and neck injuries.)
- Immobilize with cervical collar and spineboard as soon as possible. Severe contractions may have injured the spinal cord.
- Treatment of entry and exit wounds should be as for other thermal burns.
- Treat for shock and maintain body heat.
- If necessary assist ventilations and administer CPR.
- Call for emergency medical aid as soon as possible.
- Continually monitor respiration and pulse.

## Work Exercises

Complete the following figures by the Rule of Nine estimation, to determine the percentage of the body that is burned.

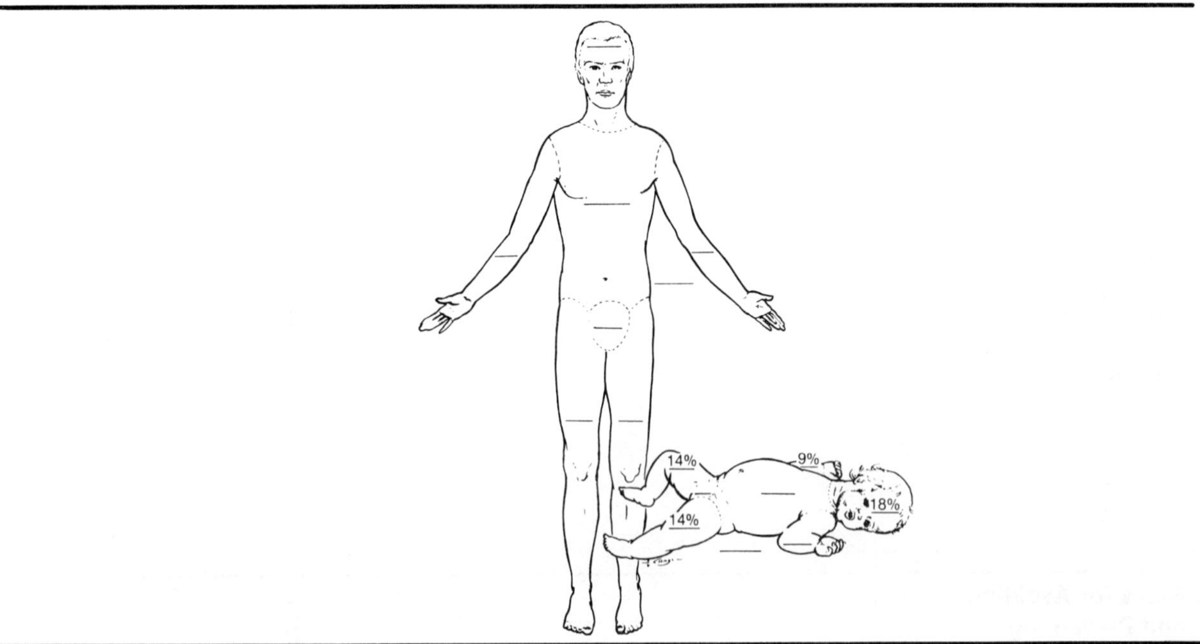


Complete the following table by listing emergency care for chemical burns.

### Chemical Burns

| | |
|---|---|
| **General Emergency Care** | |
| **Emergency Care for Eye Burns** | |
| **Exceptions to the above General Care** | |

Complete the following table by listing emergency care for thermal burns and electrical burns.

## Thermal Burns

| | |
|---|---|
| **General Emergency Care** | |

## Electrical Burns

| | |
|---|---|
| **Emergency Care** | |
| **Rules for Avoiding and Preventing Electrical Burns To Yourself** | |

## SELF-TEST

### Part I: True and False

If you believe the statement is true, circle the T. If you believe the statement is false, circle F.

T F 1. A burn is an injury that results from contact with heat, chemical agents, or electricity.

T F 2. Cold applications should be used on extensive moderate burns.

T F 3. Electrical burns are often more serious than they appear.

T F 4. Major electrical burns should NOT be immersed in cool running water.

T F 5. Second-degree burns are usually very painful because nerve endings have been destroyed.

T F 6. The First Aider should not elevate the burned area.

T F 7. Avoid ointments on burns, especially if the burn is bad enough to require hospitalization.

T F 8. A victim can get a second-degree burn from exposure to the sun.

T F 9. Third-degree burns, characterized by charring of all skin layers, are the most painful kinds of burns.

T F 10. In treating second-degree burns, you should gently break any blisters and apply antiseptic ointment to prevent infection.

T F 11. The best treatment for chemical burns is to remove the victim's clothing from the area, wash the burned area with running water, and cover the area with a sterile dressing.

T F 12. The nerve endings would not be destroyed in a third-degree burn.

T F 13. A burn on the front of each arm and leg of an adult would result in approximately an 18 percent burn.

T F 14. Cold-water application is probably the best emergency care for most burns.

T F 15. Immediate cooling of a burn will help alleviate pain. It will also reduce the burning effect in the deeper tissues.

T F 16. Infection is usually not a complicating factor in burns.

T F 17. First-degree burns will heal more quickly if treated with some type of petroleum jelly or suntan lotion.

T F 18. Chemical burns should always be neutralized with other chemicals.

T F 19. The best care for chemical burns is flushing the affected area with copious amounts of water.

T F 20. CPR should be started in electrocution victims even if six minutes has elapsed.

T F 21. If blisters develop from a burn, it is best to puncture them as you would a friction blister.

T F 22. The higher the amperage, the greater the damage in an electrical burn.

T F 23. The amount of moisture on the victim can affect the severity of electric shock.

T F 24. The amount of insulation (clothing, rubber shoes, and so on) worn by an electrical shock victim will help reduce the severity of electric shock.

T F 25. Dazed and confused behavior may be signs of electrical shock.

T F 26. Artificial ventilation and circulation are the most important first aid treatments for electrical shock.

## Part II: Multiple Choice

For each question, circle the answer that best reflects an accurate statement.

1. A burn that reddens the skin but does not cause blistering is a:
   a. 1st-degree burn
   b. 2nd-degree burn
   c. 3rd-degree burn
   d. electrical burn

2. What type of burn appears charred, white, or brown?
   a. 1st degree
   b. 2nd degree
   c. 3rd degree
   d. electrical

3. Third-degree burns involve which of the following?
   a. bone
   b. organs
   c. muscles
   d. all of the above

4. A victim who has suffered a third-degree burn will likely:
   a. be in severe pain
   b. be in severe pain but experiencing a numbing effect
   c. not experience pain
   d. feel nothing at all below the burn site

6. According to the "Rule of Nines," which of the following areas is estimated to comprise 9% of the body area?
   a. one leg
   b. back of trunk
   c. front of trunk
   d. one arm

7. What percentage of the body would a burn of the entire left leg and left arm be?
   a. 18%
   b. 22½%
   c. 27%
   d. 36%

8. In reference to the "Rule of Nines," the infant's head area represents what percent of total body area?
   a. 4½%
   b. 9%
   c. 15%
   d. 18%

9. A "partial-thickness" burn:
   a. only partially burns underlying muscle tissue
   b. burns all skin layers but not muscles, bones, or organs
   c. goes through only part of skin layers
   d. is the equivalent of a third degree burn

10. A victim with which of the following burns should be considered "critical?"
    a. 3rd-degree burns of the face
    b. 3rd-degree burns covering more than 10% of the body surface
    c. 2nd-degree burns covering more than 30% of the body surface
    d. all of the above

11. Hoarseness, increased respiratory rate, and carbon particles in the victim's sputum may indicate:
    a. bronchial asthma
    b. pneumonia
    c. electrical burns
    d. respiratory burns

12. Second-degree burns are characterized by:
    a. blisters
    b. redness and mottling
    c. considerable swelling
    d. all of the above

13. Particularly critical burn locations include all *except:*
    a. face
    b. hands
    c. genitalia
    d. chest

14. What treatment should be given if clothing or debris is sticking to a burn that is not severe:
    a. remove it carefully
    b. soak the involved area in cool salt water
    c. leave it alone
    d. scrub the involved area with a soft brush and water

15. What effect does cold water have on burns?
    a. speeds up blister formation
    b. reduces tissue destruction
    c. increases tissue swelling
    d. relaxes the victim

16. In a serious burn case, pain is best relieved by the exclusion of air from a burn through the application of a:
    a. burn spray
    b. thick, clean, dry dressing
    c. thick petroleum-based burn ointment
    d. soybean oil-base burn ointment

17. Which of the following causes the most damage in inhalation injury accompanying burns?
    a. heat
    b. noxious chemicals
    c. carbon monoxide gas
    d. smoke

18. Immersion of second-degree thermal burn areas in cold water can:
    a. reduce swelling
    b. relieve pain
    c. prevent infection
    d. a and b are correct

19. What should be done when treating most chemical burns?
    a. neutralize the area with alkali or acid solutions
    b. remove clothing while flushing the area with water
    c. locate an antidote before treating; water may intensify the reaction
    d. cover the area with a dry, sterile gauze

20. In cases of *extensive* third-degree burns, do the following:
    a. gently remove adhered clothing or other debris from the burn
    b. apply ice water compresses to the burn
    c. cover the entire burned area with a thick, sterile dressing
    d. all of the above

21. To treat a first-degree burn:
    a. cover the burned area with butter
    b. submerge the burned area in cold water
    c. apply salve to the burned area
    d. any of the above

22. What should a First Aider do if he/she comes across a downed power line lying across a wrecked vehicle?
    a. instruct conscious victims to attempt to jump from the vehicle
    b. tell conscious victims to stay inside the vehicle and wait for a power company crew
    c. tell victims to turn on the ignition and move the vehicle
    d. throw a blanket or jacket over the line, and instruct conscious victims to leave the vehicle

23. If an accident results in a downed power line, what is an indication the area is energized?
    a. hair will stand on end
    b. there is a tingling feeling at the back of the neck
    c. soles of the feet tingle when entering an area
    d. a popping sound can be heard in the area

24. Which of the following comes first in emergency care of an electrical burn victim?
    a. separate the victim carefully from the electrical source
    b. CPR
    c. opening an airway
    d. locating an entrance and exit wound

25. Possible effects of electric shock include:
    a. ringing in the ears
    b. visual disorders
    c. kidney failure
    d. all of the above

26. What serious condition frequently accompanies or follows electrical burns?
    a. cardiac arrest
    b. permanent scarring
    c. epilepsy
    d. chronic infection

27. Immediate care in the case of a lightning strike victim should consist of:
    a. determine the victim's reaction to pain
    b. treatment for shock
    c. getting the victim under cover
    d. restoring and maintaining breathing and heartbeat

Corresponds with:
**American Red Cross**
**Standard First Aid & Personal Safety**
Chapter 10, pages 160-165 and
Chapter 11, pages 166-169
and
**Advanced First Aid & Emergency Care**
Chapter 11, pages 147-150 and
Chapter 12, pages 151-154

# 16 Heat and Cold Emergencies

Heat and cold produce a number of injuries. Critical to your ability to care for those injuries is a basic understanding of the way in which the body maintains its temperature and how it physiologically adjusts to extremes in heat and cold.

## HOW THE BODY LOSES HEAT

The body loses heat through several different processes: radiation, **conduction** and convection, and the evaporation of moisture.

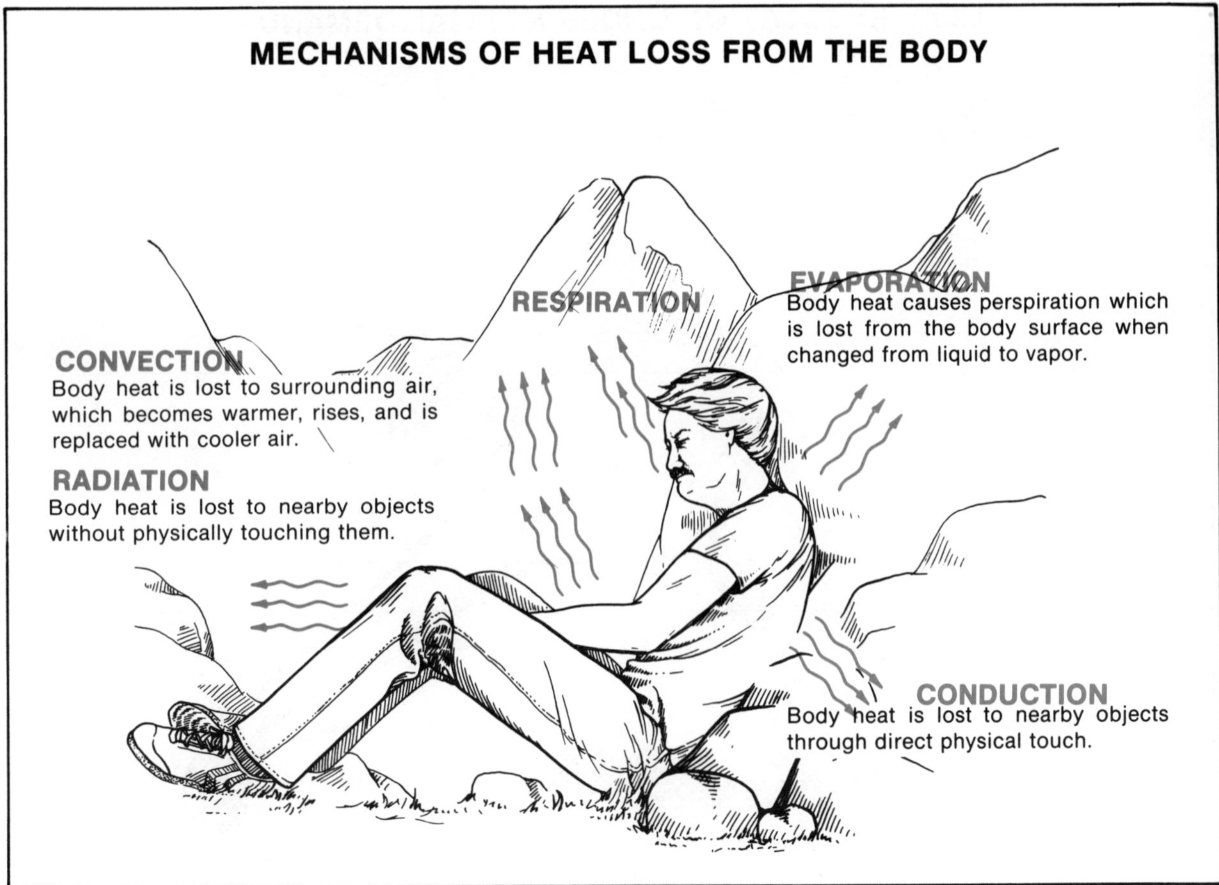


The illustration assumes that a wet, poorly dressed climber has taken shelter in a crevasse or among cold, wet rocks.

1. Radiation, the most important method of heat loss, involves the transfer of heat from one surface of one object to another without physical contact between the two. Heat loss from radiation varies considerably with environmental conditions. In a temperate climate and under normal conditions, a person loses about 60 percent of his heat production by radiation. Most heat is lost from the head. At temperatures of 90° F., though, radiation loss will probably drop to zero; in subzero temperatures, radiation loss of heat will skyrocket.

2. Conduction and convection, less important methods of heat loss in temperate climates, are major considerations in polar climates. By conduction, the cold air in immediate contact with the skin is warmed. The heated **molecules** move away, and cooler ones take their place. Those, in turn, are warmed, and the process starts all over again. Any process that speeds movement of the air — such as wind — also speeds the cooling process.

The phenomenon of conduction has been incorporated into the concept of **windchill**. A unit of windchill is defined as the amount of heat that would be lost in an hour from a square meter of exposed skin surface that has a normal temperature of 91.4° F. In essence, the windchill factor combines the effects of the speed of the wind and the temperature of the environment into a number that indicates the danger of exposure. When the windchill factor is 1200, the temperature is bitterly cold; at 1400, exposed flesh may freeze; at 2000, exposed flesh will freeze in less than one minute; and at 2300, exposed flesh will freeze in less than thirty seconds. For instance, flesh will freeze in less than one minute in only ten-mile-per-hour winds if the temperature is forty degrees below zero.

## HEAT REGULATION UNDER NORMAL DEMAND

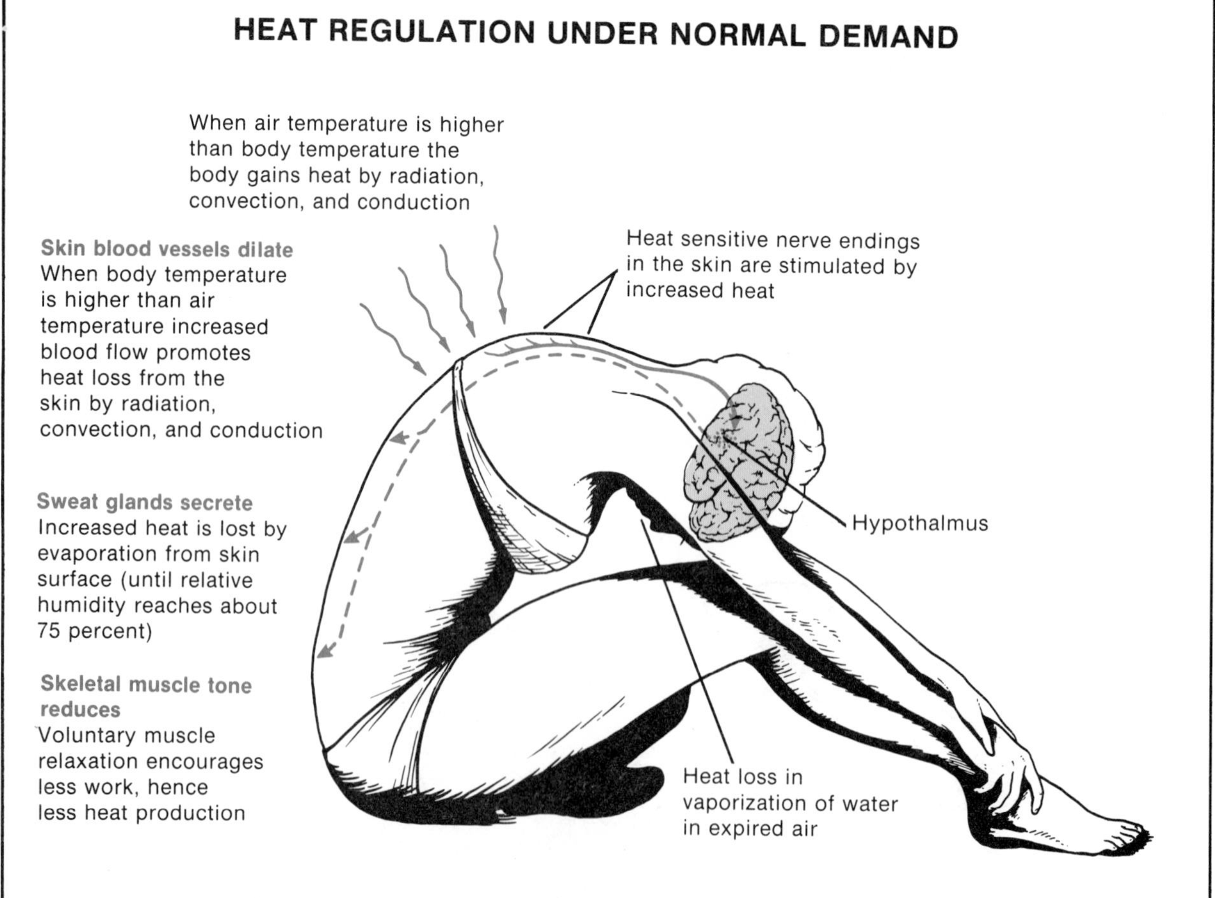


Adapted with permission of PATIENT CARE magazine. 

Conduction is also the method of heat loss in **waterchill**. Water conducts heat 240 times more intensely than air does. This means that wet clothing conducts heat away from the body at a rate 240 times greater than dry clothing. A person whose clothing is wet, then, is in exceptional danger of losing heat — the wet clothing pulls heat away from the body more rapidly than the body can produce the heat.

Heat loss by conduction also occurs from transfer of heat to air as it is warmed in the respiratory passages and lungs (a person inhales cold air and exhales warm air), from water and food taken into the digestive tract, and from waste materials (urine and feces) as they are eliminated.

3. Loss of heat by **vaporization** (evaporation) of perspiration is usually more massive in hot weather; it slows down when the air is humid. In polar climates, the only loss from perspiration is due to wearing improper clothing. When the temperature of the air equals or exceeds the temperature of the skin, body heat must be eliminated through vaporization.

## HYPERTHERMIA (HEAT-RELATED INJURY)

Heat-related injuries fall into three major categories: **heatstroke, heat exhaustion**, and **heat cramps**. Heat emergencies are most frequent on days when the temperature is 95° to 100° F., when the humidity is high, and when there is little or no breeze. Most highly susceptible to heat injuries are athletes, workers who labor outdoors or near to furnaces or ovens, people who are in poor physical condition, and the elderly. Most heat injuries occur early in the summer season, before people have acclimated themselves to the higher temperatures.

### Heatstroke

Heatstroke (sometimes called **sunstroke**, although the sun is not required for its onset) results when the heat-regulating body mechanisms break down and fail to cool the body sufficiently. The body becomes overheated, the body temperature rises to between 105° to 110° F., and no sweating occurs. Because no cooling takes place, the body stores more and more heat, the heat-producing mechanisms speed up, and eventually the brain cells are damaged, causing permanent disability or death.

Emergency care of heatstroke is aimed at immediate cooling of the body — and cooling should be your first priority after establishing an airway.

1. Establish an airway.
2. At minimum, remove the victim from direct sunlight, undress the victim, wet down his/her body thoroughly with cold water, and fan him/her as briskly as possible. Wrap the victim in cold, water-soaked sheets, and call for medical assistance or transport him/her as quickly as possible. Keep the victim wrapped in cold, wet sheets during transport, and instruct someone to fan him/her briskly during transport. Run the air conditioner, if available, to maximum capacity.
3. Ideal, immediate care is to immerse the victim's entire body in a cold water bath and to vigorously rub the skin with ice.
4. Where immersion is not feasible, ice massage is the best alternative. Put ice cubes or chunks in a plastic bag, wet down the victim's body, and rub him/her briskly all over with the ice bag in the air current from an electric fan or room air conditioner. Place cold packs under the victim's arms, around the neck, and around the ankles to cool the large surface blood vessels. Simple ice packs will not effectively lower temperature when used alone; you should employ a variety of methods. If necessary, use a cold shower or garden hose. Wrapping a wet sheet around the victim's body and then directing an electric fan at the victim is also a good means of cooling.
5. When the victim's body temperature has dropped to 102° F., take measures to prevent chilling. Keep working until you have lowered the core temperature to below 100° F. If the victim's temperature does not drop below 100°, the hyperthermia could recur.

6. Elevate the victim's head and shoulders slightly during cooling, and make sure that he/she is comfortable.
7. **Never give the victim stimulants or hot drinks.**
8. Because heatstroke involves the entire body, a number of complications may result from the ailment itself or from necessary care. Be prepared to care for the following complications as cooling proceeds:
   - **Convulsions.** Tremors and convulsions tend to accompany and retard cooling.
   - **Aspiration of vomit.** Vomiting commonly accompanies convulsions caused by cooling techniques. Position the victim for easy drainage.
9. If you succeed in lowering the core body temperature at least 2° C. (about 4° F.) over a thirty-to-sixty-minute period, discontinue active cooling measures; the body will usually continue to cool spontaneously.

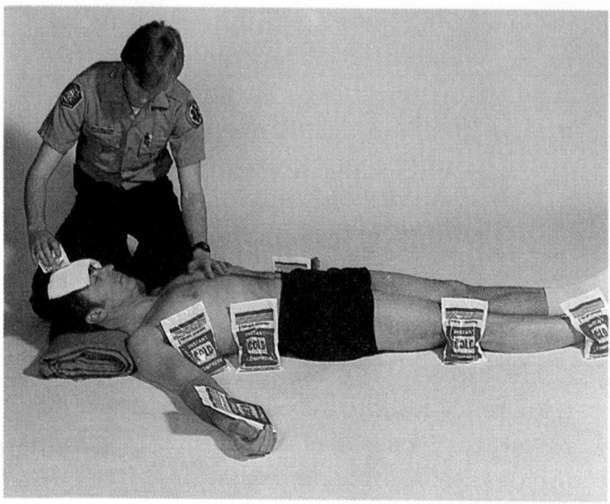

Use cold applications on the head and body to cool a heatstroke victim.

10. Watch the victim closely and maintain normal body temperature.
11. Always call for medical aid as soon as possible.

## SIGNS AND SYMPTOMS OF HEAT STROKE

The commonest victims of heat stroke include drug abusers, the elderly, the physically disabled, and persons with alcoholic intoxication, chronic illness, fever or malnourishment.

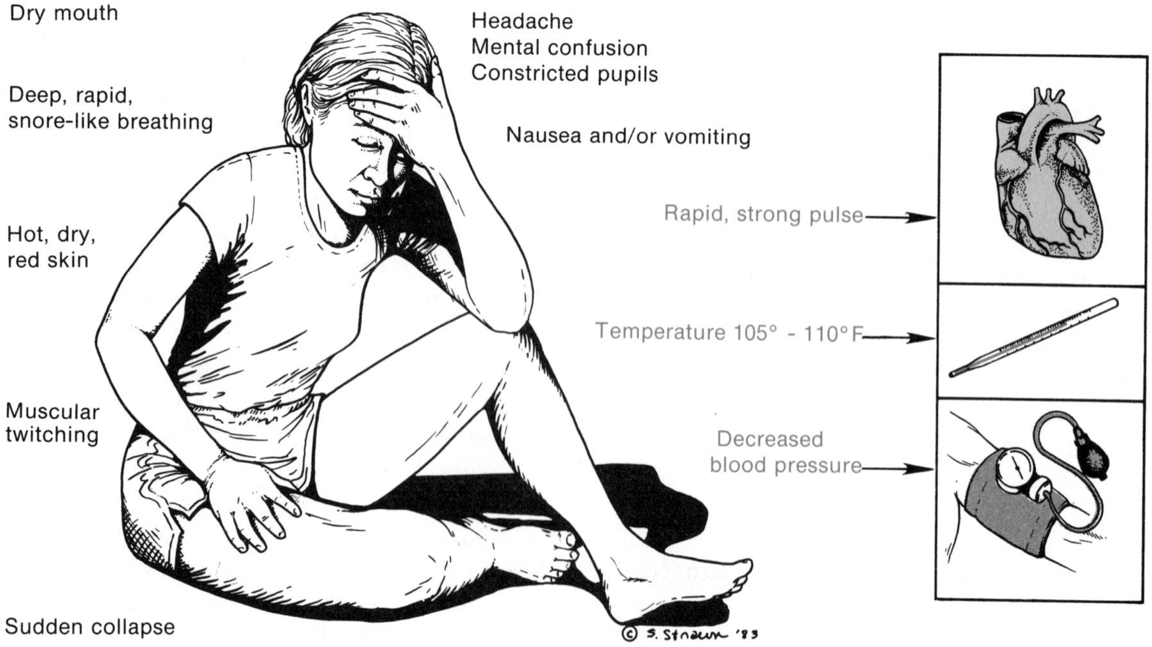

Dry mouth

Deep, rapid, snore-like breathing

Hot, dry, red skin

Muscular twitching

Sudden collapse

Headache
Mental confusion
Constricted pupils

Nausea and/or vomiting

Rapid, strong pulse

Temperature 105° - 110° F

Decreased blood pressure

© S. Strauss '83

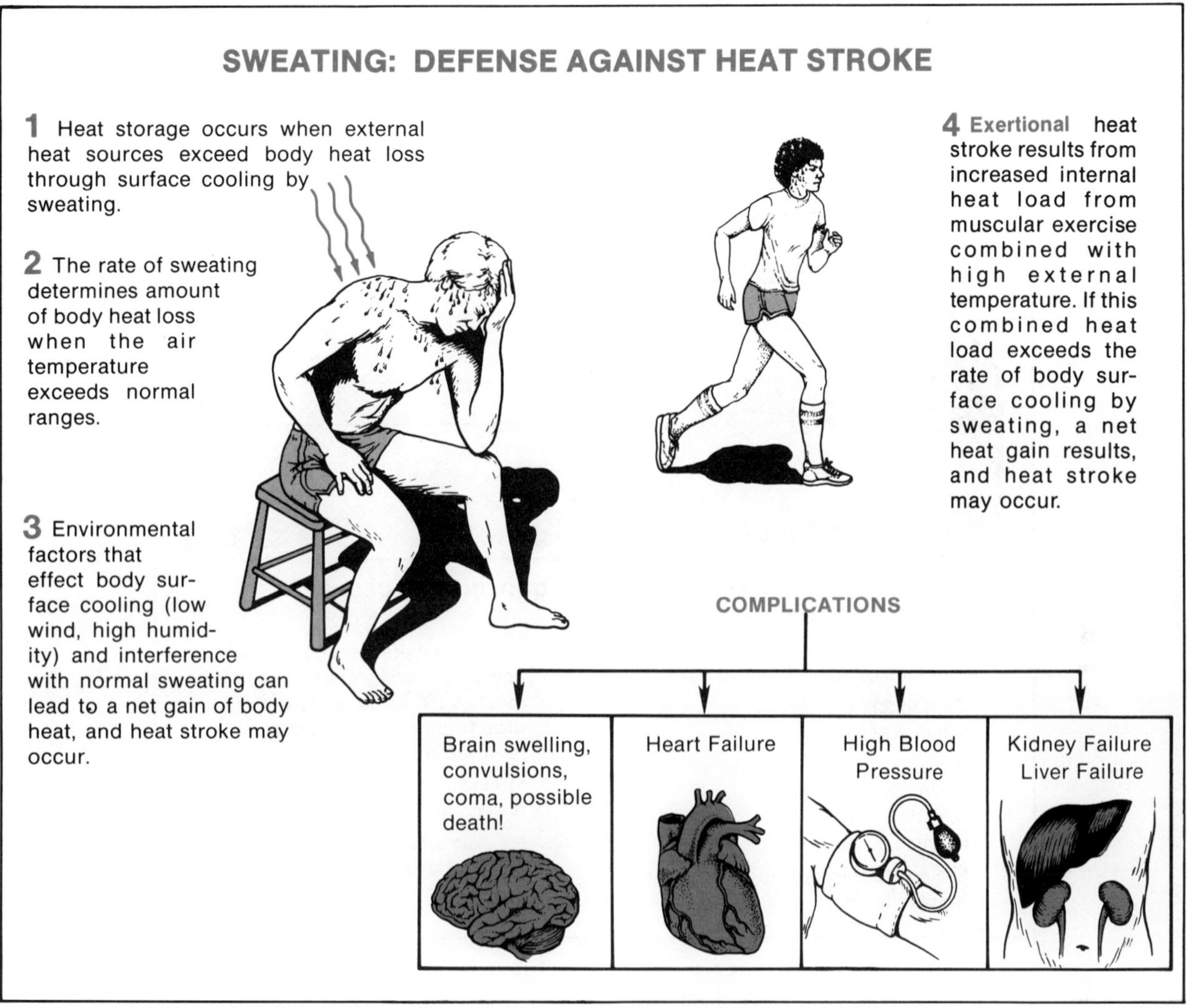


## Heat Exhaustion

Heat exhaustion occurs in an otherwise fit person who is involved in extreme physical exertion in a hot environment and is a result of a serious disturbance of the blood flow, similar to the circulatory disturbance of shock. Heat exhaustion is, in fact, a mild state of shock brought on by the pooling of blood in the vessels of the skin, causing blood to flow away from the major organs of the body. Due to prolonged and profuse sweating, the body loses large quantities of salt and water. When the water is not adequately replaced, blood circulation diminishes, and brain, heart, and lung functions are affected. Heat exhaustion is sometimes — though not always — accompanied by heat cramps due to salt loss.

While the signs and symptoms of heat exhaustion are similar to those of heatstroke — especially to the casual observer or to an uninformed victim — there are some distinct differences that will help you make the correct evaluation.

The two most reliable and distinct differences are the condition of the skin and the body temperature. In heatstroke, the skin is flushed, dry, and fiery hot to the touch. Victims experiencing heat exhaustion usually have wet or clammy, cool, and pale skin. Body temperature with heatstroke can soar to above 106° F.; it usually stays at normal or sometimes dips below normal in the heat exhaustion victim.

The most critical problem in heat exhaustion is salt loss. Heat exhaustion normally strikes at those who are usually sedentary or who are poorly acclimatized and who suddenly participate in strenuous exercise in a hot climate. The water and salt levels become unbalanced: either the salt depletion is greater than the

## HEAT STROKE: EMERGENCY CARE

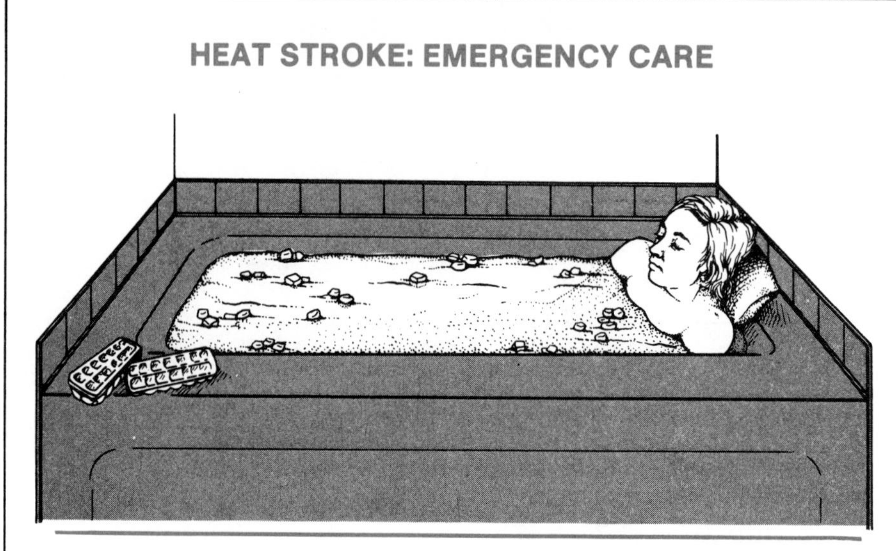

**MONITOR PULSE, RESPIRATION, and TEMPERATURE**

Begin cooling immediately with fans or applications of ice.

Cool to 39° C (102° F) within 30-60 minutes.

Immerse in tub of ice water if in circumstances where transportation to a hospital is not possible or is delayed.

Immediate transport to a hospital is crucial.

**COOLING PROCEDURES**

Check temperature continuously and stop cooling when temperature reaches 39° C. Temperature will drop further when victim is removed from ice bath.

Monitor respiration and pulse. If necessary, begin resuscitation.

Be alert and care for possible seizures.

water depletion, or the water depletion is greater than the salt depletion.

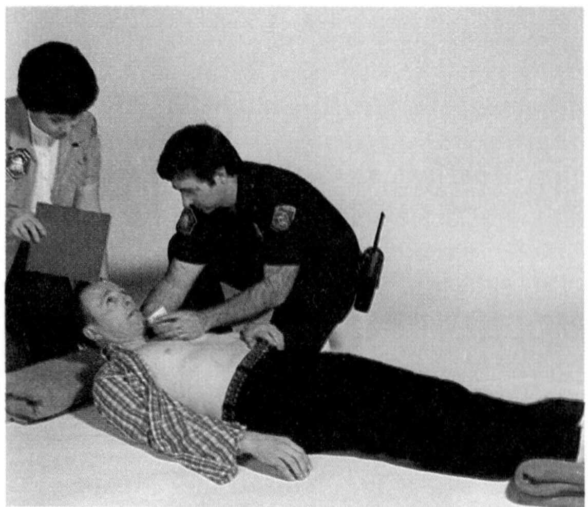

For heat exhaustion, loosen clothing, keep victim in a lying position, and keep him as comfortable and cool as possible.

To relieve a victim experiencing heat exhaustion:

1. Move the victim to a cool place, but make sure that he/she does not become chilled. Apply cold, wet compresses to the skin, and fan the victim lightly.
2. Have the victim lie down. Raise the feet eight to twelve inches, and lower the head to help increase blood circulation to the brain. Remove as much of the victim's clothing as possible, and loosen what you cannot remove. Help make the victim as comfortable as possible.
3. Administer saltwater (one teaspoon per quart) at the rate of one-half glassful every fifteen minutes for one hour.
4. If the victim vomits — which he/she may do because of the saltwater — stop giving fluids immediately. Transport to a hospital, or call for emergency medical assistance.

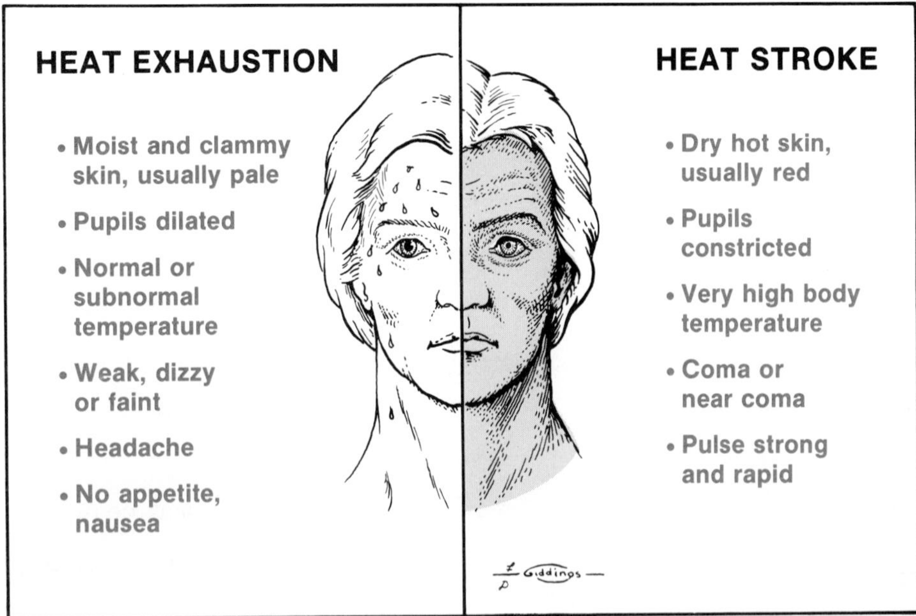


5. If no vomiting occurs and a victim declines to be transported, instruct family members or friends to keep the victim quiet and resting for two to three days and to protect him/her from hot temperatures.

## Heat Cramps

Heat cramps are muscular pains and spasms that occur when the body loses too much salt during profuse sweating or when inadequate salt is taken into the body. When the body becomes low on salt and water, the victim interprets it as thirst. To quench his thirst, the victim consumes large quantities of water without replacing the salt. Heat cramps usually occur in the arms, legs, or abdomen and are often a signal of approaching heat exhaustion.

Hot weather is not necessarily a requisite to heat cramps. A person who exercises strenuously in cold weather and who perspires and fails to replace salt may develop heat cramps.

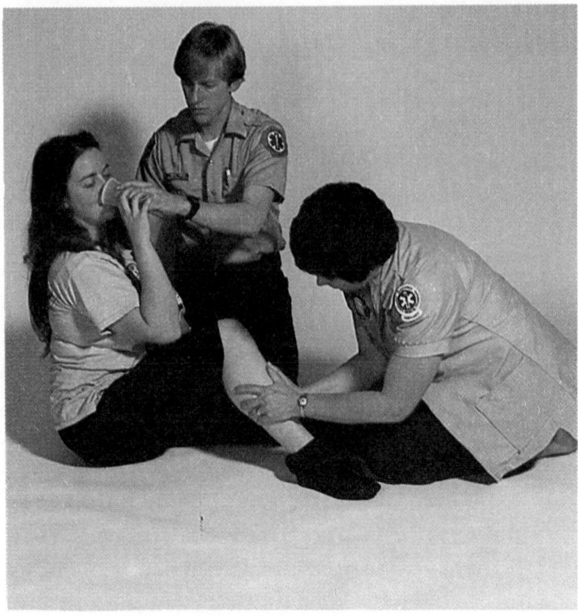

A victim with heat cramps can be given sips of cool saltwater.

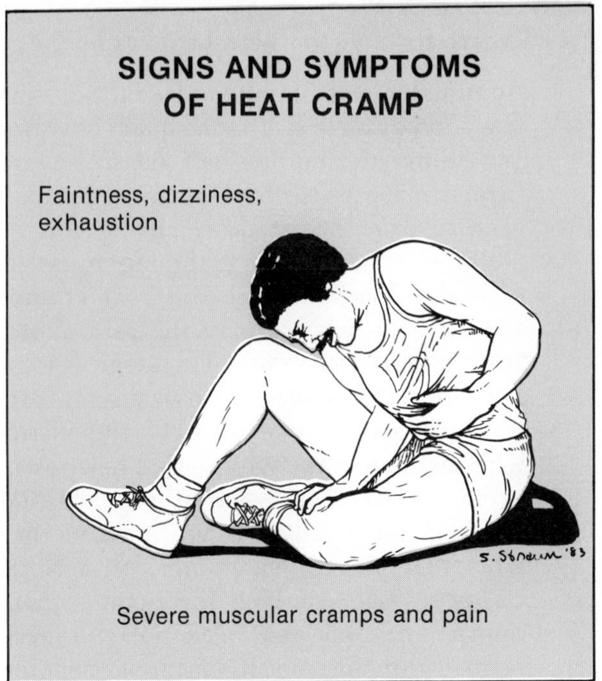

**Emergencies Due to Heat Exposure: Summary**

| Characteristics | Heat Cramps | Heat Exhaustion | Heat Stroke |
|---|---|---|---|
| Pathophysiology | salt and water loss | salt and water loss<br>peripheral blood pooling | failure of heat-regulating mechanism |
| Cramping | present | may be present | absent |
| Mental state | clear | may be disoriented | stupor or coma |
| Skin | cool, moist | cool, pale, moist | hot, flushed, dry |
| Temperature | normal | normal or low | markedly high |
| Pulse | rapid | rapid, weak | rapid, bounding |
| Blood Pressure | may be low | may be low | may be high early |
| Emergency Care | salt and water if tolerated | salt and water<br>cooling | RAPID COOLING |

In order to function properly, the muscles need a strict balance of water and salt. Whenever that balance is disrupted, regardless of the temperature, muscular contraction malfunctions, and heat cramps result.

The mental status and consciousness level of heat cramp victims remain normal. Victims will experience severe muscular cramps and pain — especially of the leg, calf and abdomen — and will suffer from faintness, dizziness, and exhaustion.

To care for a victim with heat cramps:

1. Administer sips of saltwater, diluting one teaspoon of table salt in one quart of water and administering one-half glassful every fifteen minutes (or a commercial product such as *Gator-Ade* or *Take Five*).
2. Do not massage the cramping muscles. Massage does not cure the heat cramps and may actually increase the pain. **Note: Some experts recommend massage as long as it does not increase pain or discomfort.**
3. It is important to explain to the victim what happened and why so that he/she can avoid a recurrence. Assure the victim that nothing is critically wrong. Some victims who suffer severe leg cramps fear a blood clot or muscle tear. Help the victim remain calm and relaxed, since relaxation will speed recovery of the muscle spasm. The victim should avoid exertion of any kind for twelve hours.

## HYPOTHERMIA (COLD-RELATED INJURY)

Major injuries related to extreme cold temperatures are **general hypothermia** and **frostbite. Snowblindness, trenchfoot,** and **immersion foot** are common cold temperature injuries that are not as serious.

### General Hypothermia

General hypothermia, the most life-threatening cold injury, affects the entire body system with general severe body cooling. Once the body temperature is lowered to 95° F., thermal control is lost, and the body is no longer in thermal balance. Coma occurs, when the core temperature reaches approximately 79° F.

General hypothermia is usually due to immersion in extremely cold water or to overall exposure without ensuing frostbite. Extremely low temperatures are not necessary to induce hypothermia — it can occur in temperatures as high as 65° F., depending on the windchill factor, and can occur at temperatures well above freezing. Most cases occur

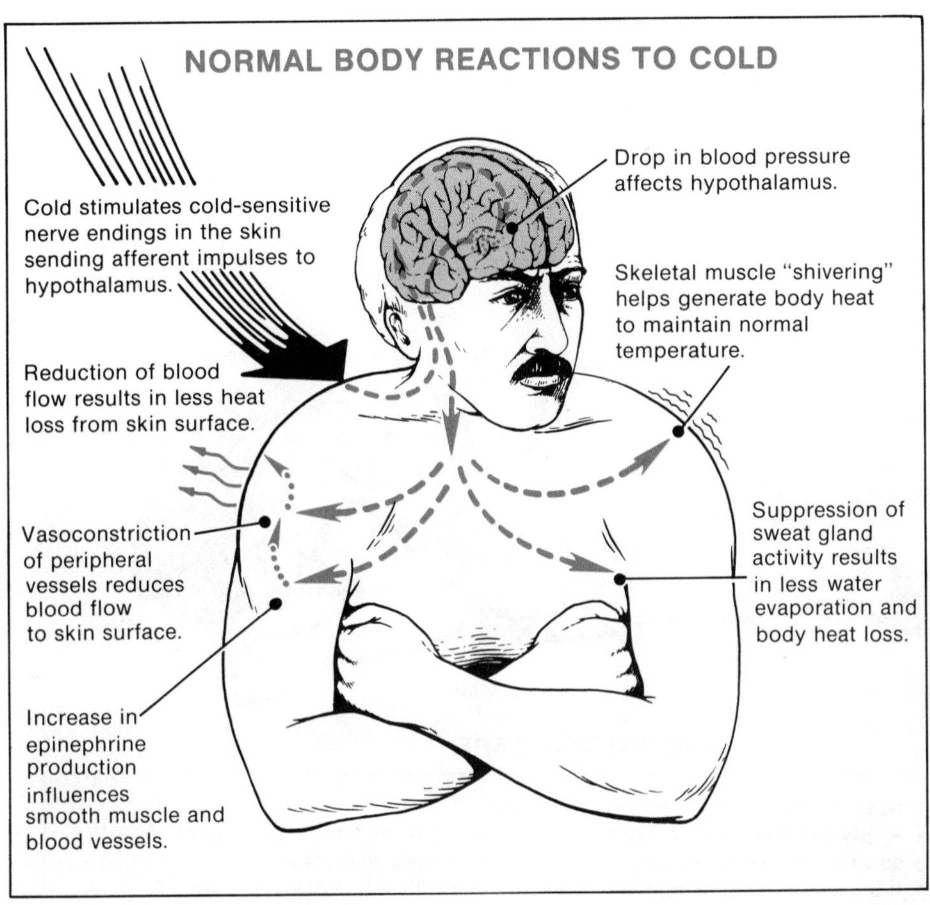


## WIND CHILL INDEX

| WIND SPEED MPH | WHAT THE THERMOMETER READS (degrees F.) | | | | | | | | | | | |
|---|---|---|---|---|---|---|---|---|---|---|---|---|
| | 50 | 40 | 30 | 20 | 10 | 0 | −10 | −20 | −30 | −40 | −50 | −60 |
| | WHAT IT EQUALS IN ITS EFFECT ON EXPOSED FLESH | | | | | | | | | | | |
| CALM | 50 | 40 | 30 | 20 | 10 | 0 | −10 | −20 | −30 | −40 | −50 | −60 |
| 5 | 48 | 37 | 27 | 16 | 6 | −5 | −15 | −26 | −36 | −47 | −57 | −68 |
| 10 | 40 | 28 | 16 | 4 | −9 | −21 | −33 | −46 | −58 | −70 | −83 | −95 |
| 15 | 36 | 22 | 9 | −5 | −18 | −36 | −45 | −58 | −72 | −85 | −99 | −112 |
| 20 | 32 | 18 | 4 | −10 | −25 | −39 | −53 | −67 | −82 | −96 | −110 | −121 |
| 25 | 30 | 16 | 0 | −15 | −29 | −44 | −59 | −74 | −88 | −104 | −118 | −133 |
| 30 | 28 | 13 | −2 | −18 | −33 | −48 | −63 | −79 | −94 | −109 | −125 | −140 |
| 35 | 27 | 11 | −4 | −20 | −35 | −49 | −67 | −82 | −98 | −113 | −129 | −145 |
| 40 | 26 | 10 | −6 | −21 | −37 | −53 | −69 | −85 | −100 | −116 | −132 | −148 |
| | Little danger if properly clothed | | | | Danger of freezing exposed flesh | | | Great danger of freezing exposed flesh | | | | |

Source: U.S. Army

**STAGES OF HYPOTHERMIA**
(General Body Cooling)

1. **Shivering** (an attempt by the body to generate heat) does not occur below a body temperature of 90°F
2. **Apathy** and decreased muscle function, first fine motor and then gross motor functions.
3. **Decreased level of consciousness** with a glassy stare and possible freezing of the extremities.
4. **Decreased vital signs** with slow pulse and slow respiration rate.
5. **Death**

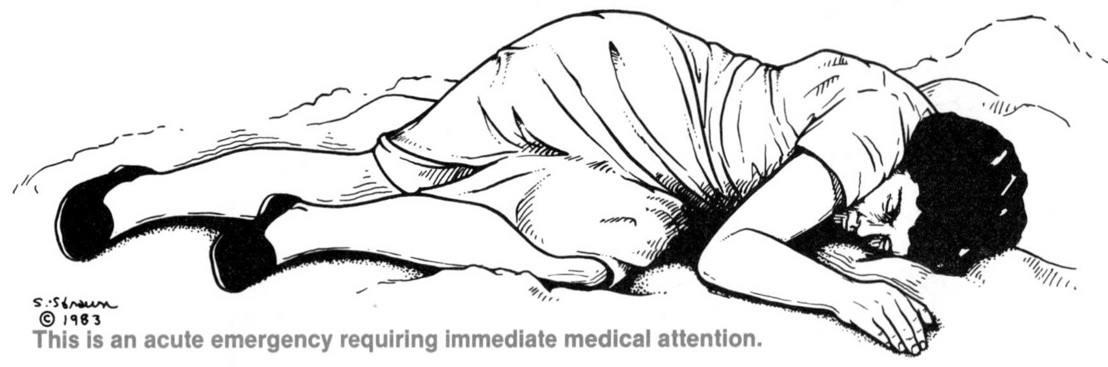


**This is an acute emergency requiring immediate medical attention.**

**EMERGENCY CARE**

- Keep the victim dry; replace wet clothing.
- Apply external heat to both sides of the victim using whatever heat sources are available including the body heat of rescuers.
- If the victim is conscious and in a warm place have him breathe warm, moist air if available.
- Monitor respirations and pulse and provide ventilations and cardiopulmonary resuscitation as required. No one is dead until warm and dead.
- Do not give hot liquids by mouth.
- Do not allow victim to exercise.
- Handle the victim gently.

| If more than 30 minutes from a medical facility: | If less than 30 minutes from medical facility: |
|---|---|
| 1. Prevent further heat loss. | 1. Prevent further heat loss. |
| 2. Handle with care. | 2. Handle with care. |
| 3. Add heated, moist air to breathe. | 3. Add heated, moist air to breathe. |
| 4. Rewarm victim. | 4. Transport or call for medical assistance. |
| 5. Prepare for CPR. | |
| 6. Transport or call for medical assistance. | |

There is disagreement among some experts regarding the temperature used for rewarming cold injuries. It is important that you follow local protocol.

when the temperature is about 60° F. or less. Wetness — either from water or from perspiration —always compounds the problem; exhaustion also affects any case of hypothermia.

As body cooling progresses, hypothermia makes itself manifest in five stages:

1. Shivering (an attempt by the body to generate heat).
2. Indifference, sleepiness, apathy, and listlessness.
3. Unconsciousness, usually accompanied by a slow respiratory rate and a slow pulse rate.
4. Freezing of the extremities.
5. Death.

## Emergency Care for Hypothermia

Hypothermia is an acute emergency: the basic principles of emergency care include preventing heat loss, rewarming the victim as quickly and safely as possible, and remaining alert for complications. Follow these general guidelines:

1. Care for very gently.
2. Remove wet clothing. Replace with dry clothing or dry coverings of some kind.
3. Add heat gradually and gently by applying warm objects to the groin, chest, neck, and head; use warm rocks wrapped in towels, chemical heatpacks (monitor carefully to prevent skin burns), hot water bottles, warmed blankets, or other bodies.
4. Have the victim breathe warm, moist air. Do not rub or manipulate the extremities.
5. Do not give coffee or alcohol.
6. Warm fluids can be used only after uncontrollable shivering stops and the victim has a clear level of consciousness and can swallow.
7. Keep the temperature even during emergency care procedures.
8. Transport the victim to a medical facility as soon as possible.

If the victim is cold and has any of the following signs or symptoms:

1. Body core temperature less than 86° F., oral temperature 90° F. or less.
2. Breathing, heart rate, and blood pressure low.
3. No shivering, even though the victim is extremely cold (remember that a person who is intoxicated may not shiver even with severe hypothermia).
4. Altered state of consciousness, including slurred speech, staggering gait, decreased mental skills.
5. Associated illness or injury that may have permitted the hypothermia to develop —

he/she is considered to have severe hypothermia, and the following guidelines should be followed:

1. Rewarming must be slow to avoid a shock to the system; more than 65 percent of all

## SIGNS AND SYMPTOMS OF HYPOTHERMIA

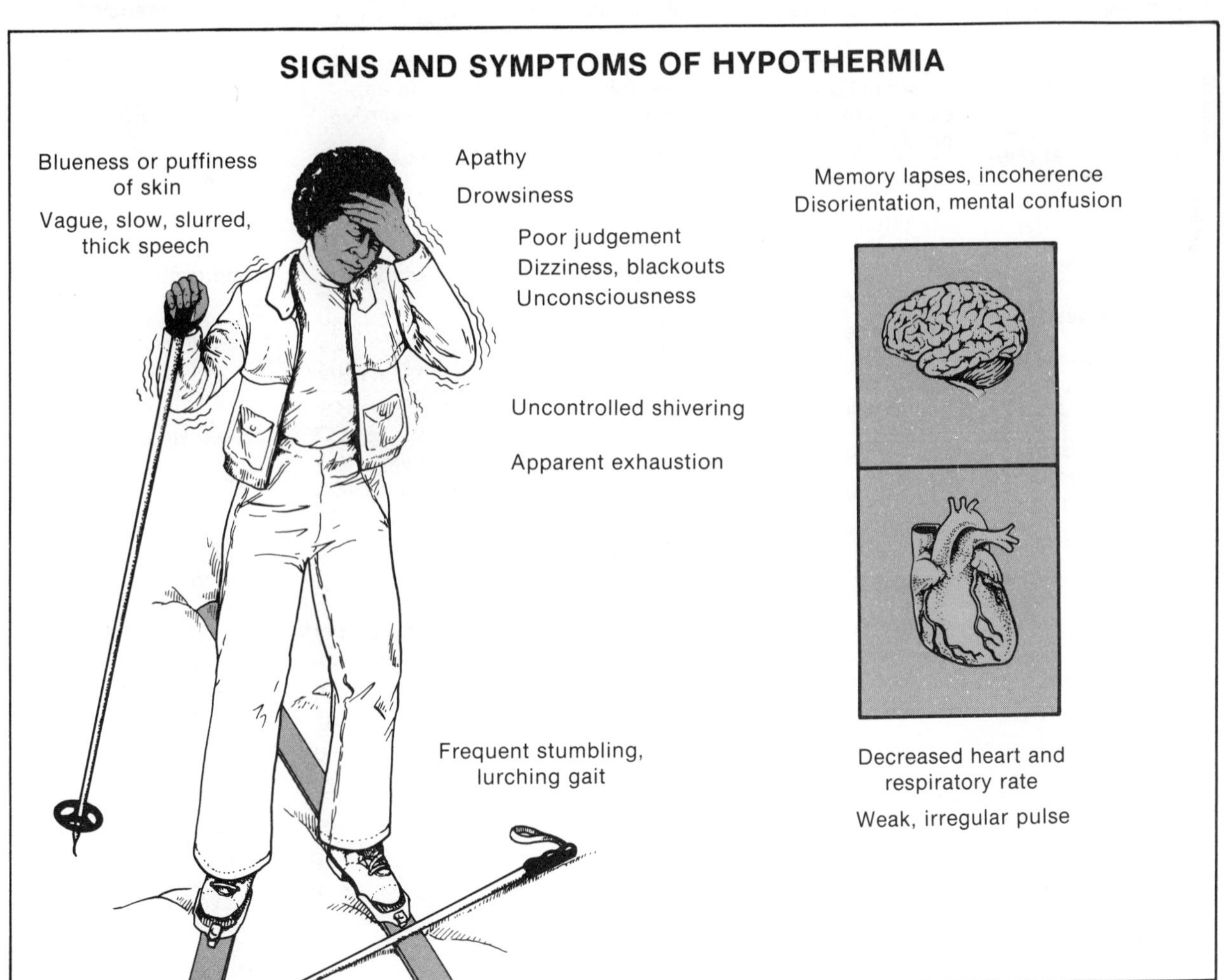

victims of severe hypothermia die during rewarming because of improper care. Be very gentle with the victim.

2. Follow the general emergency care guidelines described above.
3. Assess presence or absence of pulse and respiration over a two-minute period.
4. Initiate CPR if pulse or respiration are absent.
5 If you are less than fifteen to thirty minutes from a medical facility, do not take the time to add heat except what can be done during transport or while waiting for an ambulance.
6. Continually monitor vital signs.
7. Always have victim transported to a hospital.

In cases of hypothermia where the victim can be immediately transported to a hospital, do the following:

1. Establish an airway, but do not **hyperventilate**.
2. Call for emergency medical aid or move the victim immediately to a vehicle, and turn on the heaters full-blast to raise the temperature to optimal level. If possible, maintain optimal temperature while preparing for transport.
3. If the victim is unconscious, care for him/her as you would for any other unconscious victim.
4. Remove any wet clothing from the victim.
5. Cover the victim with blankets. If hot-packs are available, place them over the

**Accidental Hypothermia**

| Predisposing Factors | Signs Others See | Symptoms Patient Feels | Prevention | Emergency Care |
|---|---|---|---|---|
| Poor physical condition<br><br>Failure to eat and drink enough<br><br>Little body fat<br><br>Inadequate clothing (wool is best)<br><br>Lack of shelter from snow, rain, wind<br><br>Wetness (from perspiration or precipitation<br><br>Exhaustion | Coordination loss; slow, stumbling pace<br><br>Speech distortion<br><br>Forgetfulness<br><br>Lack of judgment; irrational ambition<br><br>Overactive imagination; possible hallucinations<br><br>Blue, puffy skin<br><br>Dilated pupils of eyes<br><br>Slow, shallow breathing<br><br>Confusion, stupor, possible unconsciousness | Violent shivering, with muscle tension<br><br>Fatigue<br><br>Feeling of extreme cold or numbness<br><br>Loss of coordination; stumbling, thick speech, disorientation<br><br>Rigidity of muscles after shivering stops<br><br>Blue, puffy skin<br><br>Pulse slow, irregular, or weak | Rest and eat before exertion<br><br>Nibble on high-energy food continuously while on trail<br><br>Wear windproof outer clothing, wool underneath<br><br>Carry emergency camping equipment<br><br>Make camp immediately if storm, injury, or loss of direction occurs<br><br>Keep moving; this keeps the body producing heat; if camped, use isometric exercises | MINIMIZE HEAT LOSS:<br><br>Protect victim from cold<br><br>Place insulating pad between victim and ground<br><br>Remove wet clothing; wrap in dry clothing and/or blankets<br><br>Keep victim dry<br><br>ADD HEAT:<br><br>Have victim get into sleeping bag with another person<br><br>Give warm liquids<br><br>Apply heat, using warmed stones wrapped in cloth, heat packs, or hot water in a canteen<br><br>Keep physical contact with others for body heat<br><br>Have victim breathe warm, moist air |

Adapted from: Brent Q. Hafen and Brenda Peterson, *First Aid for Health Emergencies*, West Publishing Co., 1980, p. 248.

chest and abdomen, not over the extremities.

6. If cardiac arrest should occur, initiate CPR. Resuscitation of these victims often takes a long time and must be carried out in conjunction with rewarming procedures. So get the victim to a hospital fast, performing CPR as needed.

In cases of hypothermia where the victim cannot be immediately transported, such as in disaster, rescue efforts, and camping excursions, the first priority is to protect the victim from further heat loss. Get the victim out of the cold and the rain, especially if the wind is blowing. If you have to construct a temporary shelter or build a fire, do so. You could use a sleeping bag as long as it is dry and you can insulate it from the ground. Remove all of the victim's clothing, and put him/her in a prewarmed sleeping bag or bed with another person who is also completely stripped. If you have a double sleeping bag or bed, place the victim between two warm bodies (skin-to-skin contact is the most effective care). Build a fire if you are not near facilities that are equipped with heaters.

**Never give alcohol to a hypothermia victim.** Even though alcohol produces a feeling of heat, it actually causes a loss in body temperature and will serve to further reduce core temperature.

## Hypothermia in the Elderly

The elderly probably account for nearly one-half of all victims of accidental hypothermia. Signs and symptoms of hypothermia in the elderly include:

1. Bloated face; skin color pale and waxy, at other times oddly pink.
2. Trembling on one side of the body or in one arm or leg, but no shivering.
3. Irregular and slowed heartbeat; slurred speech; shallow, very slow breathing that may be barely discernible.
4. Low blood pressure.
5. Drowsiness, perhaps lapsing into a coma. The lower the body temperature, the more likely the victim will be unconscious.

## Immersion Hypothermia

Immersion hypothermia — a lowering of body temperature that occurs as a result of immersions in cold water — should be considered in all cases of accidental immersion. When the water is 50° F. or lower, death can occur within a few minutes, so emergency care is vital and consists of getting the victim out of the water immediately.

Once the victim is out of the water, follow these guidelines:

1. Keep the victim still and quiet.
2. Remove the victim's wet clothing carefully and gently; do not let the victim struggle to help you, or otherwise use his/her muscles.
3. Handle the victim very gently; **never** rub or massage the victim.
4. Dress the victim in dry clothing; if none is available, any insulation material, including dry newspapers, will help. Then cover the insulation with a waterproof material such as plastic.
5. Protect the victim from the wind; if no shelter is immediately available, position rescuers' bodies around the victim to keep him/her sheltered from the wind.
6. Do not give hot liquids by mouth, and **never** give alcoholic beverages.
7. Use gentle rewarming techniques.
8. Have the victim transported immediately.

## Frostbite (Local Cooling)

Frostbite, the literal freezing of body tissue, often accompanies hypothermia. In those cases, care of hypothermia **always** takes precedence. The three general stages of frostbite are detailed in the illustration.

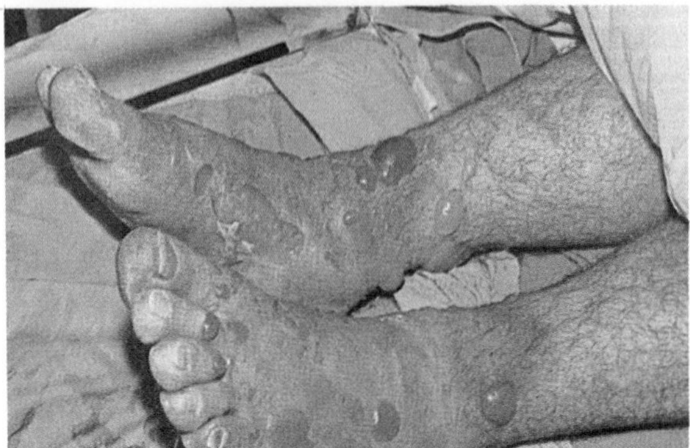

Frostbite.

## STAGES OF FROSTBITE

**1. INCIPIENT** (Frost Nip)
Affects tips of ears, nose, cheeks, fingers, toes, chin - skin blanched white, painless

FROSTBITE is local cooling of the body.
- 70% of the body is composed of water.
- When the body is subjected to excessive cold, the water in the cells will freeze; resulting ice crystals may even destroy the cell.
- Never rub any condition of frostbite; the ice crystal in the tissue can cut and destroy cells.

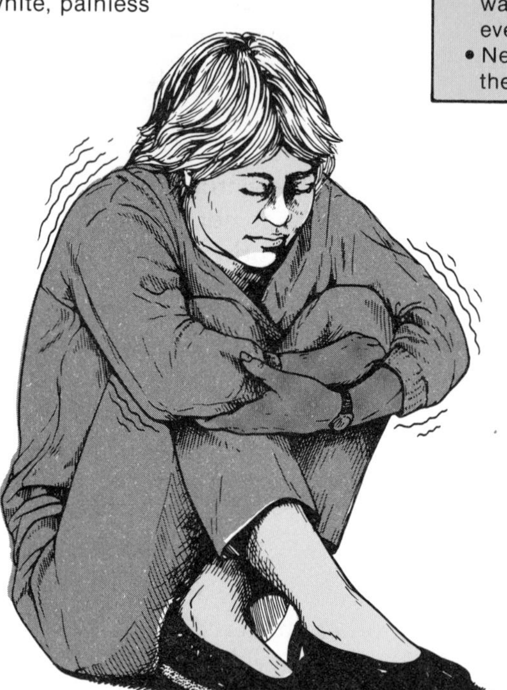

**2. SUPERFICIAL**
Affects skin and tissue just beneath skin; skin is firm and waxy, tissue beneath is soft, numb, then turns purple during thawing.

**3. DEEP**
Affects entire tissue depth; tissue beneath skin is solid, waxy white with purplish tinge.

**1. Emergency care for Incipient Frostbite:**
The skin can be warmed by applying firm pressure with a hand (no rubbing) or other warm body part, by blowing warm breath on the spot or by submerging in warm water.

**2. Emergency care for Superficial Frostbite:**
Treatment includes providing dry coverage and steady warmth. Submerging in warm water is also helpful.

**3. Emergency care for Deep Frostbite:**
This victim needs immediate hospital care. Dry clothing over the frostbite will help prevent further injury. Submerging in warm water can help thaw. Rewarm by immersion in water 105° F, and maintain body core temperature. The frostbitten part should not be rubbed or chaffed in any way. The part should not be thawed if the victim must walk on it to get to the medical facility. Do not delay transport to a medical facility for rewarming.

Emergency procedures for frostbite consist of the following:

1. If the tissue is still frozen, **keep the tissue frozen until you can initiate care**. Also, never initiate thawing procedures if there is any danger of refreezing — keeping the tissue frozen is less dangerous than submitting it to refreezing.
2. It is a mistake to thaw frostbitten tissue gradually. Thaw the tissue **rapidly** in water at 105° to 110° F. Check the water temperature with a thermometer and keep the water warm by adding warm water. Slower rewarming leads to tissue loss, and water hotter than 110° may add burn injury to the frostbite.

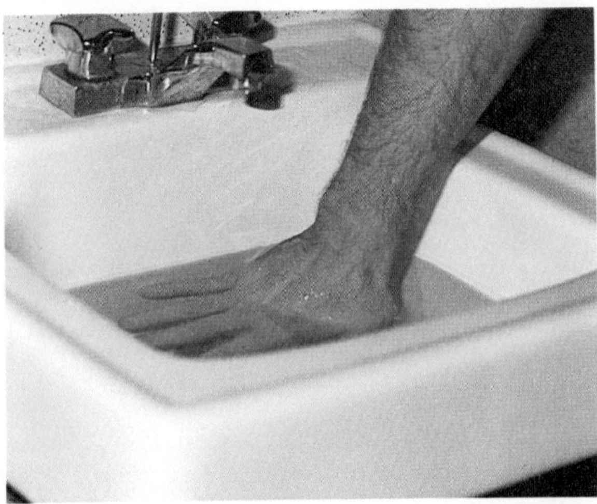

Rewarming frostbitten fingers in water maintained at 105-110° F.

3. If the frostbitten tissue is a nose or ear, pour the warm water over the affected area instead of attempting submersion.
4. Continue the rewarming process until the affected area turns deep red or bluish; the rewarming to this point may require as long as thirty minutes. Never attempt to rewarm the area by rubbing or massaging.
5. **All victims of frostbite should be seen by a physician.** Call for emergency medical aid as quickly as possible, preferably while conducting the rewarming process.
6. Bandage thawed areas gently with sterile dressings; place cotton between affected toes and fingers. Leave blisters unopened. Move victim with the extremity elevated.
7. Get medical assistance as quickly as possible; keep the victim warm, and take measures to prevent shock. Avoid refreezing.
8. **Do not delay seeking emergency medical aid.**

## Work Exercises

1. A constant body temperature is maintained when heat ______________ equals heat ______________.

2. What four processes allow the body to lose heat?

   1.

   2.

   3.

   4.

3. Fill in the following table with the proper signs and symptoms for skin, perspiration, and temperature.

**SIGNS AND SYMPTOMS OF HEAT-CAUSED EMERGENCIES**

| | Heat Cramps | Heat Exhaustion | Heat Stroke |
|---|---|---|---|
| Skin | | | |
| Respiration | Rapid and unusually shallow breathing | Normal | Initial deep, rapid breathing (snoring). Later shallow and almost absent breathing, dry mouth |
| Perspiration | | | |
| Pulse | Weak | Weak and rapid | Initial rapid and strong pulse later |
| Blood pressure | Normal | Elevated | Elevated, then decreased |
| Temperature | | | |
| Pupils | Normal (equal and reactive) | Dilated | Initial — constricted<br>Later — dilated |
| Consciousness and Mental State | Faintness<br>Dizziness<br>Exhaustion<br>Victim easily remains conscious | Headache<br>Weakness<br>Dizziness<br>Collapse<br>Briefly unconscious | Headache<br>Dizziness<br>Weakness<br>Convulsions<br>Sudden collapse<br>Possible unconsciousness |
| Other Signs and Symptoms | Possible convulsions | | |

4. List the major differences between heat exhaustion and heat stroke by filling in missing items.

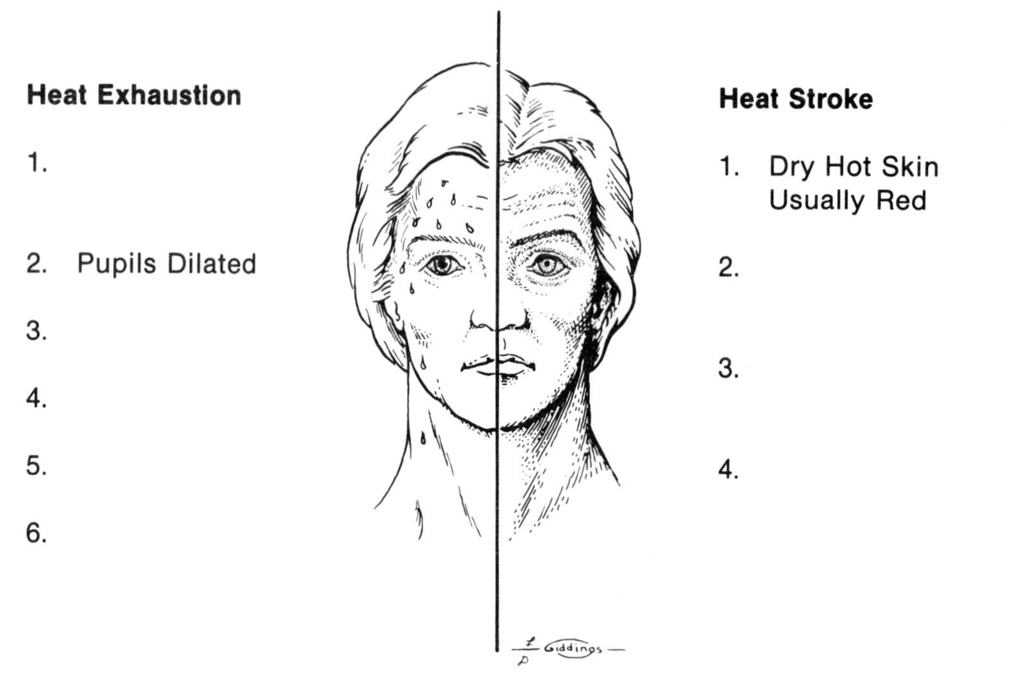


5. Complete the following table by listing the proper emergency care:

**EMERGENCIES DUE TO HEAT EXPOSURE — EMERGENCY CARE**

| Emergency Care | Heat Stroke | Heat Exhaustion | Heat Cramps |
|---|---|---|---|
| Cause | Failure of Heat Regulating Mechanism | Salt and Water Loss Peripheral Blood Pooling | Salt and Water Loss |
| Care | 1.<br>2.<br>3.<br>4.<br>5.<br>6. | 1.<br>2.<br>3.<br>4.<br>5.<br>6. | 1.<br>2.<br>3.<br>4.<br>5.<br>6. |

## Hypothermia

6. Hypothermia manifests itself in five stages or steps. Fill in the missing steps:

   1. Shivering
   2.
   3.
   4.
   5. Death

7. List five things you can do for a hypothermia victim.

   1.
   2.
   3.
   4.
   5.

## Frostbite

8. Frostbite, the literal freezing of body tissue, often accompanies hypothermia. Complete the following table by listing the proper emergency care.

**SEVERITY OF FROSTBITE**

| Stage of Frostbite | Signs, Symptoms and Complications | Emergency Care |
|---|---|---|
| Incipient | Injury to surface skin, somewhat like sunburn. The affected part will show redness, swelling, burning and tingling.<br>No blister formation.<br>No tissue loss usually | |
| Superficial | Similar in appearance to first degree frostbite with a grey-white color.<br>Blisters occur minutes to hours after cold injury.<br>Undue redness of skin on rewarming.<br>Edema or swelling. | |
| Deep | Damage to deep tissues; necrosis.<br>Much of the frozen part lost, possibly all of it.<br>Usually no blisters. | |

9. Match the following heat and cold emergencies with the appropriate signs/symptoms and emergency care.

**HEAT & COLD EMERGENCIES**

| Type of Emergency | Signs/Symptoms and Emergency Care |
|---|---|
| A. Heat Stroke | ________ 1. Pale and clammy skin |
| B. Heat Exhaustion | ________ 2. Firm, waxy white skin |
| C. Heat Cramps | ________ 3. Apply firm pressure with a hand or other warm body part |
| D. Frostbite | ________ 4. A dangerous medical emergency |
| E. Hypothermia | ________ 5. Hot, flushed, dry skin |
| | ________ 6. Painful abdomen |
| | ________ 7. Body temperature can reach 106° F |
| | ________ 8. Do not rub or chafe |
| | ________ 9. Give sips of cool salt water |
| | ________ 10. Keep victim dry and replace wet clothing |
| | ________ 11. Slow, slurred, thick speech |
| | ________ 12. Immerse in cold bath |
| | ________ 13. Sweating mechanisms fail |
| | ________ 14. General cooling of entire body |
| | ________ 15. May require CPR |

## SELF-TEST

### Part I: True and False

If you believe the statement is true, circle the T. If you believe the statement is false, circle F.

T F 1. Heat stroke represents a failure of the heat-regulating mechanisms of the body.

T F 2. Heat exhaustion is usually caused by an excessive loss of salt and water following strenuous exercise and profuse sweating.

T F 3. Heat cramps only occur in hot weather.

T F 4. A heat exhaustion victim's skin feels hot and dry.

T F 5. In heat stroke sweating has stopped and the temperature rarely exceeds 100° F.

T F 6. The pulse is rapid in heat stroke and heat exhaustion.

T F 7. Victims of heat exhaustion usually require hospitalization.

T F 8. As with heat cramps, the skin of a heat exhaustion victim is pale, cool, and moist.

T F 9. The key to the care of heat cramps is salt replacement, but salt tablets should usually not be used because they may increase nausea.

T F 10. A heat exhaustion victim may be disoriented or confused.

T F 11. Emergency care for heat stroke is usually limited to moving the victim to a cool place and administering a salt-water solution.

T F 12. The elderly, small children, and alcoholics are more susceptible to the effects of heat.

T F 13. In heat stroke, the body temperature may be 106° F. or higher.

T F 14. The skin is red and moist in heat stroke.

T F 15. You should elevate the feet of a victim of heat exhaustion.

T F 16. The extent of injury caused by exposure to abnormally low temperatures depends on such factors as wind velocity and humidity.

T F 17. Smoking and drinking alcoholic beverages may intensify the harmful effects of cold.

T F 18. The effects of frostbite are more severe if the injured area is thawed and then refrozen.

T F 19. First aid for frostbite should include rapid rewarming of the affected part.

T F 20. The frostbitten part should be vigorously massaged to aid circulation.

T F 21. If a person with frozen feet must walk to get medical aid, he should first attempt to thaw his feet.

T F 22. After a frostbitten part has been warmed, the First Aider should encourage the victim to move the part gently to aid in the restoration of circulation.

T F 23. A person suffering from hypothermia may have poor coordination and thickness of speech.

T F 24. The two most important objectives in administering first aid for hypothermia are to reduce heat loss and to add heat.

T F 25. To promote circulation, you should rub snow on the frozen part.

T F 26. The victim of frostbite should exercise thawed body parts as soon as they are rewarmed.

T F 27. Even though wind and humidity increase the sensation of cold, they have no effect on the speed at which the body freezes.

## Part II: Multiple Choice

For each question, circle the answer that best reflects an accurate statement.

1. Which of the following is *not* a means for the body to lose heat?
   a. evaporation
   b. osmosis
   c. convection
   d. radiation

2. The phenomenon of conduction has been incorporated into the concept of ______________________.
   a. windchill
   b. evaporation
   c. perspiration
   d. hyperthermia

3. Heat emergencies are most frequent under *all but one* of the following conditions:
   a. there is little or no breeze
   b. the temperature is 95-100 degrees Fahrenheit
   c. the humidity is high
   d. the temperature is 80-95 degrees Fahrenheit

4. What heat exposure injury results from a breakdown of the body's ability to sweat?
   a. heat exhaustion
   b. heat stroke
   c. heat cramps
   d. sun poisoning

5. What is the most important characteristic of heat stroke?
   a. profuse perspiration
   b. dizziness
   c. very hot and dry skin
   d. painful muscle cramps or spasms

6. Which of the following is the most important emergency care procedure for victims of heat stroke:
   a. treat for shock
   b. replace lost body fluids
   c. cool body any way possible
   d. give victim salt and sugar water

7. What is the ideal way to cool the body of a heat stroke victim?
   a. hyperthermia blankets
   b. immersion in an ice water bath
   c. water soaked sheets
   d. ice massage

8. The body's core temperature must drop below ______________ and stay that low before the danger period has passed for a heat stroke victim.
   a. 96 degrees Fahrenheit
   b. 98 degrees Fahrenheit
   c. 100 degrees Fahrenheit
   d. 102 degrees Fahrenheit

9. What is *not* a sign and symptom of heat exhaustion?
   a. profuse perspiration
   b. dilated pupils
   c. deep, rapid, snore-like breathing
   d. normal or subnormal temperature

10. The victim suffering from heat exhaustion can be identified by which of the following:
    a. hot, dry, flushed skin
    b. cool, moist skin, shallow breathing
    c. cool, dry skin, dizziness, headache
    d. hot, moist skin, labored respirations, slow pulse

11. Who is most susceptible to heat exhaustion?
    a. someone who rarely perspires
    b. persons accustomed to hot weather
    c. individuals who are underweight
    d. a person on diuretics

12. What may cause heat cramps?
    a. drinking liquids in too large quantities or too quickly
    b. working in a hot environment and not perspiring
    c. excessive amount of salt intake
    d. all of the above

13. The proper care for heat cramps is:
    a. massage the cramping muscles even if it causes pain
    b. administer sips of salt water or Gator-Aid
    c. exercise the muscle until cramping ceases
    d. all of the above

14. Which of the heat-related emergencies listed below is the most serious?

a. heat exhaustion
b. heat stroke
c. heat cramps
d. all are equally serious

15. Hypothermia is:

a. warm body core temperature but very cold skin temperature
b. severe body core cooling with an inability to rewarm itself
c. a temporary cooling of the body as it conserves heat
d. cold body core temperature but very warm skin temperature

16. The first stage of hypothermia is:

a. shivering
b. sleepiness, apathy
c. indifference
d. exhaustion

17. Victims of accidental hypothermia are extremely prone to:

a. respiratory arrest
b. ventricular fibrillation
c. infections
d. irreversible shock

18. In cases where the hypothermia victim cannot be transported immediately, the first priority is to:

a. administer CPR
b. monitor vital signs
c. prevent further heat loss
d. rewarm the patient as quickly as possible

19. A good way of rewarming a hypothermia victim in the field is to:

a. give alcohol because it will give the victim a feeling of heat due to increase in body temperature
b. rub or massage the victim's skin
c. give hot liquids
d. remove a victim's clothes and put him/her in a prewarmed sleeping bag with another person who is completely stripped

20. Which of the following is *not* a procedure for care of an immersion hypothermia victim?

a. do not give hot liquids by mouth
b. encourage the victim to walk around to increase circulation
c. remove the victim's wet clothing
d. protect the victim from the wind

21. Incipient frostbite:

a. involves the skin and the tissue just beneath the skin
b. is a second-degree frostbite
c. is a third-degree frostbite
d. is sometimes called frostnip

22. Superficial frostbite is characterized by:

a. the involvement of only the tips of the ears, the nose, the cheeks, the tips of toes and fingers, and the chin.
b. the skin is solid to the touch
c. a firm, white, waxy appearance
d. the condition is painless

23. For which of the following reasons should a frostbitten part be left frozen?

a. diagnosis has not been confirmed
b. pain becomes severe as thawing takes place
c. there is a possibility of refreezing
d. acclimatization needs to be increased

24. A frostbitten part should be rewarmed:

a. by rubbing it with snow
b. with water between 105 and 110 degrees Fahrenheit
c. with heat from a fire or stove
d. with water between 75 and 85 degrees Fahrenheit

25. If the frozen skin has been thawed and refrozen, treat it by:

a. submerging it in cool water to thaw it slowly
b. warming it at room temperature
c. submerging it in hot water
d. wrapping it thoroughly in sterile dressings

26. During camping excursions, which of the following is the most readily available method for treating a victim of hypothermia?

    a. engine exhausts
    b. rewarming tubs
    c. "buddy warming"
    d. artificial heat

27. When frostbite initially begins, the skin is:

    a. slightly reddened
    b. white and blistered
    c. gray and glossy
    d. yellow and blistered

Corresponds with:
**American Red Cross**
**Advanced First Aid & Emergency Care**
Chapter 15, pages 245-246

# 17 Psychological Emergencies and Disasters

## PRINCIPLES OF PSYCHOLOGICAL EMERGENCY CARE

Physical emergency care is tangible — it is bandaging wounds, splinting bones, or restoring breathing. Psychological emergency care does not benefit from tangible properties. You cannot readily see the comfort that you provide to a husband who loses his wife in an apartment building fire. It is hard to immediately gauge the results of caring for a child who is depressed because a flood destroyed her home.

Stating the principles behind psychological emergency care — tangible principles that should guide First Aiders — can help make emotional emergency care more understandable.

1. Every person has limitations. In an emergency situation involving psychological crises, remember that every person there — including yourself — is susceptible to emotional injury.
2. Each person has a right to his/her own feelings. Each person reacts individually to the environment. Each person has a *right* to feel that way. A person who is emotionally or mentally disturbed does not want to feel that way, but at that particular time, those feelings are valid and real. Those suffering an emotional crisis simply need help to pull themselves together. Psychological care means that you are accepting and helpful, not critical or judgmental.
3. Each person has more psychological resilience than it seems. For every manifestation of crazed emotion, some strength is probably left within.
4. Everyone feels some emotional disturbance when involved in a disaster or when injured. A relatively minor hand injury may seem of little consequence to you, but it could ruin the career of a concert violinist.
5. Emotional injury is just as real as physical injury. Unfortunately, physical injury is visual, so people more readily accept it as being real. You would not expect a man to walk one month after having his leg amputated in an industrial accident, yet too many times, the victim suffering emotional trauma is expected to act normal immediately.

## EMOTIONAL RESPONSES OF VICTIMS

Although victims' reactions to critical illness or injury are largely determined by mechanisms that they already have developed, most of these reactions will follow common patterns. Victims usually become aware of painful or unpleasant sensations, and sometimes of decreased energy and strength, when they become ill. The common response to this awareness is anxiety.

Feelings of loss of control are common among ill or injured persons. They may feel helpless in knowing that they are completely dependent on someone else, often a stranger,

## SIGNS AND SYMPTOMS OF PSYCHOLOGICAL EMERGENCIES

**FEAR**
May be afraid of a person or persons, activity or place.

**ANXIETY**
Not related to any specific person, place or situation.

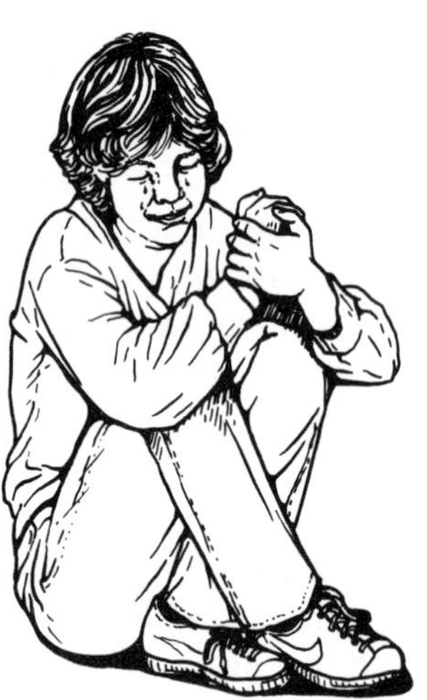

**CONFUSION**
May be preoccupied with fears or imaginary attacks.

**BEHAVIORAL DEVIANCE**
Radical changes in lifestyle, values, relationships, etc.

**ANGER**
Inappropriate anger directed at an inappropriate source usually brief but destructive.

**MANIA**
Unrealistically optimistic — unwarranted risks and poor judgement.

**DEPRESSION**
May range from crying to inability to function to threatened suicide. Often has feelings of hopelessness, helplessness, unworthiness, and guilt.

**WITHDRAWAL**
Loses interest in people or things that were previously considered important.

**LOSS OF CONTACT WITH REALITY**
Has trouble distinguishing or identifying smells, sounds, and sights in the real world from those in an imaginary world.

One or more of the above symptoms may indicate a psychological emergency. These may also be accompanied by physical signs and symptoms such as sleeplessness, loss of appetite, loss of sex drive, constipation, crying, tension, irritability.

whose experience in medical care and whose ability they cannot evaluate easily. Victims whose self-esteem depends on their being active, independent, and aggressive are particularly prone to anxiety.

Victims often respond to discomfort or limitation of activity by becoming resentful and suspicious. They may vent this anger on the First Aider by becoming impatient, irritable, or excessively demanding. Remember that the victim's anger stems from fear and discomfort, not from anything you have done. The First Aider must be aware that once victims begin to see themselves as ill or injured, the signs and symptoms depicted in the accompanying illustration may occur.

In addition, victims usually will have uncomfortable feelings about being helped by a stranger. Some victims may consider the physical assessment a humiliating invasion of privacy. Therefore, try to establish a relationship with the victim during an initial interview, and then conduct the physical assessment. Conduct the assessment in an efficient, businesslike manner, and continue talking with the victim during the entire procedure.

### Functions of Psychological Emergency Care and Crisis Intervention

Psychological emergency care should be planned and developed with four goals in mind.

- To help the injured person begin functioning normally again as soon as possible.
- Even when the victim cannot be returned to normal quickly, to minimize as much as possible his psychological disability.
- To decrease the intensity of his emotional reaction until professional medical help is available.
- To keep the victim from hurting himself or others.

## VICTIM ASSESSMENT IN PSYCHOLOGICAL EMERGENCIES

The assessment should begin as soon as the First Aider begins talking with the victim. The victim's general appearance and clothing should be noted, and it should be observed whether the victim appears neat or disheveled. The victim's rate of speech also should be noted. If it is slowed, it may suggest depression or some kind of intoxication. If it is rapid and pressured, it may suggest mania or the presence of amphetamines. The following questions should be kept in mind when assessing these victims:

1. Is the victim easily distracted?
2. Are the victim's responses appropriate?
3. Is the victim alert and able to communicate coherently?
4. Is the victim's memory intact?
5. What is the victim's mood?
6. Does the victim seem abnormally depressed, elated, or agitated?
7. Does the victim appear fearful or worried?
8. Does the victim show evidence of disordered thought, such as disturbances in judgment, delusions (false ideas), or hallucinations (seeing or hearing things that are not there)?

Initial questions should be direct and specific to establish whether the victim is alert, oriented, and able to communicate. Only information that is crucial to immediate management should be collected.

In general, seriously disturbed victims should be seen by a physician who can decide whether they need to be hospitalized.

## MANAGEMENT OF CRISES AND PSYCHOLOGICAL EMERGENCIES

There are a number of general guidelines for dealing with the emotionally disturbed:

1. Be prepared to spend time with the victim. You must be able to talk to the person and learn what is bothering him/her.
2. Be as calm and direct as possible. Most emotionally disturbed individuals are terrified of losing self-control. You will elicit the best cooperation possible if you show the victim through your actions that you have confidence in his/her ability to maintain control.
3. Identify yourself clearly. Tell the victim exactly who you are and what you are trying to do.
4. Do not rush the victim to the hospital unless some medical emergency dictates the need for life-saving care. Instead, take your time.
5. Talk to the victim alone. Often, a victim hesitates to talk in front of relatives or friends because he/she is ashamed and does not want to lose their respect. Sometimes *they* may be the source of the problem — a fact that the victim cannot divulge in their presence.
6. Sit with the victim while you talk to him/her. Never tower above the victim. Most victims with psychological disorders have problems relating to others, especially authority figures, and may have become suspicious.
7. Be interested in the victim's story, and empathize, but do not be oversympathetic. Treat the victim as if you expect him/her to improve and recover.
8. Never be judgmental. The victim is convinced that his/her feelings are accurate. They are real to the victim, no matter how ridiculous they may appear to you.
9. Be honest. Reassure the victim sincerely; give supportive information that is truthful. Do not make promises that you cannot keep.

## Communicating in Psychological Emergencies

The main consideration in giving psychological emergency care is to develop confidence and rapport with the victim by:

- Identifying yourself.
- Expressing your desire to help.
- Using understandable language.
- Maintaining eye contact.
- Listening intently and being empathetic.
- Acting interested and concerned.
- Giving calm and warm reassurance.
- Not invading victim "space" until it is comfortable.
- Never using any physical force unless the victim is a threat to himself or others.
- Never lying to or misleading the victim.
- Not engendering false hope.
- Not judging, criticizing, arguing, or being overly sympathetic.
- Explaining the situation to the victim and your plan of action, letting him know that you are in control.
- Avoiding stock phrases like "everything will be o.k."

### VICTIMS WITH SPECIAL COMMUNICATION NEEDS

#### Geriatric

- Do not assume senility or lack of understanding.
- Use victim's name.
- Check for hearing deficiency.
- Allow extra time for response.
- Ask victim what makes him most comfortable.

#### Pediatric

- May be frightened.
- May be modest.
- Move slowly.
- Explain procedures.
- Use simple terms.
- Allow child to keep toy, blanket, etc.
- Be honest about pain caused by procedure.
- Dolls may be useful to demonstrate procedure.
- Parents and siblings may be useful to help calm and explain

#### Deaf

- Determine if victim can read lips.
- Position self properly.
- Use interpreter if necessary and possible.
- Use common signs:
  - sick
  - hurt
  - help
  - etc.
- Use written messages.

#### Blind

- Determine if victim has hearing impairment.
- Do not shout.
- Explain incident and procedures in detail.
- Lead victim if ambulatory, alerting to obstacles.

#### Non-English Speaking

- Use interpreter if available.
- Use gestures.
- Refer to illustrated charts.

#### Confused and/or Developmentally Disabled

- Determine level of understanding.
- Speak at appropriate level.
- Wait for delayed response.
- Speak as you would to any adult.
- Evaluate understanding and re-explain if necessary.
- Listen correctly.

10. Make a definite plan of action, a technique that helps to reduce the victim's anxiety.
11. Do not require the victim to make decisions.
12. Encourage the victim to participate in some motor activity, a technique that further reduces anxiety. Let the victim do as many things as possible.
13. Stay with the victim at all times.
14. Never assume that it is impossible to communicate with a victim until you have tried.
15. When you talk to the victim, ask questions that are direct and specific. This will enable you to measure his/her level of consciousness and contact with reality. Do not confuse the victim by asking complicated questions.
16. If a victim is extremely fearful or violent, skip the physical assessment unless you have serious suspicions of a physical problem that will require immediate attention.
17. Do not be afraid of silences. They may seem intolerably long, but maintain an attentive and relaxed attitude.
18. As you talk to the victim, encourage him/her to communicate. Let the victim know that you are interested in what he/she has to say and that you would like to learn more.
19. As you talk to the victim, point out something in his/her behavior or conversation that will help you direct the conversation in ways helpful to you. Do this only if the victim seems to be wandering; never interrupt while he/she is trying to express a thought.
20. Make your questions nondirective. Avoid asking questions that can be answered with a "yes" or "no."
21. Do not foster unrealistic expectations. For instance, do not listen to the story and then say, "You have nothing whatsoever to worry about." Instead, find out what the victim's strengths are, and reinforce them.
22. Respect the victim's personal space. Some patients will be able to tolerate you if you sit close and touch them; others prefer to maintain a distance and do not like to be touched.
23. Do not abuse or threaten.
24. Do not let the victim get you angry. Remain kind and calm. You may be upset by what the victim says to you, but do not react in any way.
25. Avoid any kind of excitement.
26. If the victim is severely disturbed and has become violent, call the police. Never attempt physical restraint; wait for professional help.
27. If the environment or the scene of the accident is especially hectic, remove the victim from the scene before you try to question or calm him/her. The victim will probably remain disturbed as long as the environment is chaotic.
28. Communicate confidence in yourself. Move with assurance.
29. If the victim disagrees with you, do not argue. Instead, point out that there are many different ways to view a situation; admit that you might be wrong.
30. Always call for professional help in a serious psychological emergency.

## VICTIMS WHO ARE CHILDREN

A child may be unable to talk about problems directly. You might be able to work around to the problem through techniques such as storytelling, game-playing, or picture-drawing, which help to establish rapport. If the child refuses to talk, watch as he/she interacts with others, and try to ascertain the extent of the problem.

1. Make sure that the child has food (if appropriate). The child will feel friendlier toward you.
2. Make the assessment short — a child's concentration span is short.
3. Even though you want to protect the child or shield him/her from unpleasant facts, do not lie. If you have to tell him something unpleasant, do it gently and gradually.
4. Since you are dealing with a child, you will probably need to help him/her articulate feelings. You may need to suggest some probable feelings before he/she will be able to tell you exactly how he/she does feel.
5. Do not think that the capacity for violence is absent. Children can be especially prone to suicide and homicide; many mistakenly

## SUICIDAL EMERGENCIES

| MISCONCEPTION | FACT |
|---|---|
| People who talk about suicide don't commit suicide | Eight out of ten people who commit suicide have given definite warnings of their intentions. Almost no one commits suicide without first letting others know how he feels. |
| You can't stop a person who is suicidal. He's fully intent on dying. | Most people who are suicidal can't decide whether to live or die. Neither wish is necessarily stronger. |
| Once a person is suicidal, he's suicidal forever. | People who want to kill themselves are only suicidal for a limited time. If they're saved from feelings of self-destruction, they often can go on to lead normal lives. |
| Improvement after severe depression means that the suicidal risk is over. | Most persons commit suicide within about 3 months after the beginning of "improvement," when they have the energy to carry out suicidal intentions. They also can show signs of apparent improvement because their ambivalence is gone — they've made the decision to kill themselves. |
| If a person has attempted suicide, he won't do it again. | More than 50% of those who commit suicide have previously attempted to do so. |

### ASSESSING LETHALITY

**Age and sex:** incidence of suicide is highest in adolescents (ages 15 to 24) and in persons age 50 and over. Men succeed at suicide more often than women.

**Plan: Remember these points:**
Does the victim have a plan? Is it well thought out?
Is it easy to carry out (and be successful)?
Are the means available? (For example, does the victim have pills collected, or a gun?
A detailed plan with availability of means carries maximum lethality potential.

**Symptoms:** What is the victim thinking and feeling?
Is he in control of his behavior? (Being out of control carries higher risk.)
Alcoholics and psychotics are at higher risk.
Depressed people are most at risk at the onset and at decline of depression.

**Relationships with significant others:** Does the victim have any positive supports? Family, friends, therapist? Has he suffered any recent losses? Is he still in contact with people? Is he telling his family he's made his will? Is he giving away prized possession?

**Medical history:** People with chronic illnesses are more likely to commit suicide than those with terminal illnesses. Incidence of suicide rises whenever a victim's body image is severely threatened — for example, after surgery or childbirth.

The goal is to shift the intensity of a suicidal act from a desire to commit suicide to conflict over the need to commit suicide. The following guidelines can help:

- Specifically talk to the victim about his intent.
- Ask the victim how serious he/she is about killing himself.
- Ask what his concerns are about taking his life. He will probably have some conflict.
- Ask why he thinks suicide is the answer to his problems.
- Ask what other alternatives the victim has considered and what problems block the choice of the other alternatives.
- Ask what hope the victim has — even if it seems remote or blocked.
- By this time you may have helped decrease the intensity of the victim's need to commit suicide, even though it may be temporary.
- Always get professional help.
- A suicidal victim should be transported to the hospital for evaluation even though he says everything is okay. Police assistance may be necessary.

Source: **Assessment,** Nurses Reference Library, Intermed Communications, Inc. Springhouse, PA, 1982, p. 116.

## Disruptive and Aggressive Victims
## Assessing the Situation

Any behavior that presents a danger to the victim or others or that delays or prevents appropriate care is disruptive and may precipitate a psychological emergency. Common causes of disruptive behavior include stress-induced hysteria; aggression; alcohol or drug problems; neurological trauma; metabolic imbalances; organic brain syndromes; psychological disorders.

**Assessing the Situation**

- What information do you have from the situation — what happened?
- Is the environment (emotional, social, and/or physical) dangerous to you and/or others?
- Does the victim seem agitated, elated, depressed, or restless?
- Has he already demonstrated aggressive or violent behavior?
- Does he talk loudly and in a sarcastic way?
- Does he use vulgar language?
- Is he easily provoked to anger?
- Does he have a limited attention span?
- Does one victim seem to be out of control or disoriented?
- Does he seem to be afraid or panicky?
- Does he have a weapon?
- Is there evidence of alcohol or drug use?
- Is a domestic disturbance involved?
- Has criminal activity occurred?

If you answer **yes** to several or most of the above questions, use extreme caution. If possible, try not to control or suppress the victim's behavior. Rather, allow him to express his feelings. Remember — the most effective way to deal with a victim who exhibits aggressive and/or violent behavior is to reduce the crisis and prevent further disruptive behavior. **Probably the safest thing to do in these situations is to call the police.**

brush off a child's destructive tendencies with the glib, "He'll grow out of it." Take any such tendencies or threats seriously.

## PHYSICAL DISORDERS THAT RESEMBLE PSYCHOLOGICAL DISTURBANCES

Occasionally, you will encounter a victim who displays the signs and symptoms of a psychological disturbance but who is in fact suffering from a physical illness. It is critical that you assess each victim (an exception, of course, would be the extremely paranoid or violent victim who obviously does not have a life-threatening problem), because ignoring a life-threatening problem or serious illness could cause the victim to die while you are trying to care for a nonexistent psychological disorder.

Just because you smell alcohol on a victim's breath, do not automatically assume that he/she is drunk. Persons in diabetic coma may appear to be drunk, and you may, indeed, smell alcohol on their breath. A victim who appears to be drunk could have hit his/her head on something.

It is critical that you take care in determining a victim's physical well-being before you begin the long and sometimes tedious procedure of handling the psychological emergency.

Another way in which psychological trauma is related to physical condition is the fact that psychological trauma often follows (or is a result of) physical injuries.

Diabetes, seizure, severe infections, metabolic disorders, head injuries, hypertension, stroke, alcohol, and certain drugs all may cause disturbed behavior.

## MASS CASUALTIES AND DISASTERS

When the situation involves multiple casualties, such as an automobile accident with several victims or a natural disaster (tornado, flood, earthquake), people may become dazed, disorganized, or overwhelmed. The American

## Disruptive and Aggressive Victims Management Guidelines

### Remember — your first task is to protect yourself and others.

| Don'ts | Do's |
|---|---|
| • Don't put yourself in a position of danger. | • If danger exists, create a safe zone and wait for assistance (police and/or emergency units). |
| • Don't attempt to diagnose, judge label, or criticize the victim. | • Keep bystanders outside of safe zone. |
| • Don't isolate yourself from other helpers. | • Remove any person or object from the environment that seems to be triggering the victim's aggression. |
| • Don't isolate yourself with a victim who has a record of potential violence. | • Convey a sense of helpfulness rather than hostility or frustration. |
| • Don't disturb a victim with treatments or taking vital signs any more than is necessary. | • Establish voice control by asking bystanders what the problem is loud enough so that the victim can hear you. |
| • Don't turn your back on the victim. | • Identify yourself. |
| • Don't position yourself between the victim and the only doorway. | • Let the victim know what you expect. |
| • Don't forget that disturbed victims' moods can fluctuate rapidly. | • Present a comfortable, confident, and professional manner. |
| • Don't reject any of the victim's complaints — acknowledge them. | • Ask the victim his name and what the problem is. |
| • Don't threaten, lie, bluff, or deceive the victim. | • Listen to, but do not take personal or respond to insults and abusive language. |
| • Don't take insults personally. | • Be honest. |
| • Don't rush into action. | • Speak in short sentences with simple ideas and explanations. |
| • Don't show hostility toward the victim's words or actions. | • Remain relaxed and confident. |
| • Don't appear aggressive or defensive. | • Adjust your physical distance from the victim to a safe range — at first no closer than approximately ten to fifteen feet — move closer only after adequate assessment and it appears that it's safe to do so. |
| • Don't be overly friendly. | • Respect the victim's difficulty in self-control. Tell him that you are aware of the problem of dealing with it, and acknowledge the victim's attempt to deal with it. |
| • Don't sound authoritarian or demanding when you speak to the victim. | • Acknowledge the victim's complaints — you do not have to agree, but acknowledge that he has a reason to be upset. |
| • Don't attempt to restrain a victim unless you have adequate assistance to do so safely. It is best to call the police. | • Use gestures and other nonverbal messages carefully. They may communicate the opposite of what you intend. A disturbed victim may interpret friendliness and smiling as an attempt to trick him. |
| | • If your preventive actions fail to reduce hostile, violent, and combative behavior, the victim is in control and it may be necessary to restrain the victim to protect him and others. |
| | • Assess the victim's strengths. |
| | • Make certain that you have a plan and sufficient help to prevent injury to the victim and yourself. |

**Note:** If you help at the scene of a criminal act, your first concern is to care for the injured victim(s).

- Always cooperate with law enforcement personnel.
- Disrupt or touch as little evidence as possible.
- If the victim is moved, mark the original body position.
- Provide reassurance and emotional support. Common victim responses include outrage, disbelief, withdrawal, hysteria, and depression.

## Emotional Reactions In Mass Casualties and Disasters

| Reaction | Signs and Symptoms | Do's | Don'ts |
|---|---|---|---|
| **Normal** | Fear and anxiety<br>Muscular tension followed by trembling and weakness<br>Confusion<br>Profuse perspiration<br>Nausea, vomiting<br>Mild diarrhea<br>Frequent urination<br>Shortness of breath<br>Pounding heart<br>These reactions usually dissipate with activity as the person organizes himself | Normal reactions usually require little emergency care<br>Calm reassurance may be all that is necessary to help a person pull himself together<br>Watch to see that the individual is gaining composure, not losing it<br>Provide meaningful activity<br>Talk with the Person | Don't show extreme sympathy |
| **Panic (blind flight of hysteria)** | Unreasoning attempt to<br>Loss of judgment — blindness to reality<br>Uncontrolled weeping or hysteria often to the point of exhaustion<br>Aimless running about with little regard for safety<br>Panic is contagious when not controlled. Normally calm persons may become panicked by others during moments when they are temporarily disorganized | Begin with firmness<br>Give something warm to eat or drink<br>Firmly, but gently, isolate him from the group. Get help if necessary<br>Show empathy and encourage him to talk<br>Monitor your own feelings<br>Keep calm and know your limitations | Don't brutally restrain him<br>Don't strike him<br>Don't douse him with water<br>Don't give sedatives |
| **Overactive** | Explodes into flurry of senseless activity<br>Argumentative<br>Overconfident of abilities<br>Talks rapidly — will not listen<br>Tells silly jokes<br>Makes endless suggestions<br>Demanding of others<br>Does more harm than good by interfering with organized leadership<br>Like panic, overactivity is contagious if not controlled | Let him talk and ventilate his feelings<br>Assign and supervise a job that requires physical activity<br>Give something warm to eat or drink | Don't tell him he is acting abnormally<br>Don't give sedatives<br>Don't argue with him<br>Don't tell him he shouldn't act or feel the way he does |
| **Underactive (daze, shock, depression)** | Cannot recover from original shock and numbness<br>Stands or sits without talking or moving<br>Vacant expression<br>Emotionless<br>"Don't care" attitude<br>Helpless, unaware of surroundings<br>Moves aimlessly, slowly<br>Little or no response to questioning<br>Pulls within self to protect from further stress<br>Puzzled, confused<br>Cannot take responsibility without supervision | Gently establish contact and rapport<br>Get him to ventilate his feelings and let you know what happened<br>Show empathy<br>Be aware of feelings of resentment in yourself and others<br>Give him warm food or drink<br>Give and supervise a simple, routine job | Don't tell him to "snap out of it"<br>Don't give extreme pity<br>Don't give sedatives<br>Don't show resentment |
| **Severe physical reaction (conversion hysteria)** | Severe nausea<br>Conversion hysteria — the victim converts his anxiety into a strong belief that a part of his body is not functioning (paralysis, loss of sight, etc.). The disability is just as real as if he had been physically injured | Show interest<br>Find a small job for him to take his mind off the injury<br>Make him comfortable and summon medical aid<br>Monitor your own feelings | Don't say, "There's nothing wrong with you" or, "It's all in your head"<br>Don't blame or ridicule<br>Don't call undue attention to the injury<br>Don't openly ignore the injury |

Source: American Psychiatric Association.

Psychiatric Association has identified five possible types of reactions in such situations:

1. Normal reaction. In multiple casualty situations, the normal reaction consists of signs and symptoms of extreme anxiety, including sweating, shaking, weakness, nausea, and sometimes vomiting. Individuals experiencing this type of response may recover completely within a few minutes and can be helpful if given clear instructions.
2. Blind panic. In this type of reaction, the individual's judgment seems to disappear completely. Blind panic is particularly dangerous because it may lead to mass panic among others.
3. Depression. The individual who remains motionless and looks numbed or dazed is depressed. It is important to give such a person a task to perform in order to bring him back to reality.
4. Overreaction. The person who talks compulsively, jokes inappropriately, and races from one task to another, usually accomplishing little, is overreacting.
5. Conversion hysteria. The person's mood may shift rapidly from extreme anxiety to relative calmness. The person may convert anxiety to some bodily dysfunction. This reaction can result in hysterical blindness, deafness, or paralysis.

First Aiders should observe the following guidelines in dealing with mass casualty situations:

1. Identify themselves. Strive to remain self-assured and sympathetic, and conduct themselves in a businesslike manner.
2. Care for serious physical injuries immediately, and reassure anxious victims or bystanders.
3. Keep spectators away from the victims, but do not leave the victims alone. If all rescue personnel are busy dealing with physical injuries, assign a responsible bystander to stay with any person showing unusual behavior.
4. Assign tasks to bystanders to keep them occupied. Feeling that they are useful and responsible will lessen their anxiety greatly.
5. Respect the right of victims to have their own feelings. First Aiders should make it apparent that they understand the victims' feelings so that they can help. First Aiders

## General Guidelines For Disaster Management

While each disaster presents individual problems, there are some guidelines that are general and that will usually apply to any disaster you may be called to respond to:

**1** Don't let yourself become overwhelmed by the immensity of the disaster. Administer aid to those who need it. Carefully evaluate the injuries, and determine which victims should be treated first. Then set about admistering the aid, treating victims one by one. This will help you maintain some calm and feel that you are making progress, despite the immensity of the disaster.

**2** Obtain and distribute information about the disaster and the victims. The families of victims deserve accurate information about both the disaster and the victims themselves.

**3** Reunite the victim with his family as soon as possible. There are two benefits of this: first, emotional stress will be lessened once the victim is with family members. Second, family members may be able to provide you with critical medical history that may affect your ability to treat the victim.

**4** Encourage victims who are able to do necessary chores. Work can be therapeutic, and should be used to help the victim get over his own problems. Help the victim devise a schedule to perform his own daily routines like he did before the disaster.

should not try to tell the victims how they should feel.

6. Accept victims' physical and emotional limitations. Fear and panic are as disabling as physical injuries, and some people are able to deal with anxiety better than others. Do not try to force victims to deal with more than they seem able to cope with. Help victims to recognize and use their remaining strength and lessen their anxiety.
7. Accept personal limitations. In mass casualty situations, realize that there are limits as to what can be done. First Aiders should not overextend themselves and should provide more effective care by establishing priorities.

## REACTIONS OF RESCUE WORKERS

First Aiders are not immune to the stresses of emergency situations. When dealing with the critically ill and injured, they may experience a wide range of feelings, some of which are unpleasant. The First Aider may feel irritated by the family or the victim's demands, be anxious when faced with life-threatening injuries, become defensive at implications that he/she is not competent to handle emergencies, and become sad in response to tragedy. Although these feelings are natural, it is best for the First Aider not to express them during an emergency. Furthermore, if the First Aider gives an outward appearance of calmness and confidence, it will help to relieve the anxiety of those on the scene. Helping others to remain calm is part of the First Aider's therapeutic role.

## TRIAGE

All the medical knowledge in the world, and all the finest care by a First Aider, is of no avail if priorities are not properly ordered. It is critical that the First Aider know which victims of multiple-victim accident or disaster require emergency care first. The First Aider's ability to save lives depends upon his/her evaluation of the victims and upon **triage** — the ability to classify which victims require attention and care the most desperately, and which victims can wait without being endangered.

### Conducting the Triage

Triage should be completed by the most experienced First Aider as soon as the scene is secured (that is, traffic is controlled, the fire is out, and so on). The key is for the Triage First Aider to not stop at one victim and become preoccupied with a bloody wound or shock, but to move through the victims to complete the triage. This sets the stage for the next arriving rescuers, who can focus on caring for salvageable victims. Many victims experience an injury (such as a blunt trauma injury) that does not show on the surface but that is more devastating to life than many observable injuries.

The triage rescuer should quickly evaluate each victim's condition, categorizing and prioritizing for care and applying the **ABCs** (airway/breathing/circulation) on a limited

### Three-Level Triage Method

| Injury Priority | Injury Description |
|---|---|
| **LIFE-THREATENED (Highest Priority)** | Critically injured but can recover if treated immediately. |
| **URGENT (Second Priority)** | Seriously injured; may die without further treatment. |
| **DELAYED (Lowest Priority)** | Noncritical injuries or minor wounds. |
| **Note: DEAD** — morgue in different location | Victims requiring vigorous care for cardiac arrest should be treated as dead. |

# TRIAGE SUMMARY

Triage means sorting multiple casualties into priorities for emergency care or for transportation to definitive care. Priorities are usually given in three levels as follows: In a two-level system, the Lowest and Second Priorities would be in the delayed category and the Highest Priority maintains that immediate status.

### LOWEST PRIORITY

- Fractures or other injuries of a minor nature
- Obviously mortal wounds where death appears reasonably certain
- Obvious dead
- Cardiac arrest (if sufficient personnel are not available to care for numerous other victims)
- Follow local protocol

### SECOND PRIORITY

- Burns
- Major or multiple fractures
- Back injuries with or without spinal cord damage

### HIGHEST PRIORITY

- Airway and breathing difficulties
- Cardiac arrest if sufficient personnel available
- Uncontrolled or suspected severe bleeding
- Severe head injuries
- Severe medical problems: poisoning, diabetic and cardiac emergencies, etc.
- Open chest or abdominal wounds
- Shock

## PROCEDURES

1. The most knowledgeable First Aider arriving in the first ambulance must become triage leader.
2. Primary survey should be completed on all victims first. Correct immediate life-threatening problems.
3. Ask for additional assistance if needed.
4. Assign available manpower and equipment to priority one victims.
5. Arrange for transport of priority one victims first.
6. If possible, notify emergency personnel and/or hospital(s) of number and severity of injuries.
7. Triage rescuer remains at scene to assign and coordinate manpower, supplies and vehicles.
8. Victims must be reassessed regularly for changes in condition.

## Two-Level Triage Method

| Injury Priority | Injury Description |
|---|---|
| **IMMEDIATE (First Priority)** | Includes those who have critical injuries that threaten life but are salvageable; those requiring immediate medical care (within five to fifteen minutes) to survive. |
| **DELAYED (Second Priority)** | Includes those who are seriously injured but are not life-threatened; those whose injuries are minor and treatment can be delayed; and those who are very critically injured — non-salvageable or dead. Also includes those with no injuries or only minor injuries requiring emergency care. |

basis (depending on the availability of triage and emergency care personnel) until triage is completed. The following evaluation order should be followed:

1. Ask a **conscious** victim the following questions:
   - Where do you hurt? A response may indicate if the victim can hear and understand and may reveal the condition of his/her thought processes.
   - Are you allergic to anything, and have you had any serious illness recently? This tests the victim's recall and thinking processes.
   - Were you unconscious at any time? This question may reveal possible head injuries and help to recall the immediate past.
   - Do you have any medical illnesses, such as diabetes? Have you taken any medication or drugs/alcohol within the past six hours? Do you hurt anywhere specifically? Are you experiencing any vision, hearing, balance, or other abnormal problems? Do you have feeling in your arms and legs? (Pinch each limb prior to asking.) How long since you last ate?
2. The **unconscious** victim needs the following specific priority assessment. Perform it within thirty seconds.
   - Open **airway** by tilting back the head or lifting the chin and supporting the neck.
   - Listen for breathing and any possible airway obstruction.
   - If airway obstruction is present, perform the **manual thrust** with the victim lying on his/her back.
   - Check chest movement and mouth for breathing.
   - If breathing is absent, perform **mouth-to-mouth resuscitation**.
   - Check the **carotid pulse** for heartbeat and circulation. If you find no pulse, tag the victim and move on to the next triage victim unless other triage personnel are available.
   - **Hemorrhage** should be quickly controlled by **direct pressure** or a dressing/**pressure bandage** and elevation. Remember you give only limited treatment. You cannot afford to wait six to seven minutes for the blood to clot.
   - The victim now needs to be marked or tagged according to the seriousness and kinds of injuries involved.

## Work Exercises

Effective emergency care requires not only an understanding of the nature and care of psychological emergencies, but also of the normal and natural emotional responses to illness and injury and their consequent psychological care.

List five principles of psychological emergency care that should give direction to First Aiders.

1.

2.

3.

4.

5.

Match the following definitions with the appropriate type of reaction and list general guidelines for dealing with disaster.

**MASS CASUALTIES AND DISASTERS**

| Types of Reactions | Definitions | Guidelines for Dealing with Mass Casualties/Disasters |
|---|---|---|
| _______ 1. Normal Reaction | A. Mood may shift rapidly from extreme anxiety to relative calmness. | 1. |
| _______ 2. Blind Panic | B. The individual remains motionless and looks numbed and dazed. | 2. |
| _______ 3. Depression | C. Extreme anxiety, including sweating, shaking, weakness, nausea, and sometimes vomiting. | 3. |
| _______ 4. Overreaction | D. Judgment seems to disappear completely. | 4. |
| _______ 5. Conversion hysteria | E. Person talks compulsively, jokes inappropriately, and races from one task to another, usually accomplishing little. | 5. |

In the right-hand column, write the injury descriptions listed below beside the appropriate triage level.

**THREE LEVEL TRIAGE METHOD**

| Injury Priority | Injury Description |
|---|---|
| Highest | |
| Second | |
| Lowest | |

**TWO LEVEL TRIAGE METHOD**

| Injury Priority | Injury Description |
|---|---|
| Immediate | |
| Delayed | |

## Injury Descriptions

a. Noncritical or minor wounds and injuries
b. Critically injured — won't recover unless treated immediately
c. DOA (Dead on Arrival)
d. Seriously injured
e. Hyper or hypothermia
f. Uncontrolled bleeding
g. Back injuries without spinal cord damage
h. Cardiac disease
i. Seizures
j. Multiple fractures
k. Obstetrical problems
l. Burns
m. Severe head injuries
n. Open chest or abdominal wounds
o. Breathing difficulties

## SELF-TEST

### Part I: True and False

If you believe the statement is true, circle the T. If you believe the statement is false, circle F.

T F 1. Sit while talking to a victim with a psychological disorder.

T F 2. When talking to a victim, the First Aider should ask questions that are direct and specific to measure the victim's level of consciousness and contact with reality.

T F 3. Do NOT allow silences when talking with psychological victims.

T F 4. Do NOT leave a victim of psychological emergencies alone.

T F 5. When dealing with children, story-telling, game-playing, or picture-drawing will help establish rapport.

T F 6. It is appropriate to lie to a child to protect him from unpleasant facts.

T F 7. Suicidal threats from children don't need to be taken seriously.

### Part II: Multiple Choice

For each question, circle the answer that best reflects an accurate statement.

1. First Aiders should observe all of the following guidelines when dealing with mass casualty situations EXCEPT:
   a. strive to remain self-assured and conduct themselves in a businesslike manner
   b. recognize the responsibility to provide care to every victim and overextend themselves to see it is provided
   c. assign tasks to bystanders to keep them occupied
   d. make it apparent that victims' anxious feelings are understood and reassure them

2. How should the First Aider handle emotional reactions in mass casualties and disasters?
   a. show extreme sympathy
   b. douse the person with water
   c. firmly but gently isolate the person from the group
   d. administer mild sedatives

3. Which of the following is NOT a general guideline for disaster management:
   a. obtain and distribute information about the disaster and the victims
   b. reunite the victim with his family as soon as possible
   c. help the victim devise a schedule to perform his daily routines
   d. treat every victim you come to before going on to someone else

4. A victim who is crying uncontrollably is exhibiting which type of emotional reaction?
   a. normal
   b. panic
   c. overactivity
   d. conversion reaction
   e. underactivity

5. Which guideline for psychological first aid is *not* correct?
   a. establish rapport with the victim
   b. encourage the victim to talk out feelings and fears
   c. use the slapping technique to bring an emotionally distraught victim around
   d. encourage an exhausted person to rest and sleep

6. Which of the following is *not* a symptom of mental disturbance?
   a. constant outbursts of temper
   b. insomnia
   c. nausea and vomiting
   d. serious juvenile delinquency

7. In dealing with a mentally disturbed person, you should:
   a. use strong physical force to restrain the victim before something serious happens
   b. do whatever you can to calm the victim down
   c. lie to the victim if you have to to calm him
   d. not let the victim talk too much — he may get more upset

8. All of the following are signs of the mentally disturbed EXCEPT:
   a. does the victim experience strange losses of memory
   b. does the victim have grand ideas about himself
   c. does the victim complain of body ailments that are not possible
   d. does the victim become more anxious about the future effects of the injury than the immediate pain

9. In giving psychological emergency care, how can the First Aider develop confidence and rapport with the victim?
   a. be overly sympathetic to show you care
   b. listen intently and be empathic
   c. criticize the victim's emotional responses
   d. lie to the victim about the extent of the injury

10. Why is it important to identify yourself clearly?
    a. so the victim will be more trusting and cooperative
    b. so the victim will know who to contact if the wrong treatment is given
    c. to protect yourself legally

11. What is a sound practice when dealing with suicidal individuals?
    a. trust rapid recoveries
    b. try to shock the victim out of a suicidal act
    c. show the person you are disgusted with his/her actions
    d. ask the victim directly about suicidal thoughts

12. What physical illness is most likely to lead the First Aider to suspect a psychological disturbance?
    a. cardiac arrest
    b. epilepsy
    c. diabetic coma
    d. shock

13. All of the following are good skills to use while talking to a victim with psychological disorders *except:*
    a. direct the conversation by asking the victim questions that are unrelated to what he/she is talking about.
    b. offer a soft drink to promote a relaxed atmosphere
    c. talk to the victim alone
    d. never be judgmental

14. Which guideline for communicating in a psychological emergency is *not* correct?
    a. maintain eye contact
    b. give warm and calm reassurance
    c. be overly sympathetic to show you care
    d. do not judge, criticize, or argue with a victim

15. Which of the following is *not* true for children experiencing a psychological emergency:
    a. may be unable to talk about the problem directly
    b. may be especially prone to homicide or suicide
    c. will probably outgrow destructive tendencies
    d. may not be responsible for own care and actions

16. Which of the following is *not* a management guideline for the disruptive victim?
    a. position yourself between the victim and the only doorway
    b. present a comfortable, confident, professional manner
    c. adjust your physical distance from the patient to a safe range.
    d. let the victim know what you expect

17. To evaluate an unconscious victim for purposes of triage classification, check the following:
    a. breathing, bleeding, burns
    b. bleeding, pulse, head injury
    c. breathing, pulse, shock
    d. breathing, pulse, bleeding

18. Triage specifically means:
    a. giving emotional support and reassurance to victims
    b. mobilizing available rescue personnel and services at the disaster site
    c. establishing a general plan for the community to follow in case of a disaster
    d. assessment of the injured and separation into categories according to the severity of injuries so treatment can proceed.

Corresponds with:
**American Red Cross**
**Standard First Aid & Personal Safety**
Chapter 15, pages 225-251
and
**Advanced First Aid & Emergency Care**
Chapter 17, pages 254-284

# 18 Lifting and Moving Victims

After receiving first aid care, an injured person often requires transportation and handling. It is the responsibility of the First Aider to see that the victim is transported in such a manner as to prevent further injury and is not subjected to unnecessary pain or discomfort. Improper handling and careless transportation often add to the original injuries, increase shock, and endanger life. If at all possible, handling and transportation should be left to the professional emergency teams.

Under normal circumstances, a victim should not be moved until a thorough assessment has been made and first aid care has been rendered. A seriously injured person should be moved in a position that is least likely to aggravate injuries. Various methods for carrying a victim can be used in emergencies, but the stretcher is the preferred method of transportation. When a stretcher is unavailable or impractical, other means of transportation may be employed.

While speed is important in a few cases, it is always more important to accomplish the handling and transfer in a way that will not injure the victim further.

The following photo series will review the various lifts and moves.

## MOVING VICTIMS — GENERAL GUIDELINES

1. All necessary emergency care should be provided first. Fractures, including neck and back, should be splinted.
2. A victim should be moved only if there is an immediate danger, that is:
   - There is a fire or danger of fire.
   - Explosives or other hazardous materials are involved.
   - It is impossible to protect the accident scene.
   - It is impossible to gain access to other victims in a vehicle who need life-saving care.

   Only in a "threat to life" situation should a victim be moved before the ABCs are completed.
3. If it is necessary to move a victim, the speed with which he/she is moved will depend on the reason for moving him/her, for example:
   - Emergency move. If there is a fire, the victim will be pulled away from the area as quickly as possible.
   - Non-emergency move. If a victim needs to be moved to gain access to others in a vehicle, due consideration will be given to his/her injuries before and during movement.
4. Victims are usually transported in a lying-down position.

## USING A BACKBOARD

Short and long backboards are standard rescue equipment and are often available at the site of accidental injury. Their purpose is

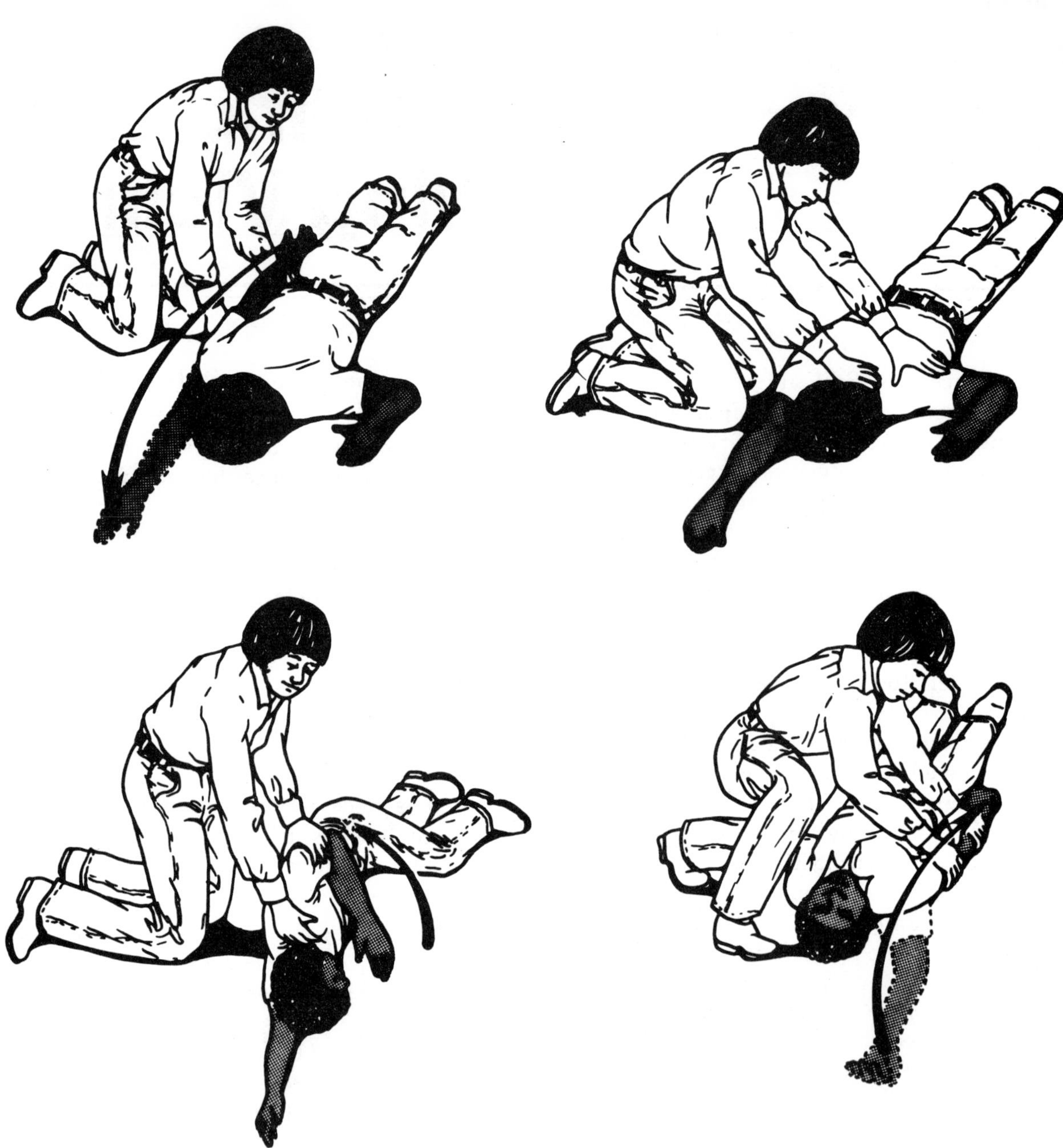

Moving victim from a face-down position to an assessment position after doing the ABC assessment and checking for possible neck injury. First, the First Aider moves the victim's nearer arm above the head; he then places one hand behind the victim's head and neck and the other hand on the distant shoulder; he rolls the victim toward the First Aider by pulling the shoulder. Once the victim is flat, the extended arm is brought back to the side.

to stabilize the victim's body so that further injury to the neck and spinal cord will not occur. They should be used anytime injury to the neck and/or back is suspected. See Chapters 9 and 19 for further information.

## EMERGENCY MOVES

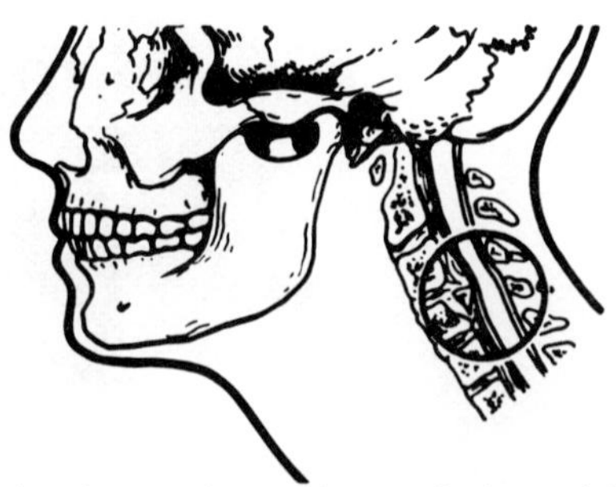

1. The major danger in moving a victim quickly is the possibility of spine injury.

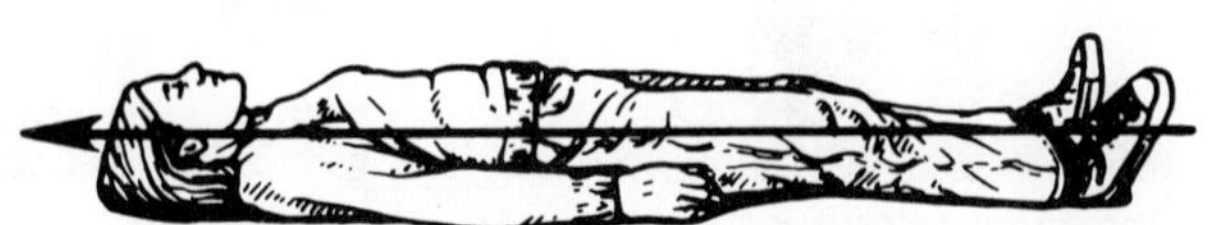

2. In an emergency, every effort should be made to pull the victim in the direction of the long axis of the body to provide as much protection to the spine as possible.

3. It is impossible to remove a victim from a vehicle quickly and, at the same time, provide protection for his spine.

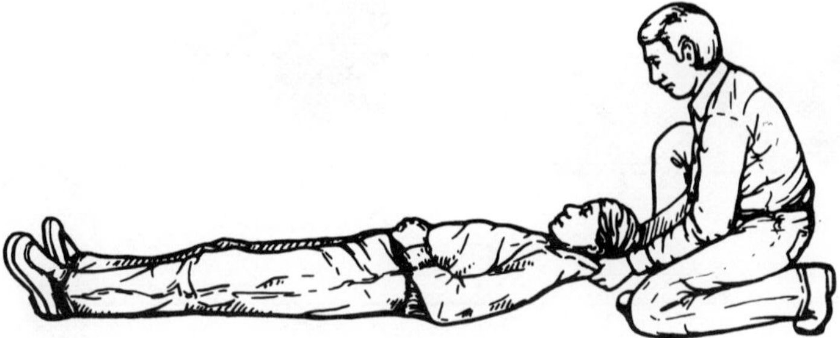

4. If the victim is on the floor or ground, he can be dragged away from the scene by tugging on his clothing in the neck and shoulder area.

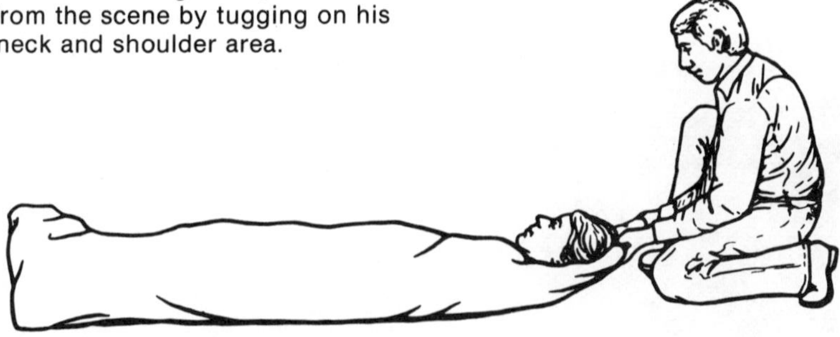

5. It may be easier to pull the victim onto a blanket and then drag the blanket away from the scene.

6. Such moves are emergency moves only. They do not really protect the spine from further injury.

7. Where possible, all injuries should be immobilized as much as possible prior to movement.

8. All injuries should be protected as much as possible during movement.

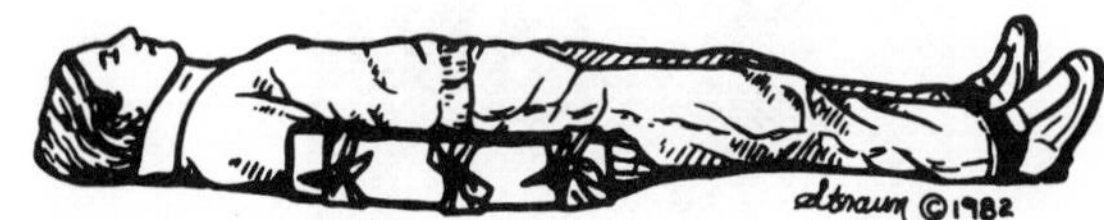

## ONE-RESCUER MOVES

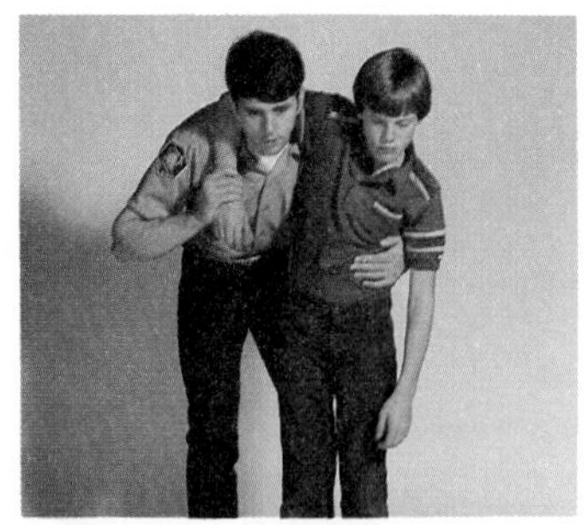

One-rescuer crutch.

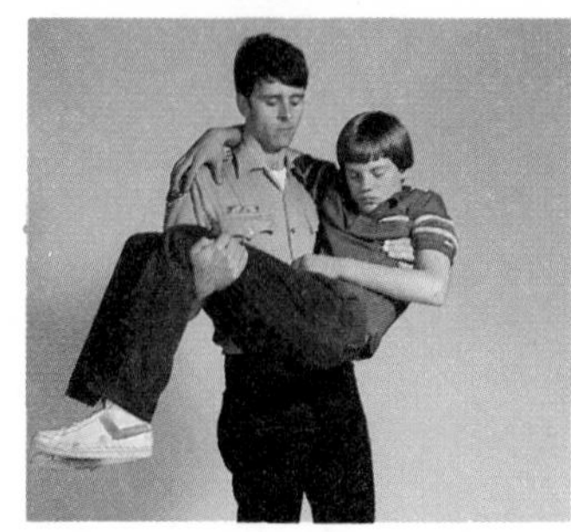

One-rescuer cradle carry.

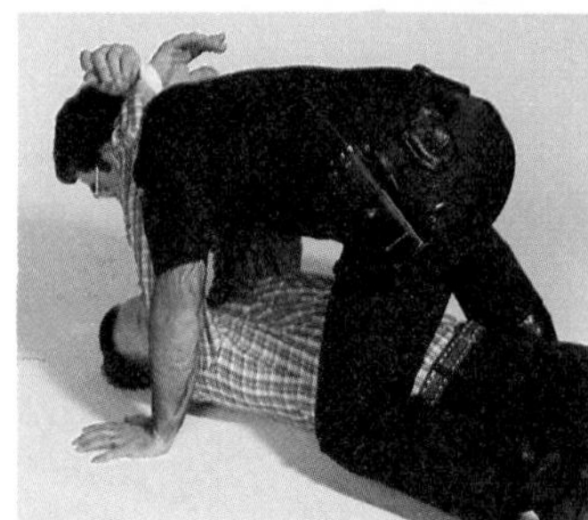

Fireman's drag.

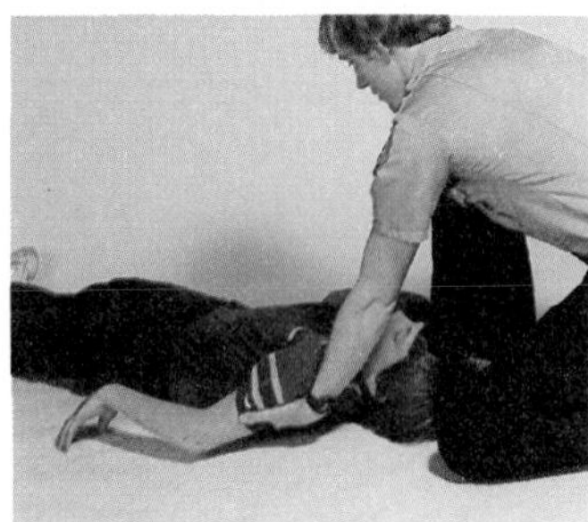

Shoulder drag.

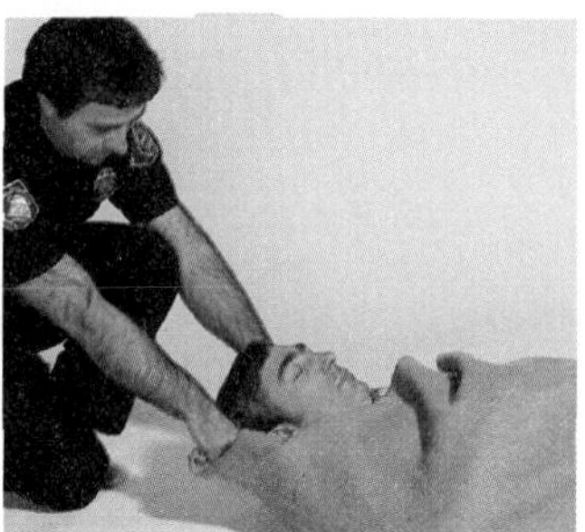

Blanket drag.

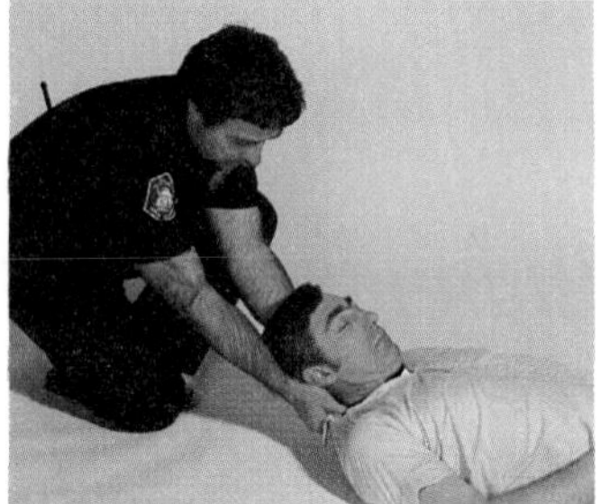

Clothes drag.

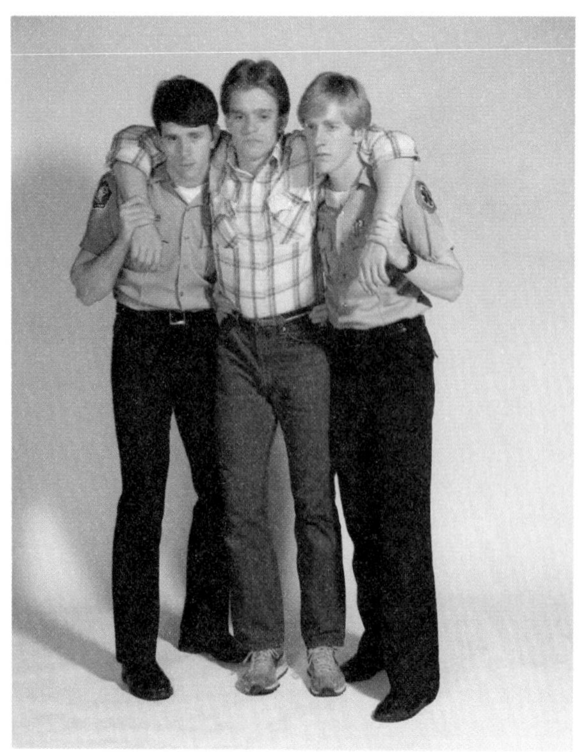

Two-rescuer crutch method for a slightly injured victim.

## THE FIREMAN'S CARRY

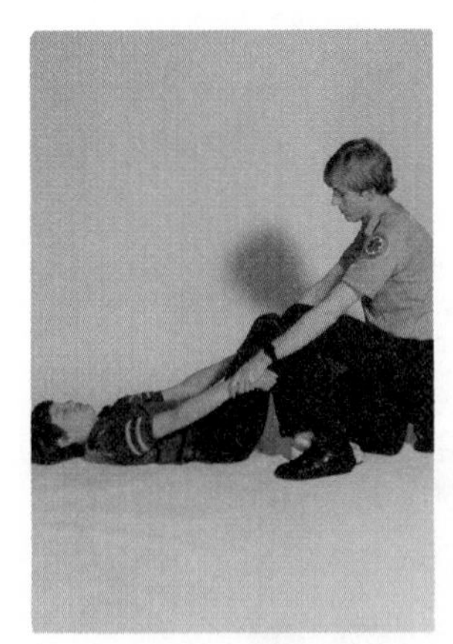
1

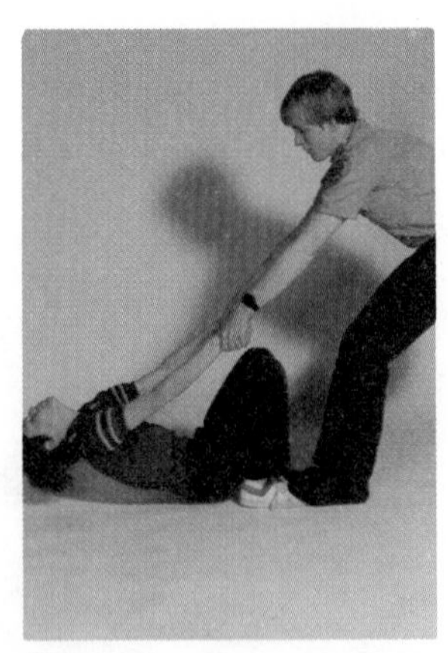
2

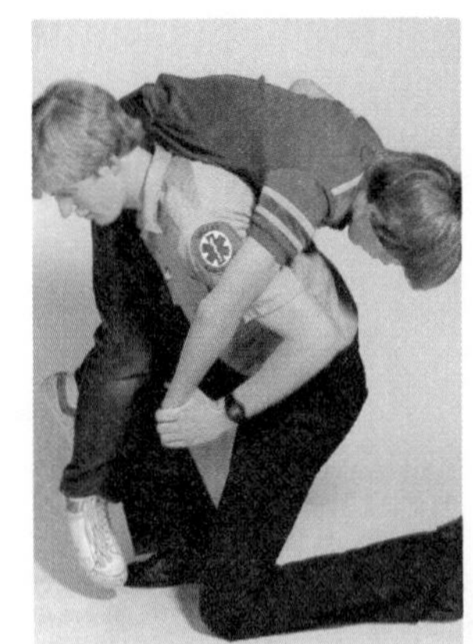
3

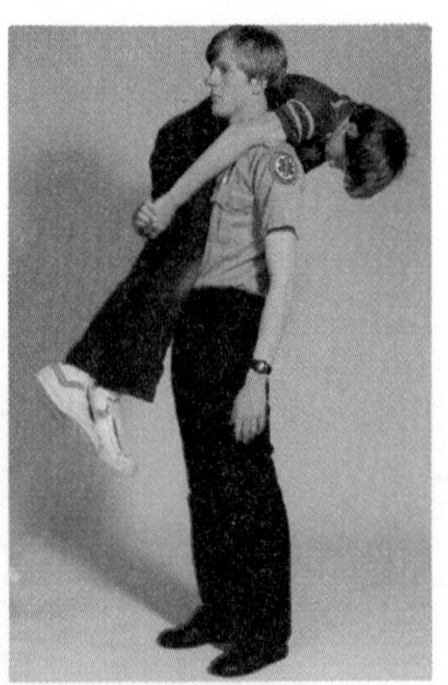
4

## PIGGYBACK CARRY

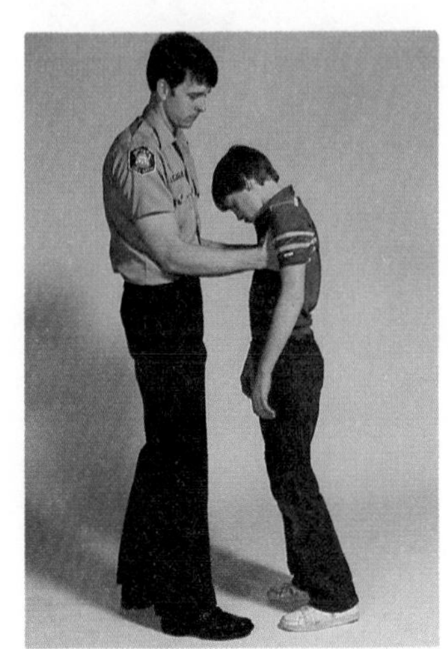
1

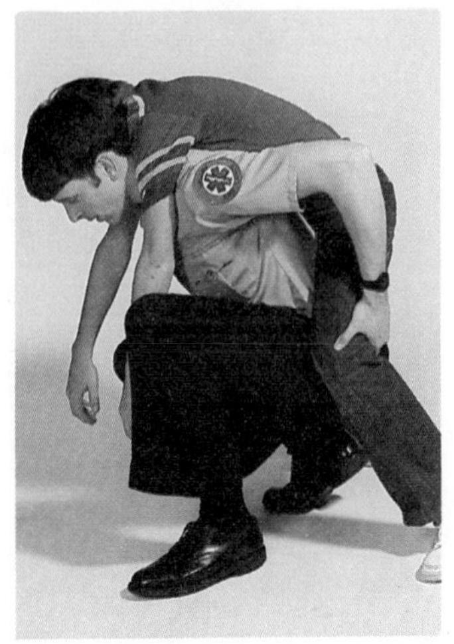
2

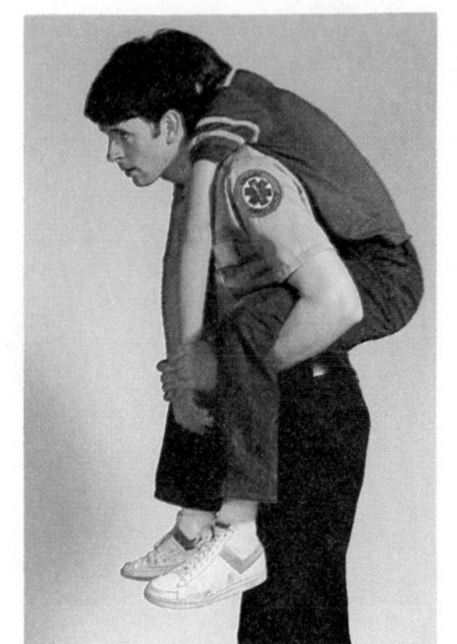
3

## EXTREMITY LIFT

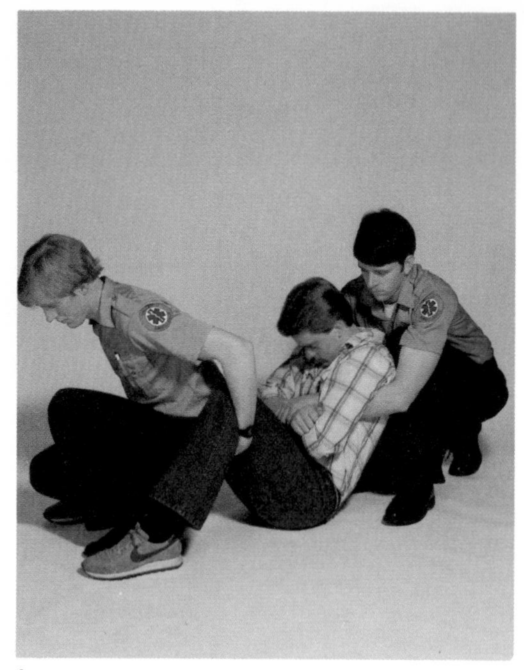
1

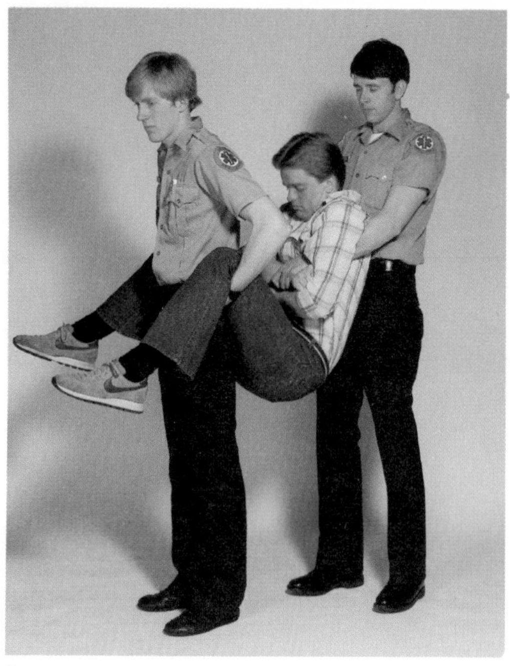
2

## SEAT CARRY

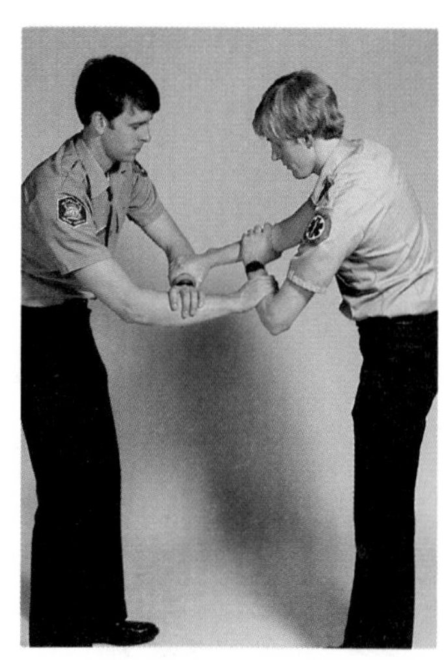
1

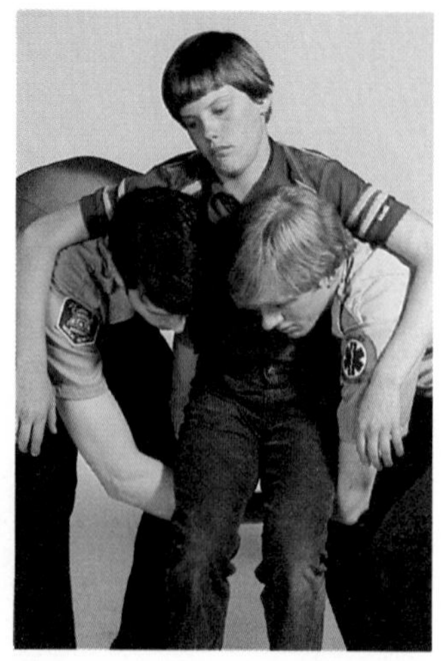
2

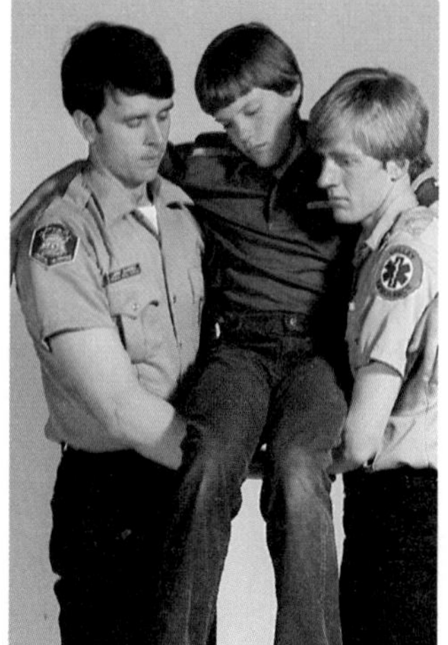
3

For a conscious victim who needs support.

## CHAIR CARRY

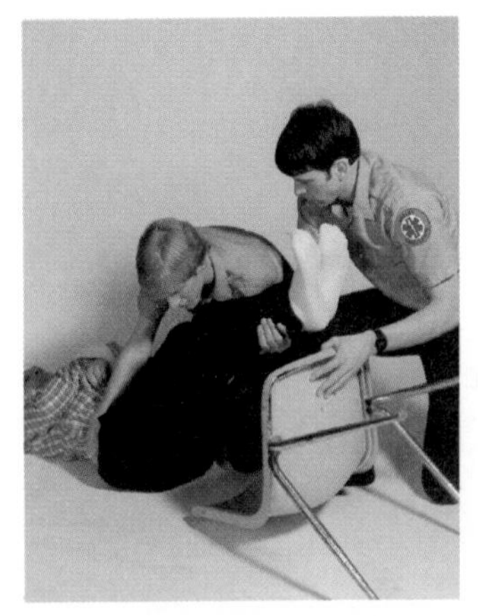
1

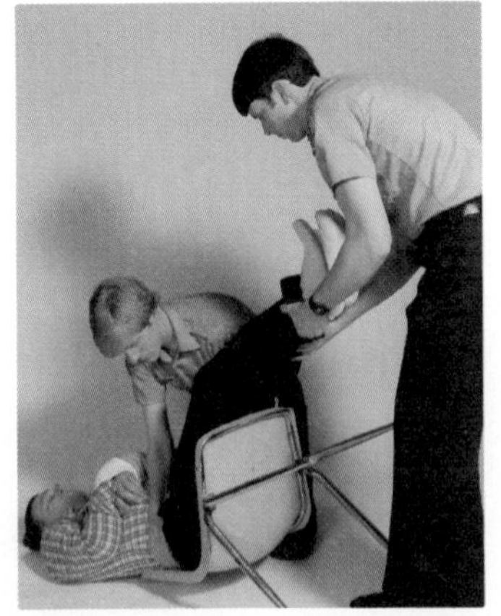
2

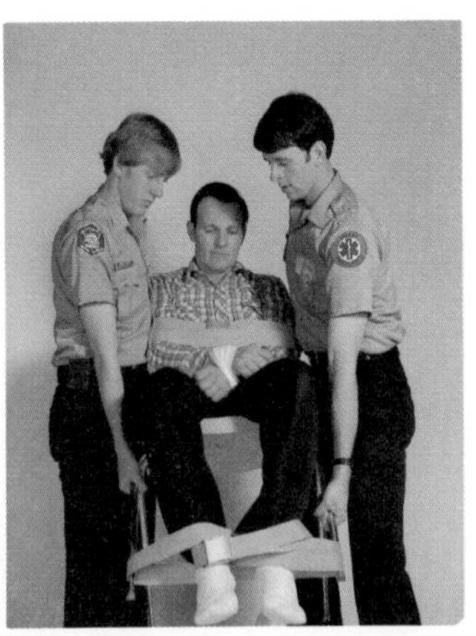
3

**Do not use if victim has neck or back injuries.**

## THREE-RESCUER LIFT AND CARRY

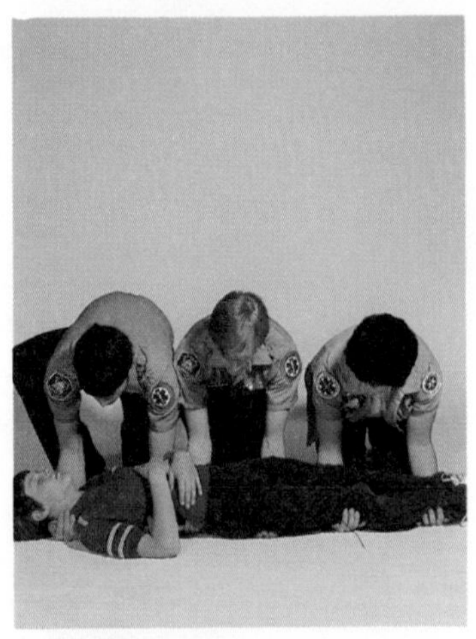
1

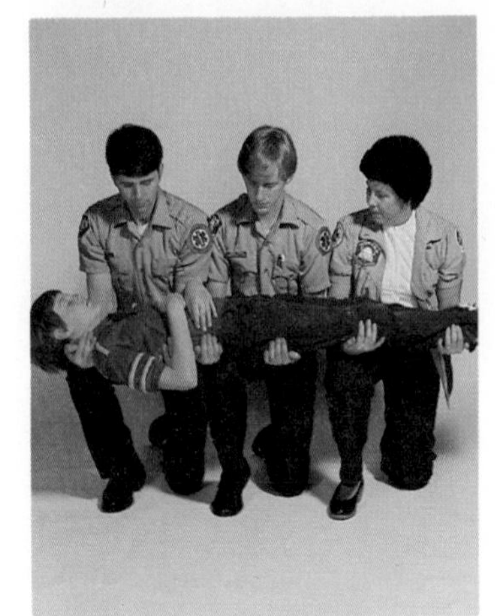
2

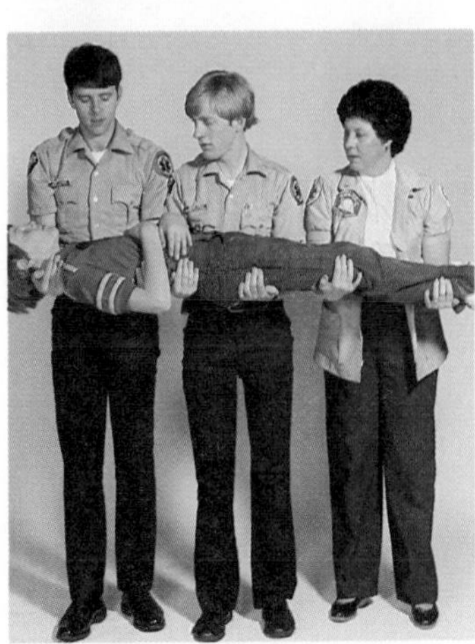
3

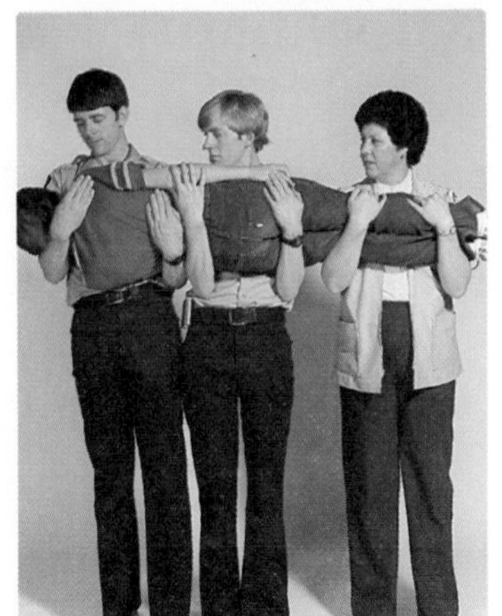
4

## Work Exercises

### General Guidelines for Moving Victims

A victim should be moved only if there is an immediate danger to him/her or others if he/she is not moved.

List four justifiable circumstances for moving a victim:

1. Fire or Danger of Fire
2. Explosives or hazardous materials involved
3. Impossible to protect accident scene
4. Can't gain access to other victims

Complete the following table by describing one specific use or situation for each of the carries listed:

| Type of Carry | Use |
|---|---|
| 1. Blanket Drag | |
| 2. Clothes or Incline Drag | |
| 3. Fireman's Drag | |
| 4. The Crutch Method | |
| 5. Two-man Seat Carry | |
| 6. Three-man Carry | |
| 7. Three-man Log Roll | |
| 8. Long Backboard. | |

## SELF-TEST

### Part I: True and False

If you believe the statement is true, circle the T. If you believe the statement is false, circle F.

T F 1. A lone First Aider who is moving a suspected broken neck victim out of a burning building should remove the victim by the clothes drag.

T F 2. Joints above and below a break should be immobilized if a victim must be moved before a fracture is splinted.

T F 3. More harm is done through improper transportation than through any other measure associated with first aid.

T F 4. A victim of an electrical emergency should be separated from the electrical current by a substance such as wood, rope, or cloth.

T F 5. A strong, straight-back chair can be used to carry a victim safely, regardless of the type of injury.

T F 6. The two-rescuer crutch method is the preferred method of transportation for a neck injury victim.

T F 7. A seat carry can safely be used for a victim with a neck injury.

T F 8. A suspected cervical spine injury victim should have his/her neck stabilized immediately.

### Part II: Multiple Choice

For each question, circle the answer that best reflects an accurate statement.

1. Two or more rescuers can use a blanket to transport an injured victim safely as long as the victim does not have:
   a. a fractured pelvis
   b. a spinal injury
   c. a skull fracture
   d. any of the above

2. When carrying a victim on a litter, how many rescuers should ideally lift and carry?
   a. two
   b. three
   c. four
   d. six

3. Why should an injured person be carried feet-first when being transported by litter?
   a. being able to see where he/she is going will calm him/her
   b. the litter bearer at the rear will be better able to observe the victim
   c. the litter bearer at the rear can protect the victim from being hit by flying debris
   d. the victim's body weight will be more evenly distributed
   e. a victim should not be carried feet-first

4. An injured person may be moved by a First Aider only if the victim's position:
   a. puts him in danger of developing shock
   b. endangers his life
   c. is inconvenient for giving first aid
   d. prevents him from receiving first aid

5. The initial step in rescuing a victim from electrical contact is:
   a. cut the contact with a wooden-handled ax
   b. look for the switch that turns off the current
   c. separate the victim from the contact by pulling on his clothing
   d. remove the wire from the victim's body with a nonconducting object

6. Immediate rescue should be undertaken in *all but which one* of the following situations?
   a. possibility of electrical injury
   b. serious traffic hazard
   c. exposure to the elements
   d. possibility of gas poisoning

7. If a victim is only slightly injured, which one-man carry would you use?
   a. fireman's carry
   b. fireman's drag
   c. crutch method
   d. extremity lift

8. Never use an extremity lift in case of ____________________ injuries.

   a. head
   b. back
   c. abdominal
   d. arm

9. A two-handed seat should be used when the victim is:

   a. conscious, but needs support
   b. unconscious
   c. suspected of having a neck injury
   d. unconscious, with unknown injuries

10. If the move is a non-emergency move, you should:

    a. treat for shock before moving the victim
    b. complete emergency care before attempting to move the victim
    c. only move the victim if it is inconvenient to give first aid
    d. if it is a non-emergency situation, do not move the victim

11. The primary consideration in an emergency move is protection of the:

    a. head
    b. extremities
    c. heart
    d. spine

12. For suspected back injuries, the ____________________________ is a good technique for moving a victim:

    a. four-man log roll
    b. blanket drag
    c. fireman's carry
    d. the crutch method

Corresponds with:
**American Red Cross**
**Advanced First Aid & Emergency Care**
Chapter 18, pages 285-301

# 19 Victim Stabilization and Extrication

Extrication is the process of removing a victim or victims from a dangerous, life-threatening situation. Two important factors to consider concerning extrication are:

1. Does the victim *really* need to be moved *now*? Is the victim's life in danger if you do not move him/her, or can you give emergency care to the trapped victim and wait for a trained rescue team with proper equipment?
2. If the victim *has* to be moved immediately, plan and prepare well, and practice safety-first for the First Aiders as well as the victim.

If you decide the victim does not need to be rescued immediately and a rescue team will be arriving soon, do the following:

- Control the hazards and stabilize the accident scene (shut off engines, put out flares, douse fires, etc.).
- Gain access to the victim, if possible, and if safe to do so.
- Give ABCs and other emergency care to stabilize the victim.
- Remain with the victim until the rescue team arrives.

Bystanders can be helpful or a hindrance. One of the First Aiders should be responsible for telling bystanders what to do. Give bystanders specific instructions on how to help you, or to stay out of the way so that they do not interfere or run the risk of becoming injured themselves.

## STABILIZING THE VEHICLE

After all possible outside hazards are controlled, make the rescue setting as safe as possible:

- Stabilize the vehicle in the position where it is found.
- Block, brace, or tie anything that might cave in, roll, slip, or fall. Increase the areas of contact with the ground as much as possible.

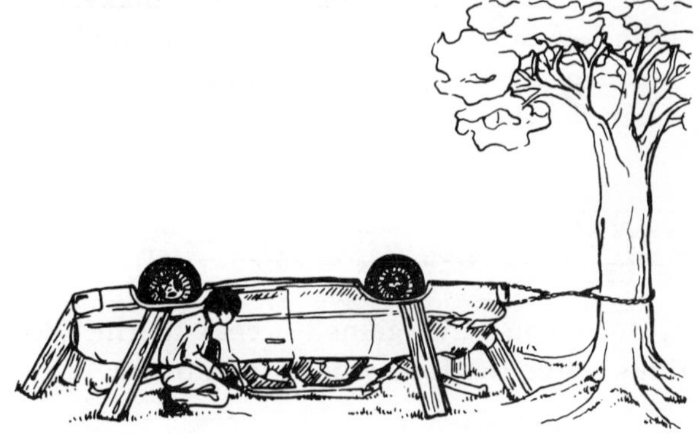

Stabilizing and bracing a car to prevent further damage.

- Use other vehicles or other heavy equipment where possible to brace the accident vehicle.

## TOOLS AND EQUIPMENT NEEDED

It is important to be prepared in case a rescue squad is not available. Basic tools which can be used include: hammer, screwdriver, chisel, crowbar, pliers, linoleum knife, work gloves and goggles, shovel, tire irons, wrenches, knives, car jacks, and ropes or chains. Ingenuity and creative thought can put these basic tools to work in a safe, effective way. Try all doors and windows you can get to for an easy entrance.

## REMOVING GLASS

It may be necessary to remove a windshield or rear window in one piece to gain access to the victim. First, cover the victim(s) with a blanket or other covering in case of glass breakage. Then:

1. Remove chrome trim.
2. Cut the top and sides of rubber moulding with a linoleum knife or other sharp tool.
3. Now begin at the top center and pry down the sides, pushing or pulling the glass out in one piece.

Once inside the damaged vehicle, the First Aider can use a folded blanket or towels as cervical supports and padding for makeshift splints. A stretcher or litter can be made from a ladder, picnic bench, surfboard, even a door taken off the hinges.

## PROPER CARE FOR VICTIMS

Once you have gained access to the victim(s), give the following care in order:

1. Urgent First Aid Care
   - Check for breathing and heartbeat.
   - Give mouth-to-mouth ventilation or CPR, if necessary. (Victim may have to be moved before effective CPR can be given.)
   - Control severe bleeding.
2. Follow-Up Care
   - Stabilize the victim(s) before you move them by:
     a. bandaging all wounds
     b. splinting all fractures
     c. giving psychological support
3. Life Support Care
   - After the victim(s) has been stabilized and moved, continue to check for:
     a. open airway
     b. breathing
     c. circulation or pulse
     d. bleeding is controlled
     e. normal victim temperature.

## PROPER SPLINTING

Very often, victims in need of extrication have possible neck and back injuries. In any accident situation, assess for neck and back injuries by:

1. Asking what happened, where does it hurt, and where is there no feeling?
2. Feel along the neck and back for muscle spasms, deformities, and painful areas.
3. See if the victim can grip your hands with his/her hands or wiggle his/her toes. Difficulty in moving the arms, legs, or head; a feeling of weakness, numbness, or no feeling below the injury; or complete paralysis all indicate neck or back injuries involving the spinal cord.

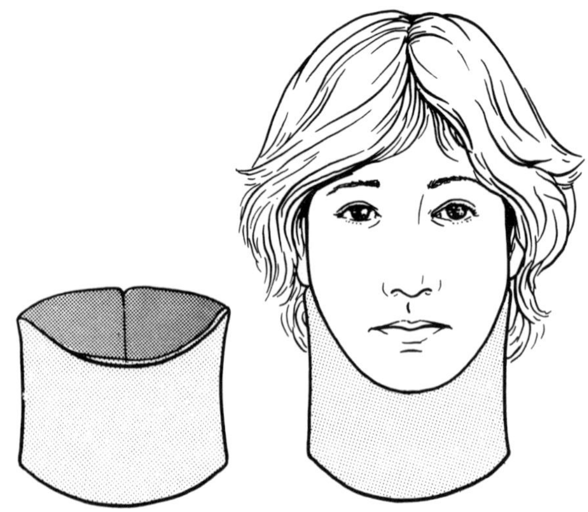

Cervical collar.

If you suspect a neck or back injury, a backboard and cervical support should be used to stabilize and transport the victim.

1. Apply a cervical support by first lifting the victim's head slightly and in a straight-up position, keeping the head and neck aligned.

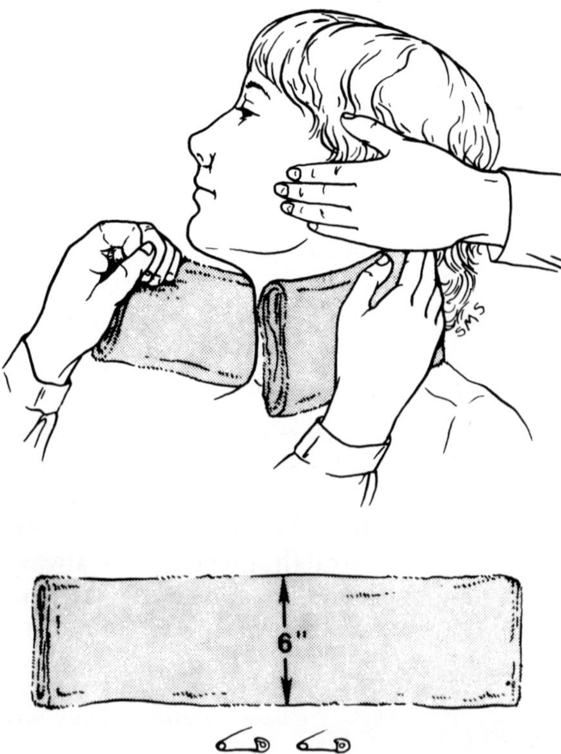


Improvised cervical support.

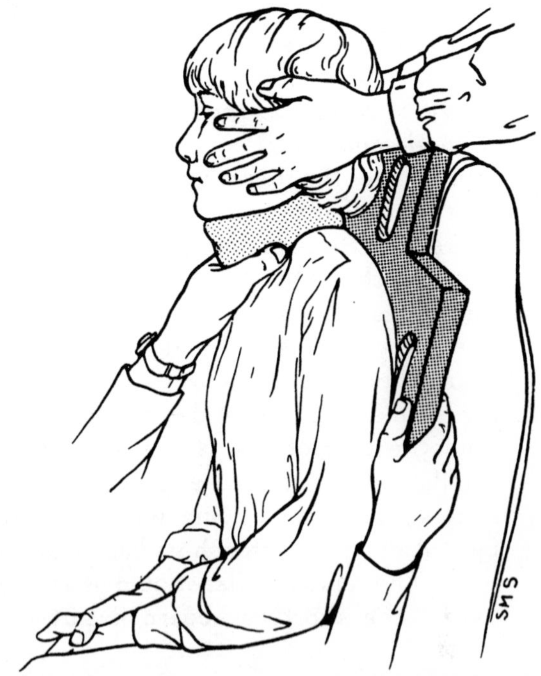

Keeping head and neck in alignment while applying short backboard.

If a cervical collar is not available, use a folded towel, blanket, or jacket.

2. Apply a short backboard if available and needed. Keep the victim straight and turn the body as a whole unit.
3. Continue to apply slight traction to the head to keep it straight. Tie the hands together, then the legs together, either to lift with or help keep the body in a straight line.
4. Lift the victim as a unit by grasping clothing. Make sure the head and neck are kept in straight alignment. DO NOT lift by feet, arms, or head. DO support them.
5. Position and fasten the victim correctly to a long backboard. Make sure the ties are snug enough so the body cannot move, but not so tight as to cut off circulation.
6. Carefully and slowly move the splinted victim. Continue to support the head and neck throughout the procedure.

## BACKBOARDS

If a victim of a suspected neck or spine injury is in a sitting position, as in an auto-

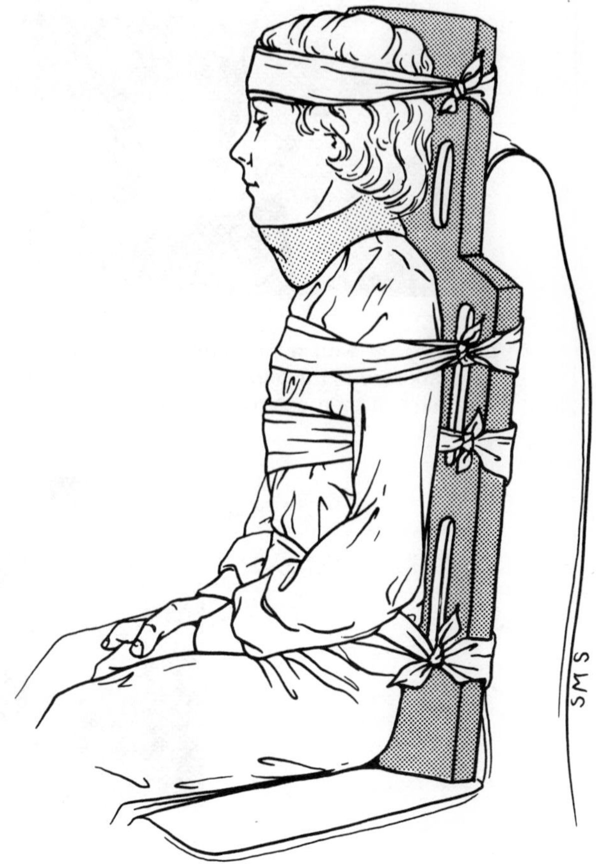

Short backboard and cervical support in place.

mobile, a short backboard needs to be used. The following steps are indicated:

1. Apply a cervical support, preferably a cervical collar.
2. Immobilize the neck and back with a short backboard.
3. Make sure there are straps or long bandages attached to the board so the victim can be easily secured.
4. Remember, the small end of the backboard should be at the top.
5. If possible, one First Aider should be behind the seat of the victim and should stabilize the victim's head and neck to keep them from moving while another First Aider places the short backboard in place. The cervical collar should be applied before the short backboard is put into place.
6. Secure the victim to the backboard with straps or bandage ties.
7. Do not place ties around the stomach.
8. The victim's head can be secured to the board with a bandage cravat across the forehead.
9. The head should not be tipped back, and if a cervical support does not provide enough immobilization, then a second tie may be needed around the chin. However, this should be watched very carefully in case of nausea or vomiting.
10. Once the cervical support and short backboard have been applied, the victim may be placed on a long backboard. This can be done by putting the victim's head, trunk, and legs in a straight line position (always holding neck and head in alignment with body) and then sliding the victim onto a long backboard.

## REMOVING A VICTIM WITH A LONG BOARD

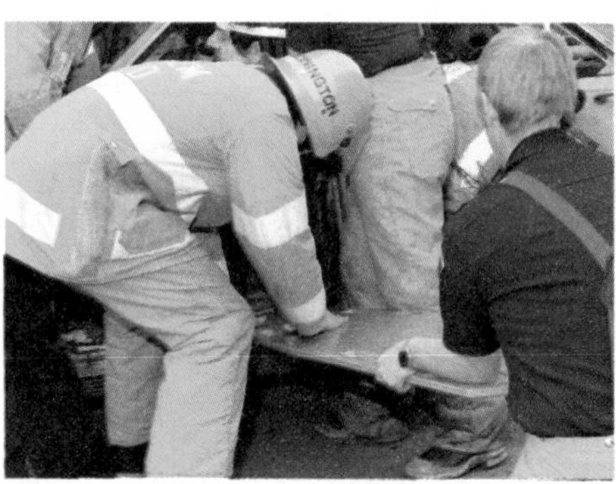

1
A victim with a possible spinal injury is stabilized in the vehicle. The end of a long board is then securely placed next to the seat.

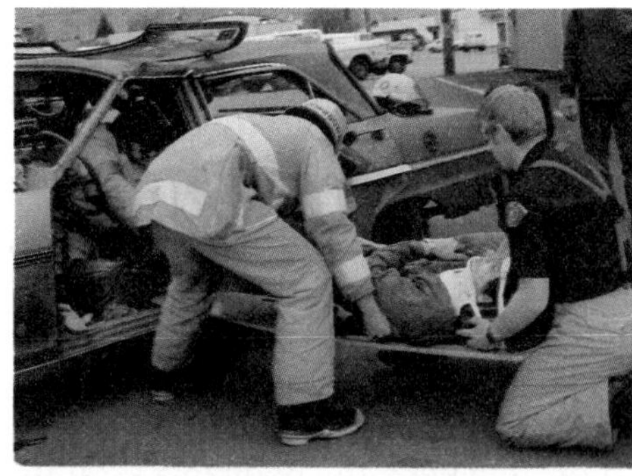

2
Slowly and carefully move victim to a prone position, and slide him onto the long board.

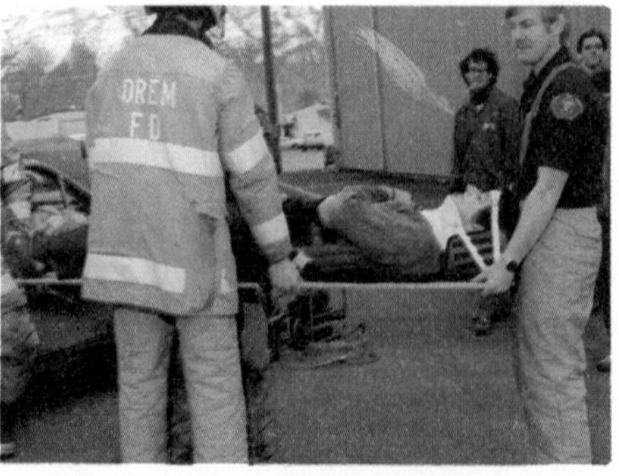


3
Carefully lift and remove victim.

## VICTIM ON SEAT OF VEHICLE

When a victim is lying down on the seat of a car, urgent first aid should be administered before moving unless there is immediate danger. The following steps should be considered:

1. One First Aider maintains a slight and gentle traction on the victim's head so that it is maintained in a normal straight line with the body.
2. A cervical collar should then be applied.
3. Another First Aider should carefully move the legs and body into alignment while head traction is still maintained. While two First Aiders maintain body alignment and head traction, another First Aider, preferably two, move the victim slightly away from the seat to allow a long backboard to be slipped beneath the victim's back.

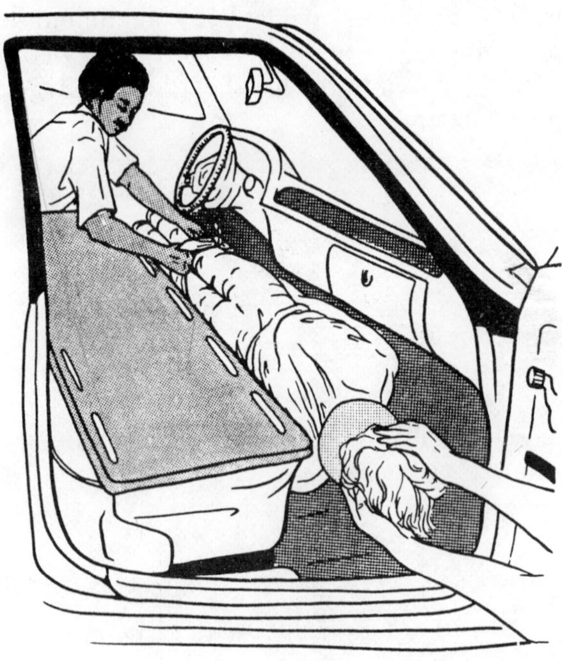

Keeping head, neck, and legs in proper alignment in preparation for applying long backboard.

4. The victim is then eased back against the backboard. When the First Aider at the victim's head gives a signal, the other First Aiders push and hold the victim snugly against the backboard until the backboard and victim are lying flat on the seat.
5. The victim is then secured to the backboard and removed from the car.
6. If a victim is found lying face down, urgent first aid should be given without moving the victim any more than necessary. If the victim must be turned over in order to administer first aid, the principles discussed in the chapter on moving and transporting victims should be carefully followed.

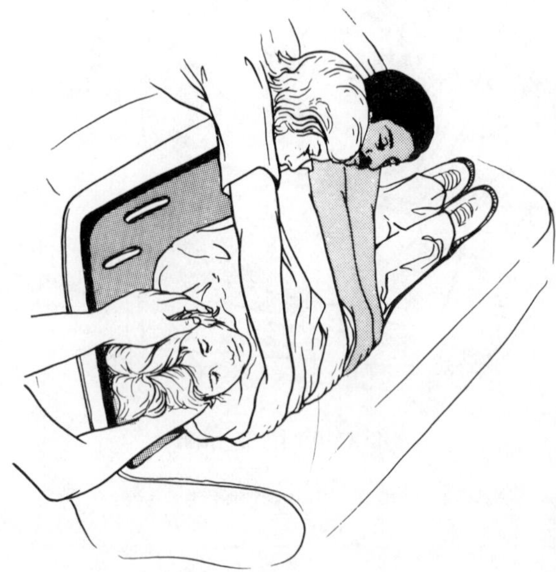

Moving the victim onto the long backboard.

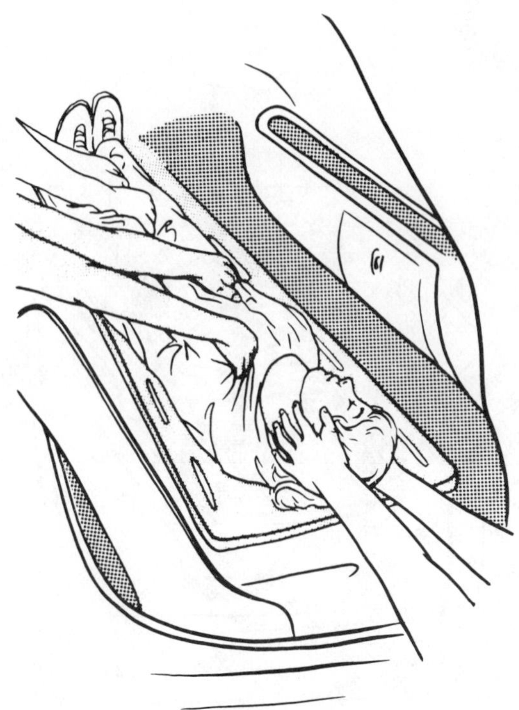

**Victim on Front Seat**

Removing a victim on the front seat.

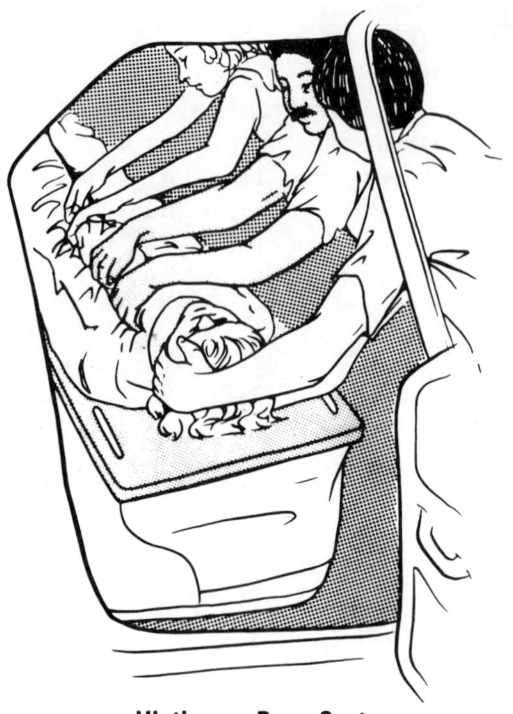

**Victim on Rear Seat**

Removing a victim on the rear seat.

## VICTIM LYING ON FLOOR OF VEHICLE

Sometimes a victim is in a space, such as under the steering wheel, dashboard, or on the floor, that does not allow for sliding a backboard into place. If this is the case, the backboard should be placed flat on the seat. One First Aider should then keep the head and neck in alignment with the body, while another First Aider maintains alignment of the feet and legs. This can be more easily accomplished if the victim's legs are secured together with a bandage. While the two First Aiders maintain the victim's body alignment, another First Aider(s) is able to reach over the seat, get a secure hold on the victim's clothing at the waist, hip, and thigh area, and then at a signal from the First Aider who is maintaining head and neck alignment, all the First Aiders lift the victim — while body alignment is maintained — onto the backboard. The victim is then secured to the backboard before being moved again.

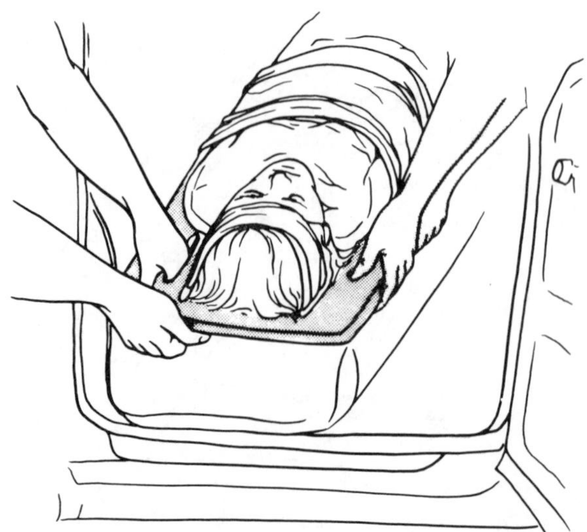

Victim is removed from the vehicle after being secured to the backboard.

## Work Exercises

Extrication is ______________________________________________

______________________________________________

What are two very important factors to consider *before* extricating a victim?

1.

2.

### Spineboards

Match the following spine immobilization devices with the correct situations (more than one device may be used):

| | |
|---|---|
| _______ 1. Unconscious person with head injuries | A. Short spineboard |
| _______ 2. Victim in large automobile. | B. Long spineboard |
| _______ 3. Victim under the dashboard. | C. Cervical collar. |
| _______ 4. Victim thrown from the vehicle. | |
| _______ 5. Victim in bucket seat. | |

Identify four common tools you could use to extricate an auto accident victim and what you would use them for:

| TOOL | USE |
|---|---|
| 1. | 1. |
| 2. | 2. |
| 3. | 3. |
| 4. | 4. |

## SELF-TEST

### Part I: True and False

If you believe the statement is true, circle the T. If you believe the statement is false, circle F.

T F 1. Bystanders are always a hazard in extrication situations.

T F 2. A vehicle should be stabilized in the position in which it is found.

T F 3. A part of stabilizing a victim is to splint all fractures.

T F 4. Slight, gentle traction should be placed on a victim's head before a cervical collar is applied.

T F 5. If a person is pinned under heavy machinery, it is best to have a medical doctor present before attempting removal.

T F 6. When a First Aider gains access to an accident victim, he should first establish an open airway.

T F 7. People with head injuries are best extricated sitting up.

T F 8. All outside hazards need to be controlled before a rescuer enters a wrecked vehicle.

T F 9. A victim's head and neck should be stabilized to the large end of a short backboard.

### Part II: Multiple Choice

For each question, circle the answer that best reflects an accurate statement.

1. Cars that are upside down or lying on their side should be:
   a. turned upright
   b. taken apart
   c. stabilized as is
   d. not touched

2. A short spineboard should be used for:
   a. immobilizing the back, neck, and pelvis
   b. immobilizing the back and neck until the victim is moved to a long board
   c. carrying the victim
   d. pelvic and femur fracture victims

3. What is the first step if a windshield or rear window must be removed to gain access to the victim?
   a. remove chrome trim around the window
   b. cover the victim with a blanket or other covering
   c. cut the top and sides of rubber moulding
   d. strike the window with a sharp instrument

4. Once the First Aider has gained access to the victim, he should next:
   a. check for breathing and heartbeat
   b. control severe bleeding
   c. splint fractures
   d. treat for shock

5. When a victim is lying down on the seat of a car, what is the first step involved in removing him?
   a. move the legs and body into alignment
   b. maintain slight and gentle traction on the victim's head
   c. apply a cervical collar
   d. move the victim slightly away from the seat

6. Extrication means:
   a. picking and sorting of the injured
   b. gaining access to an accident scene
   c. moving and transporting the injured
   d. disentangling or freeing a trapped victim

7. The major role of the First Aider in extrication is to:
   a. damage the vehicle or machinery in which the victim is trapped
   b. assure proper care of the victim
   c. use cutting and prying tools to gain access to the victim
   d. direct traffic around an automobile accident

# Glossary

**A**

**ABC's:** airway, breathing and circulation; the first three steps in the examination of any victim; basic life support.

**Abrasion:** a scraped or scratched skin wound.

**Absorption:** passage of a substance through a membrane into blood.

**Abstinence syndrome:** a complex of signs and symptoms caused by nonuse of a substance to which the body has been habituated.

**Addiction:** the state of being strongly dependent upon some agent; drugs, tobacco, for example.

**Air splint:** a double-walled plastic tube that immobilizes a limb when sufficient air is blown into the space between the walls of the tube, to cause it to become almost rigid.

**Airway:** the route for passage of air and/or gases into and out of the lungs.

**Amnesia:** loss or impairment of memory.

**Amputation:** complete removal of an appendage.

**Antigen:** any agent which, when taken into the body, stimulates the formulation of specific, protective proteins called antibodies.

**Antiseptic:** any preparation that prevents the growth of bacteria.

**Antitoxin:** an antibody produced in response to a specific toxin, which it neutralizes.

**Aorta:** the largest artery in the body, originates at the left ventricle and terminates at the bifurcation of the iliac arteries.

**Apex:** the peak, top or highest point.

**Artery:** a blood vessel, consisting of three layers of tissue and smooth muscle, that carries blood away from the heart.

**Aseptic:** sterile; free of bacteria.

**Aspirate:** to inhale foreign material into the lungs; to remove fluid or foreign material from the lungs or elsewhere by mechanical suction.

**Asthma:** a condition marked by recurrent attacks of dyspnea with wheezing due to spasmodic constriction of the bronchi, often as a response of allergens, or by mucous plugs in the bronchioles.

**Atherosclerosis:** a common form of arteriosclerosis caused by fat deposits in arterial walls.

**Avulsion:** an injury that leaves a piece of skin or other tissue either partially or completely torn away from the body.

**B**

**"Bad Trip":** a drug episode resulting in a state of intense anxiety or panic.

**Bandage:** a material used to hold a dressing in place.

**Bandage compress:** a folded cloth or pad used for applying pressure to stop hemorrhage or as a wet dressing.

**Basal skull fracture:** a fracture involving the base of the cranium.

**Biologic Death:** present when irreversible brain damage has occurred, usually after 3-10 minutes of cardiac arrest.

**Blanket splint:** a blanket used as an improvised splint.

**Blood Pressure:** the pressure exerted by the pulsatile flow of blood against the arterial walls.

**Blood volume:** the total amount of blood in the heart and blood vessels; represents 8 to 9 percent of body weight in kilograms.

**Botulism:** food poisoning caused by *Clostridium botulinum* toxin.

**Brachial:** relating to the arm.

**Brachial artery:** the artery of the arm that is the continuation of the axillary artery, that in turn branches at the elbow into the radial and ulnar arteries.

**Brachial pulse:** pulse taken at the brachial artery.

**Bruise:** an injury that does not break the skin but causes rupture of small underlying blood vessels with resulting tissue discoloration; a contusion.

**Burn:** an injury caused by heat, electrical current, and chemicals of extreme acidity or alkalinity.

- **Arcing injury:** a burn caused when an electric current jumps from one surface to another.
- **Contact burn:** a burn caused by touching either a hot surface or a live electrical circuit.
- **Flash burn:** a burn caused when an extremity is close to an electrical flash or is struck by lightning.

**Burn pad:** refer to general purpose dressing.

**Butterfly Strips:** adhesive strips used to hold the edges of a wound together.

**C**

**Capillaries:** the very small blood vessels that carry blood to all parts of the body and the skin. Capillaries are a link between the ends of the arteries and the beginning of the veins.

**Cardiac arrest:** the sudden cessation of cardiac function with no pulse, no blood pressure, unresponsiveness.

**Cardiac asthma:** a condition characterized by left heart failure and pulmonary edema with wheezing respirations; not related to bronchial asthma.

**Cardiogenic shock:** the inability of the heart to pump adequate amounts of blood to perfuse the vital organs.

**Cardiopulmonary Resuscitation (CPR):** application of artificial ventilation and external cardiac compression in patients with cardiac arrest to provide an adequate circulation to support life.

**Carotid artery:** the principal artery of the neck, palpated easily on either side of the thyroid cartilage.

**Carotid pulse:** pulse taken at the carotid artery.

**Cerebrospinal Fluid:** fluid secreted by cells in cavities within the cerebrum. It circulates through the membranes that cover and protect the brain and spinal cord.

**Chronic:** a long duration, or recurring over a period of time.

**Circulatory system:** the body system consisting of the heart and blood vessels.

**Clinical death:** a term that refers to the lack of signs of life, when there is no pulse and no blood pressure; occurs immediately after the onset of cardiac arrest.

**Closed chest injury:** an injury in which the skin is not broken.

**Closed head injury:** a head injury in which there is no open wound or break in the skin or outer tissues.

**Clostridium perfringens:** anaerobic bacteria that can cause food poisoning in cooked food held without proper refrigeration.

**Coma:** state of unconsciousness from which the patient cannot be aroused, even by powerful stimulation.

**Coma position:** the position for an unconscious patient; lying on one side with one arm tucked under the head and the face turned downward to allow free drainage of mucus or vomitus.

**Compulsive drug use:** preoccupation with the procurement and use of a drug.

**Concussion:** a jarring brain injury resulting from a head blow or fall.

**Conduction:** the transmission of a stimulus from one fiber to another within a muscle.

**Congestive Heart Failure (CHF):** excessive blood or fluid in the lungs or body tissues caused by the failure of the ventricles to pump blood effectively.

**Conscious:** capable of responding to sensory stimuli and having subjective experiences.

**Consent:** an agreement by patients to accept treatment offered as explained by medical personnel.

- **Actual consent:** informed consent in either oral or written form.
- **Implied consent:** an assumed consent given by an unconscious adult when emergency lifesaving treatment is required.

Adapted from: U.S. Government Publication No. DOT S 501207

**Informed consent:** a consent given for treatment by a mentally competent adult who understands what the treatment will involve; can also be given by parent or guardian of a child, as defined by the State, or for a mentally incompetent adult.

**Minor's consent:** the right to consent is usually given to the parent or person *in loco parentis*.

**Consent of the mentally ill:** a situation similar to that for minors.

**Constrict:** to be made smaller by drawing together or squeezing.

**Contamination:** contact with an unsterile object or infective agent.

**Continuity:** an unbroken, connected whole.

**Contusion:** a bruise; an injury which causes a hemorrhage into or beneath the skin but does not break the skin.

**Convulsion:** a violent involuntary contraction or series of contractions of the voluntary muscles, a "fit," a seizure.

**Coronary Thrombosis:** formation of a clot in a coronary artery, obstructing blood flow.

**Counterpressure:** application of external pressure to counteract the dilation of blood vessels and raise the blood pressure, as in shock.

## D

**Depressant:** an agent that lowers functional activity, a sedative.

**Depressed fracture:** a skull fracture with impaction, depression, or a sinking in of the fragments.

**Dilation:** the process of expanding or enlarging.

**Direct injury:** injury caused by a direct blow or trauma.

**Direct pressure:** force applied directly on top of a wound to stop bleeding.

**Disease:** illness; ailment.

**Dislocation:** the state of being misaligned; the displacement of the ends of two bones at their joint so that the joint surfaces are no longer in proper contact.

**Dressing:** protective covering for a wound, used to stop bleeding and to prevent contamination of the wound.

**Drug abuse:** the self-administration of a drug or drugs in a manner not in accord with approved medical or social patterns.

**Dry sterile dressing:** a sterile dressing that is free of moisture.

## E

**Ecchymosis:** blood under the skin causing a black and blue mark; bruise.

**Edema:** a condition in which fluid escapes into the body tissues from the vascular or lymphatic spaces and causes local or generalized swelling.

**Electrocution:** death caused by passage of electrical current through the body.

**Epilepsy:** a chronic brain disorder marked by paroxysmal attacks of brain dysfunction, usually associated with some alteration of consciousness, abnormal motor behavior, psychic or sensory disturbances; may be preceded by aura.

**Evisceration:** internal organs exposed to the outside through a complete break in the abdominal wall.

**Exit wound:** injury at the point where a penetrating object departed the body, such as a bullet. Usually larger than an entrance wound.

## F

**Femoral:** pertaining to the femur or thigh bone.

**Fracture:** a break or rupture in a bone.

**Comminuted fracture:** a fracture in which the bone is shattered, broken into small pieces.

**Linear fracture:** a fracture running parallel to the long axis of the bone.

**Frostbite:** damage to the tissues as a result of prolonged exposure to extreme cold.

## G

**Gangrene:** local tissue death as the result of an injury or inadequate blood supply.

**General purpose dressing:** large, thick-layered, bulky pad used to control profuse bleeding. Available in several sizes, some with waterproof covering.

**Germ:** any disease-causing organism.

**Grand Mal:** a type of epileptic attack; characterized by a short-term, generalized, convulsive seizure.

## H

**Habituation:** a situation in which a patient produces a tolerance to a drug and becomes psychologically dependent on the drug.

**Hallucinogen:** an agent or drug which has the capacity to stimulate hallucinations of any type.

**Heat cramps:** painful muscle cramps resulting from excessive loss of salt and water through sweating.

**Heat exhaustion:** prostration caused by excessive loss of water and salt through sweating, characterized by cold, clammy skin and a weak, rapid pulse.

**Heat stroke:** life-threatening condition caused by a disturbance in temperature regulation; characterized by extreme fever, hot and dry skin, delirium, or coma.

**Heimlich Maneuver:** also known as the manual thrust, a system developed by Heimlich to remove a foreign body from the airway.

**Hematoma:** localized collection of blood in the tissues as a result of injury or a broken blood vessel.

**Hemophiliac:** "bleeder", a person who has inherited a disorder that causes the blood not to clot normally, resulting in heavy bleeding even from slight cuts.

**Hemorrhage:** abnormally large amount of bleeding.

**Histamine:** a decomposition product of histidine, formed in the intestines and found in most body tissues or produced synthetically; it causes dilation and increased permeability of capillaries and stimulates gastric secretion and visceral muscle contraction.

**Hives:** red or white raised patches on the skin, often attended by severe itching; a characteristic reaction in allergic responses.

**Hyperextension:** overextension of a limb or other part of the body.

**Hyperventilation:** an increased rate and depth of breathing resulting in an abnormal lowering of arterial carbon dioxide, causing alkalosis.

**Hypoglycemia:** an abnormally diminished concentration of sugar in the blood; insulin shock.

**Hypothermia:** decreased body temperature.

## I

**Immersion foot:** painful inflammation of the foot followed by discoloration, swelling, ulcers, and numbness, due to prolonged exposure to moist cold.

**Impaled object:** an object which has caused a puncture wound and which remains embedded in the wound.

**Incised wound:** a clean cut as opposed to a laceration.

**Indirect injury:** fracture or dislocation at a distance from the point of impact, such as a hip fracture caused by the knees striking the dashboard.

**Ingestion:** intaking of food or other substances through the mouth.

**Inhalation:** the drawing of air or other gases into the lungs.

**Injection:** the forcing of a liquid through a needle or other tube into subcutaneous tissues, the blood vessel, a muscle mass, or an organ.

**Insulin:** a hormone secreted by the islets of Langerhans in the pancreas; essential for the proper metabolism of blood sugar.

**Insulin shock:** not a true form of shock; hypoglycemia caused by excessive insulin dosage, characterized by sweating, tremor, anxiety, unusual behavior, vertigo, and diplopia; may cause death of brain cells.

**Intercostal muscles:** muscles between the ribs.

**Internal bleeding:** bleeding within the body, without a visible external wound.

**Intravenous:** within or into a vein.

**Irrigation:** cleansing by washing and rinsing with water or other fluids.

## K

**Ketoacidosis:** a condition arising in diabetics where their insulin dose is insufficient to their needs; fat is metabolized, instead of sugar, to ketones; characterized by excessive thirst, urination, vomiting, and hyperventilation of the Kussmaul type.

**Kidneys:** the paired organs located in the retroperitoneal cavities that filter blood and produce urine; also act as adjuncts to keep a proper acid-base balance.

## L

**Laceration:** a wound made by tearing or cutting of body tissues.

**Log roll:** a method of rolling the body as a complete unit.

## M

**Manual thrust:** Heimlich maneuver.

**Marijuana:** a narcotic obtained from the dried leaves and flowers of the hemp plant.

**Midsternum:** the middle of the sternum.

**Mobile:** movable.

**Molecule:** the smallest particle of a substance that retains the characteristics of a compound or element.

**Mouth-to-mouth resuscitation:** the act of reviving an apneic patient by applying one's mouth and forcing air into the lungs.

**Multitrauma dressing:** refer to general purpose dressing.

**Musculature:** the muscular system of the body, or a part of the system.

## N

**Narcotic:** drug used to depress the central nervous system, thereby relieving pain and producing sleep.

**Nerve:** a cordlike structure composed of a collection of fibers that convey impulses between a part of the central nervous system and some other region.

**Neurological:** of or relating to the branch of medical science dealing with the nervous system and its disorders.

## O

**Occiput:** the back of the skull.

**Occlusion:** the closing of a tube or duct, such as a blood vessel.

**Occlusive dressing:** a watertight dressing for a wound.

**Open chest injury:** an injury in which there is a break in the skin or outer tissues.
**Open head injury:** a head injury in which there is a break in the skin or outer tissues.
**Opiate:** technically, one of several alkaloids derived from the opium poppy plant.
**Oxygenated:** perfused with oxygen.

## P

**Palm:** inner, slightly concave surface of hand between wrist and fingers.
**Paradoxical movement:** the motion of an injured section of a flail chest; opposite to the normal movement of the chest wall.
**Pathophysiology:** the study of the changes in normal body function in the presence of disease.
**Penicillin:** powerful antibiotic used in treatment of a wide variety of infections.
**Perfusion:** the act of pouring through or into; the blood getting to the cells in order to exchange gases, nutrients, etc., with the cells.
**Petroleum gauze:** sterile gauze dressing saturated with petrolatum (*Vaseline*) to prevent it from sticking to an open wound.
**Physical dependence:** habituation or use of a drug, or other maneuver, because of its physiologic support, and because of the undesirable effects of withdrawal.
**Pillow splint:** an improvised splint made by wrapping it around the injured area and securing it with several cravats.
**Plasma:** the fluid portion of the blood, retains the clotting factors, but has no red or white cells.
**Platelet:** a small cellular element in the blood that assists in blood clotting.
**Poison ivy:** any of several American sumacs with grayish berries and pointed leaves in groups of three that can cause a rash if touched.
**Poison oak:** a shrubby western variety of poison ivy.
**Poison sumac:** a swamp shrub with greenish-white flowers, grayish berries, and compound leaves of 7 to 13 leaflets that can cause a severe rash if touched.
**Pressure dressing:** a dressing with which enough pressure is applied over a wound site to stop bleeding.
**Pressure point:** one of several places on the body where the blood flow of a given artery can be restricted by pressing the artery against an underlying bone.
**Psychological dependence:** dependence of a drug, or other therapeutic maneuvers, because of its support to the patient's psyche, rather than to his physiologic function.
**Pulse:** the rhythmic expansion and contraction of an arterial wall caused by ventricular systole and diastole.
**Puncture wound:** a result of a puncture of any sharp object that pierced the skin.

## R

**Rabid:** having or pertaining to rabies.
**Rabies:** viral disease of the CNS transmitted by the bite of an infected animal, invariably fatal unless treated before symptoms appear; also called hydrophobia from a supposed aversion of the victim to water.
**Red blood cell:** an erythrocyte; the cell that carries oxygen from alveoli to cell.
**Respiratory arrest:** the cessation of breathing.
**Respiratory injury:** damage to the breathing system.
**Roller dressing:** a strip of rolled-up material used for dressings.
**Rule of Nines:** a method for estimating the amount of skin surface burned.

## S

**Salmonella:** an organism related to that of typhoid fever which produces intestinal upsets.
**Seizure:** a sudden attack or recurrence of a disease; a convulsion; an attack of epilepsy.
**Serum:** the liquid portion of the blood containing all of the dissolved constituents except those used for clotting.
**Shock:** a state of inadequate tissue perfusion that may be a result of pump failure (cardiogenic shock), volume loss or sequestration (hypovolemic shock), vasolilation (neurogenic shock), or any combination of these.
- **Anaphylactic shock:** a rapidly occurring state of collapse caused by hypersensitivity to drugs or other foreign materials (insect venom, certain foods, inhaled allergenic); symptoms may include hives, wheezing, tissue edema, bronchospasm, vascular collapse.
- **Irreversible shock:** very deep shock condition leading inevitably to death unless counterreacted by extraordinary measures.

**Skull:** the bony structure surrounding the brain; consists of the cranial bones, the facial bones, and the teeth.
**Sling:** a triangular bandage applied around the neck to support an injured upper extremity; any wide or narrow material long enough to suspend an upper extremity by passing the material around the neck; used to support and protect an injury of the arm, shoulder, or clavicle.
**Snowblindness:** obscured vision caused by sunlight reflected off snow.
**Soft tissue:** the nonbony and noncartilaginous tissue of the body.
**Spineboard:** a device used primarily for transporting patients with suspected or actual spinal injuries.
**Sprain:** a trauma to a joint causing injury to the ligaments.
**Staphylococcus:** a bacteria that causes boils and other infections.
**Status asthmaticus:** severe, prolonged asthmatic attack that cannot be broken with epinephrine.
**Sterile:** free from living organisms, such as bacteria.
**Sternum:** the long, flat bone located in the midline in the anterior part of the thoracic cage; articulates above with the clavicles and along the sides with the cartilages of the first seven ribs.
**Stimulant:** any agent that increases the level of bodily activity.
**Strain:** excessive stretching of a muscle, tendon, or ligament.
**Substernal notch:** the point where the ribs meet the sternum.
**Sunstroke:** form of heatstroke due to prolonged sun exposure.
**Syndrome:** a complex of symptoms and signs characteristic of a condition.

## T

**Tendon:** a tough band of dense, fibrous, connective tissue that attaches muscles to bone and other parts.
**Tetanus:** an infectious disease caused by an exotoxin of a bacteria, *Clostridium tetani*, that is usually introduced through a wound, characterized by extreme body rigidity and spasms, trismus, or opisthotonus, of voluntary body muscles.
**Tolerance:** the state of enduring, or of less susceptability to the effects of a drug or poison after repeated doses.
**Tourniquet:** constrictive device used on the extremities to impede venous blood return to the heart or obstruct arterial blood flow to the extremity.
**Trauma:** surgical definition: physical injury. Psychiatric definition: emotional distress, relating to a specific incident.
**Trauma pack:** refer to general purpose dressing.
**Trench foot:** a foot condition caused by exposure to cold and dampness.
**Triage:** a system used for sorting patients to determine the order in which they will receive medical attention.
**Triangular bandage:** a piece of cloth cut in the shape of a right-angled triangle; used as a sling, or folded for a cravat bandage.

## U

**Unconscious:** without awareness, the state of being comatose.
**Universal dressing:** a large (9 by 36 inches) dressing of multilayered material that can be used open, folded, or rolled to cover most wounds, to pad splints, or to form a cervical collar.

## V

**Vaporization:** conversion of a liquid or solid to a gas.
**Vascular:** relating to, or containing blood vessels.
**Vein:** any blood vessel that carries blood from the tissues to the heart.
**Venom:** a poison, usually derived from reptiles or insects.
**Vomit:** to discharge the stomach contents through the mouth; the disgorged contents.
**Vomitus:** the disgorged contents of the stomach brought up by the act of vomiting.
**Waterchill:** heat loss of a body immersed in water due to relatively high heat conductivity of water.
**Wet dressing:** a dressing that may not be sterile.
**White blood cells:** leucocytes, the white or colorless cells in the bloodstream that defend the body against infection.
**Windchill:** the cooling effect of moving air on a body, due principally to evaporation of moisture from exposed skin; expressed as the amount of heat lost per unit area per unit of time and taking into account both temperature and wind speed. Some charts give the result in degrees of equivalent still-air temperature.
**Wound:** an injury or break in the skin.
**Xiphoid process:** sword-shaped cartilage at lowest part of the breast bone.

# Index